Free Radicals in
AGING

Free Radicals in

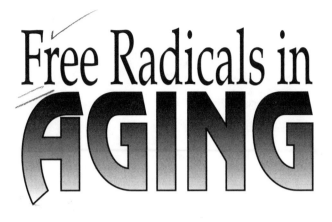

Edited by
Byung Pal Yu
Professor
Department of Physiology
University of Texas
Health Science Center
San Antonio, Texas

CRC Press
Boca Raton   Ann Arbor   London   Tokyo

Library of Congress Cataloging-in-Publication Data

Free radicals in aging / edited by Byung P. Yu.
    p. cm.
    Includes bibliographical references and index.
    ISBN 0-8493-4518-9
    1. Free radical (Chemistry)—Physiological effect. 2. Aging-
Molecular aspects. 3. Free radical reactions. I. Yu, Byung P.
    [DNLM: 1. Aging—physiology. 2. Free Radicals—metabolism. WT
104 FB527]
    RB170.F755   1993
    612.6'7—dc20
    DNLM/DLC
    for Library of Congress   92-48902
                                                      CIP

PREFACE

Advancement in the understanding of free radical biochemistry and its multifaceted effects on biological function have led to a renewed interest in studying the role of free radicals and related reactions in the biological and pathological changes occurring in aging organisms. Scientific interest and experimental inquiry into the role of free radicals in aging formally began with Denham Harman's proposal in 1956 of The Free Radical Theory of Aging. This theory has since served as a useful underlying hypothesis for the field of gerontology and has thus guided experimental gerontologists who have continuously sought the biochemical and molecular bases underlying the complex biological and pathological problems of aging.

The Free Radical Theory of Aging was neither the first nor the last to try to explain the aging process. In fact, no other discipline of science has as many theories and hypotheses as gerontology. Unfortunately, most of the theories or hypotheses of aging, proposed in the past and present, limit themselves to merely describing epiphenomena and fail to provide a means by which to be tested. Similarly, no satisfactory experimental verification of The Free Radical Theory of Aging has yet been provided, and this theory has thus been criticized on these grounds. Hopefully, our recently improved ability to better design critical experiments will now allow more direct examination of The Free Radical Theory of Aging and its implications. For example, data recently obtained from experiments in both fields have provided further insights implicating free radicals in major age-related diseases such as atherosclerosis, cancer, and diabetes.

It is the purpose of this book to bring together two diverse fields in a more comprehensive manner by discussing salient subjects ranging from the basic free radical biochemistry to future directions of the study of free radicals in aging. This will include modern variations on the theme of The Free Radical Theory of Aging, such as The Free Radical-Glycation/Maillard Theory of Aging, recently proposed by myself and my colleague, Bruce Kristal. It should be emphasized that none of the existing theories are sufficient to explain all the phenomena observed in aging organisms, but free radical-related reactions appear to have the widest implication in both primary aging processes and age-related pathological processes, as we know them today.

I wish to express my sincere thanks to my many colleagues who contributed their time and effort in making this book possible. I also thank Mrs. Kimberley Kennedy for her assistance in preparing and editing this book.

Byung Pal Yu

THE EDITOR

Byung Pal Yu, Ph.D. is a Professor of Physiology in the Department of Physiology at The University of Texas Health Science Center at San Antonio, Texas. He graduated in 1960 from Central Missouri State College, Warrenburg, Missouri with a B.S. degree in Chemistry and obtained his Ph.D. degree in 1965 from the University of Illinois, Urbana, Illinois where he studied lipid biochemistry.

Dr. Yu is a member of the American Physiological Society, the International Society for Free Radical Research, and the Oxygen Society. He is also a member and Fellow of the Gerontological Society of America for which he is a Chairman-Elect of the Biological Sciences Section. In addition, Dr. Yu is President of the American Aging Association. He has received the Research and Development Award of American Diabetes Association and the Henry L. Moss Award. He is also the Program Director of the Nutritional Gerontology Research Program funded with a $5.4 million budget by the National Institute on Aging and serves on the editorial boards of *Journal of Gerontology; Age and Nutrition; Proceedings of the Society for Experimental Biology and Medicine*; and *Aging*. He also serves as a member of the Nutrition Study Section of the National Institutes of Health.

Dr. Yu has published more than 185 papers and his current research interests are in the areas of free radicals, membranes, aging, and dietary restriction.

CONTRIBUTORS

Robert G. Allen, Ph.D.
Center for Gerontological Research
The Medical College of
  Pennsylvania
Philadelphia, Pennsylvania

Anne C. Andorn, M.D.
Department of Psychiatry and
  Human Behavior
St. Louis University School of
  Medicine and Psychiatry Service
VA Medical Center
St. Louis, Missouri

Harris Bernstein, Ph.D.
Department of Microbiology and
  Immunology
College of Medicine
University of Arizona
Tucson, Arizona

William J. Evans, Ph.D.
Human Physiology Laboratory
USDA-Human Nutrition Research
  Center on Aging at Tufts
  University
Boston, Massachusetts

Robert A. Floyd, Ph.D.
Free Radical Biology and Aging
  Research Program
Oklahoma Medical Research
  Foundation
Oklahoma City, Oklahoma

Helen L. Gensler, Ph.D.
Department of Radiation Oncology
College of Medicine
Arizona Cancer Center
University of Arizona
Tucson, Arizona

Denham Harman, M.D., Ph.D.
Department of Medicine
College of Medicine
University of Nebraska
Omaha, Nebraska

Edward J. Masoro, Ph.D.
Department of Physiology
University of Texas Health Science
  Center
San Antonio, Texas

Mitsuyoshi Matsuo, Ph.D.
Tokyo Metropolitan Institute of
  Gerontology
Tokyo, Japan

Michael B. Mattamal, Ph.D.
Geriatric Research, Education, and
  Clinical Center
VA Medical Center
  and
Departments of Internal Medicine
  and Biochemistry
St. Louis University School of
  Medicine
St. Louis, Missouri

Mohsen Meydani, D.V.M., Ph.D.
Antioxidant Research Laboratory
USDA-Human Nutrition Research
  Center on Aging at Tufts
  University
Boston, Massachusetts

Larry W. Oberley, Ph.D.
Radiation Research Laboratory
University of Iowa College of
  Medicine
Iowa City, Iowa

Terry D. Oberley, M.D., Ph.D.
Laboratory Service
William S. Middleton Memorial
  Veterans Hospital
Madison, Wisconsin

Pamela E. Starke-Reed, Ph.D.
Geriatrics Program
National Institute on Aging
Bethesda, Maryland

Randy Strong, Ph.D.
Geriatric Research, Education, and
  Clinical Center
VA Medical Center
      and
Departments of Pharmacological
  and Physiological Science and
  Internal Medicine
St. Louis University School of
  Medicine
St. Louis, Missouri

Huber R. Warner, Ph.D.
Biology of Aging Program
National Institute on Aging
Bethesda, Maryland

Richard Weindruch, Ph.D.
Department of Medicine
Institute on Aging
University of Wisconsin
Madison, Wisconsin

Simon P. Wolff, D. Phil.
Department of Clinical
  Pharmacology
University College London
London, England

Byung P. Yu, Ph.D.
Department of Physiology
Health Science Center
University of Texas
San Antonio, Texas

TABLE OF CONTENTS

Dedication

To my wife, Kyung Hi, and son, Victor

Chapter 1

CONCEPTS AND HYPOTHESES OF BASIC AGING PROCESSES

Edward J. Masoro

TABLE OF CONTENTS

0-8493-4518-9/93/$0.00 + $.50

I. INTRODUCTION

The human aging phenotype, changes in observable characteristics with advancing age, is well known. It is also recognized that similar changes occur in many species (e.g., pets and farm animals). Indeed, the aging phenotype is so familiar that many consider it to be an inevitable consequence of time, similar to the deterioration that occurs in automobiles, houses, and other inanimate objects. However, further thought makes it evident that it is not obvious in any way why the deterioration that typifies the aging phenotype should occur.

An organism, which develops from a fertilized egg into a complex structural and functional adult system, should be able to accomplish what would appear to be the less difficult task of maintaining the system, provided energy resources are available. The basic riddle is that deterioration does occur when there is no *a priori* reason for it to occur in an organism living in a thermodynamically open system.

Before considering this issue further, a formal definition of aging is in order. However, because so little is known, it is difficult to define aging in a way that is acceptable to all. Probably the following definition would not be objected to by most biological gerontologists: Aging refers to processes occurring during the lifetime which increase the vulnerability of the organism to challenges, thereby increasing the likelihood of death. Finch[1] feels that such a definition relates to senescence, and that aging refers to all changes in the organism with time, including developmental events. In this chapter, aging will be used in the sense of senescence. What the processes are that underlie this increase in vulnerability is the question that biological gerontologists have been and are addressing.

II. THEORIES OF AGING

The basic premise often unstated but held by most biological gerontologists is that there is or are primary aging processes that underlie the aging phenotype. Most of the many theories of aging are proposals regarding the nature of these primary processes. Indeed, for many years, it was felt that a single process was responsible for the aging phenotype, and The Theory of Aging was proposed.[2] Few today believe that the aging phenotype is the result of a single, primary, aging process. Most feel several such processes are involved, and others doubt the validity of the concept of primary aging processes.

It was also long held that similar primary aging processes were operating in all species. In an article published in 1977, Rockstein et al.[3] concluded that this view is unlikely. However, although primary aging processes may differ between species, there also may be important commonalities. Indeed, Sacher[4] points to the similarity in aging characteristics between mammalian species.

The number of theories of aging that have been proposed is great. It would not be possible to even briefly describe each in the space allotted to this chapter, nor would it be profitable to do so. A few examples will be presented, chosen because of their impact on gerontological research and/or their relevance to the subject matter of this book.

In 1928, Pearl[5] proposed the Rate of Living Theory of Aging, which is based on the concept that the duration of life varies inversely with the rate of energy expenditure. However, the concept of a link between metabolic rate and aging predates this theory by 20 years, when in 1908, Rubner[6] presented evidence for such a relationship from his studies with domestic animals. Over the years, many studies have supported metabolic rate hypotheses, while others have not (see Masoro[7] for a review of this literature). Economos[8] pointed out that findings not in support of this concept do not invalidate it as an important aspect of aging because other factors, including protective mechanisms, may mask the effect of metabolic rate in particular circumstances.

Another theory that has had a great impact on aging research is the Somatic Mutation Theory proposed in 1959 by Szilard.[9] This theory states that genetic mutations accumulate with time, eventually resulting in functional failure. This concept has been the subject of many studies in the ensuing years. The evidence obtained so far does not indicate that this hypothesis describes a major process of aging.[10] However, further study is warranted using the powerful tools of modern molecular genetics.

Probably the theory of aging that has been subject to most study is The Error Catastrophe Theory advanced in 1963 by Orgel.[11] This theory proposes that if an error is made in synthesis of a protein involved in the synthesis of genetic material or the protein synthesizing machinery (transcription or translation), this faulty protein could cause further errors, ultimately resulting in an error crisis. Such a crisis would be expressed in impaired functions, not unlike those observed during aging. Much effort went into testing this theory because of its conceptual attractiveness. The results of these studies provide essentially no support for it.[12] However, such studies have not totally invalidated the concept, and because of its attractiveness, there are still some advocates of this theory.

Another theory involving the structure of macromolecules is the Crosslinkage Theory proposed in 1968 by Bjorksten.[13] In this case, the alteration was proposed to occur posttranslationally. Functional deterioration was felt to be due to the cross-linking of proteins and nucleic acids. The presence of cross-linking agents in living organisms was proposed to be the cause of this change in macromolecular structure. The functional alterations envisioned were changes in elasticity, in brittleness, in swelling capacity, and in enzymatic function. Increased cross-linking of some macromolecules does indeed occur with advancing age. However, it is not established that this crosslinking plays a major role in senescence.

The concept that aging is genetically programmed has been and continues to be a popular one. Hayflick,[14] in 1968, was the first to clearly postulate this concept when he said " . . . we surmise that the aging and finite lifetime of normal cells constitute a programmed mechanism that sets an overall limit on an organism's length of life." This view was primarily based on studies of cells in culture. However, the relevance of "*in vitro* aging" to *in vivo* aging is still being debated.[7] Indeed, at this time there is little experimental support for programmed aging. Moreover, as will be discussed below, the developing concepts of the evolutionary biology of aging make programmed aging in an adaptive developmental sense unlikely.

The concept that aging is not intrinsic to most cells of complex multicellular organisms, but rather secondary to alterations in neuroendocrine pacemaker cells, has been proposed by several gerontologists during the past two decades.[15] Most of the research aimed at testing this hypothesis has been focused on the reproductive system and the adrenal-glucocorticoid system. A specific example is the Glucocorticoid Cascade Hypothesis of Sapolsky et al.[16] This hypothesis is based on the fact that neurons in the hippocampus contain a high density of glucocorticoid receptors, and the belief that these neurons are involved in the negative feedback regulation of glucocorticoid secretion. Stress-induced increases in plasma glucocorticoid concentration, an inevitable occurrence during daily living, are proposed to down-regulate the hippocampal glucocorticoid receptors, resulting in periods of glucocorticoid hypersecretion. It is further envisioned that the periods of glucocorticoid hypersecretion coupled with insults such as ischemia result with advancing age in a loss of these hippocampal neurons. As a consequence, a feed-forward cascade of sustained hyperadrenocorticism is felt to occur, which causes much of the aging phenotype, e.g., immunosuppression, osteoporosis, impaired cognition, etc. Recent findings of Sabatino et al.[17] do not support the Glucocorticoid Cascade Hypothesis as a major aspect of the aging processes. Similar experimental testing has not been done in regard to other neuroendocrine theories, except for the research showing such a role for estrogen in the aging of the female reproductive system.[15]

The Free Radical Theory of Aging, a subject covered in depth in this book, was proposed in 1956 by Harman.[18] In recent years, this concept has been related to fuel use, specifically to the generation of oxygen free radicals or reactive oxygen compounds during oxidative metabolism of fuel.[19] The recently proposed Glycation Theory of Aging[20] also relates to fuel use. Specifically, it is hypothesized that nonenzymatic reactions of glucose and other reducing sugars with amino groups of proteins and nucleic acids result in a series of events which alter protein and nucleic-acid structure and function. The altered function is viewed as a molecular basis of aging. Moreover, the Free Radical Theory and the Glycation Theory have been tied together by Wolff et al.[21] by their "autoxidative glycosylation" concept. Since these theories and related issues are discussed in depth in this book, it suffices here to briefly summarize the current state of knowledge. Both reactive oxygen molecules and glycation reactions occur in living organisms. However, whether these reactions lead to long-term, harmful effects which underlie aging has yet to be established. The research activities seeking to address this issue as well as recent findings are the subject of the other chapters of this book.

The theories just discussed, as well as others, are not mutually exclusive. In many instances, they clearly interrelate to form a continuum. For example, crosslinking, somatic mutation, errors in synthesis of genetic material and protein-synthesizing machinery could all be secondary to free radical damage. Moreover, much free radical generation may be secondary to fuel use, and therefore, related to the Rate of Living Theory of Aging. The major problem faced by gerontologists is that of separating events that cause aging from those caused by aging processes.

III. EVOLUTION AND THE THEORIES OF AGING

Evolutionary biologists have been developing concepts which provide a theoretical foundation for the study of aging. From their viewpoint, theories of aging fall into one of two classes: adaptive theories and nonadaptive theories.[22] Adaptive theories are those which are based on the concept that senescence leading to death provides the species a selective advantage. Nonadaptive theories are those which are based on the concept that senescence is detrimental to evolutionary fitness or, at best, selectively neutral.

Two fundamental concepts underlie adaptive theories of aging: (1) eliminating old individuals makes space, nutrients, and other resources available to progeny; and (2) increasing the rate of succession of generations improves the chances for a species to adapt to changes in the environment. Most programmed aging theories are examples of adaptive theories in that aging processes are viewed to be programmed for Darwinian fitness in the same strict sense as developmental events; i.e., there is direct genetic programming of primary aging processes.[23] Such theories are popular and underlie concepts such as that of a genetic aging clock. However, there is reason to believe that adaptive theories of aging are not likely to be correct. Accidental deaths are so high in most species living in the wild that senescence is an infrequent occurrence.[24] Therefore, aging cannot be viewed as needed to free up resources for progeny. Nor is aging needed to increase the succession of generations and thereby improve the chances of a species to adapt to changes in environment. Although most evolutionary biologists do not embrace the concept of adaptive programmed aging, it is a view that is held by some well-respected gerontologists. Russell[25] has recently reviewed the evidence for and against developmentally programmed aging.

The nonadaptive evolutionary view of aging has been well presented in a recent book by Rose.[26] The basic concept is that a declining force of natural selection occurs with increasing age. On the basis of this concept, Rose defines aging as a persistent decline with age in Darwinian fitness due to internal physiological deterioration.

A genetic mechanism for this nonadaptive theory was proposed by Medawar[27] in his concept of late-acting genes. Based on the observation that accidental mortality in most natural environments progressively reduces the fraction of the population surviving to old age, Medawar proposed that any new gene arising from mutation which is expressed late in life will be subject to little or no selection. This should result in an accumulation of deleterious genes expressed at late ages. In most, but not all, natural environments and species, senescence rarely occurs because most organisms die before the expression of these deleterious genes. Of course, in the protective environments that humans have developed for themselves and domestic animals, death from accidental causes is reduced, and senescence is a common occurrence. Thus, from Medawar's viewpoint senescence occurs because the force of natural selection declines with increasing age, thereby preventing the elimination of late-acting, deleterious genes.

Another genetic mechanism that is consistent with the nonadaptive evolutionary theory of aging was postulated by Williams.[28] He attributed aging to pleiotropic genes which promote Darwinian fitness in early life, but have harmful actions late in life. The early beneficial effects would be selected for, but because of the decline in the force of natural selection with age the deleterious late effects would not be removed by negative selection. There is some experimental evidence in support of a role for antagonistic pleiotropy in aging, which has been obtained primarily in studies using *Drosophila* as the animal model.[26] There is also evidence supporting a role for late-acting genes in aging.

A somewhat different nonadaptive theory of aging, but one consistent with the evolutionary views of aging just described, is the Disposable Soma Theory of Aging proposed by Kirkwood.[29] Basic to this theory is the concept of the organism as an entity, which functions to transform free energy of its environment into progeny. To do so, part of this energy must be used for somatic maintenance. This theory proposes that the force of selection results in a partitioning of this energy between processes maintaining the soma and those needed for reproduction in a fashion which maximizes Darwinian fitness. As a result, it is proposed that less energy is used for somatic repair than is needed for indefinite somatic survival. It is projected that the extent of investment in somatic maintenance will depend on the ecological niche of the species. This theory predicts that species in a niche with high rates of accidental mortality will invest little in the maintenance of the soma and, therefore, will age rapidly. The converse is predicted for species living in protected ecological niches. This theory is consistent with much that is known about aging and with many of the aging theories that have been proposed. For instance, it predicts that aging involves somatic damage, and that long-lived species will have better repair systems than short-lived species. Indeed, the disposable soma hypothesis is readily related to several of the theories discussed in this chapter, such as the cross-linking theory, the error in protein synthesis theory, the glycation theory, and the free radical theory. The disposable soma hypothesis attributes aging to wear and tear, not because deterioration due to wear and tear is inevitable in a thermodynamically open system, but because it is the consequence of the balance struck between somatic maintenance and reproduction.

IV. ENVIRONMENT AND AGING

In addition to the role of the environment on aging predicted by the disposable soma hypothesis, there is a reason to feel that there is direct interaction of environment with specific aging processes. Although such an interaction seems likely, the evidence supporting this view is scant.

Probably the strongest evidence for an interaction of aging processes and the environment comes from studies with the dietary restriction rodent models.[30] In addition to markedly increasing the mean, median, and maximum length of life of different rodent species and strains, dietary restriction increases the Mortality Rate Doubling Time (MRDT). In four rat studies involving a reduction in energy intake of about 40%, restricted rats had an MRDT which averaged 197 d (range of 187 to 210 d) compared to an average value of 102 d (range of 99 to 104 d) for *ad libitum*-fed control rats.[31] Finch[1] views the MRDT to be a good quantitative index of the rate of aging; i.e., he believes it relates inversely to the rate of aging. In addition, dietary restriction maintains a broad spectrum of physiological processes in a youthful state at advanced ages.[32] Even more strikingly, dietary restriction inhibits most age-associated disease processes (ranging from neoplasia to autoimmune disease) in many different rat and mouse strains.[30] Collectively, this evidence strongly supports the view that dietary restriction (specifically a decreased energy intake) retards the aging processes.

The only other environmental factor that has clearly been shown to influence the rate of aging is ambient temperature in the case of poikilotherms.[4] Many other environmental factors can influence aspects of the aging phenotype, but that they do so by influencing aging processes has not been established. An example is the altered appearance of human skin with age, which in the eyes of most laymen, is almost synonymous with aging. However, most of the skin changes are not due to aging per se.[33] Long-term sun exposure accounts for more than 90% of these skin changes; cigarette smoking also underlies such change in people who indulge in it. The important point is that, although photoaging and intrinsic aging of skin are strikingly similar, the two processes can be distinguished by electron microscopic analysis of skin morphology.[34]

In summary, environmental factors have effects which simulate intrinsic aging events. However, as shown for skin, these actions of the environment may differ from those of intrinsic aging. In mammals, dietary restriction is the only environmental manipulation that has clearly been shown to influence aging processes. Other environmental factors may also do so, but clear evidence of such action has yet to be obtained. As knowledge of basic aging processes increases, assessment of the role of the environment in aging processes should be facilitated.

V. SUMMARY OF CURRENT STATUS OF BIOLOGICAL GERONTOLOGY

Although the aging phenotype is well known, the basic nature of the aging processes is totally unknown. Many theories of aging have been proposed regarding the basic nature of aging, but none has been validated as even, in part, underlying intrinsic aging; however, the evolutionary biologists are beginning to provide insights on why aging occurs. These insights may provide the platform needed for an incisive study of aging mechanisms by other biologists, e.g., biochemists, physiologists, geneticists, and molecular biologists. It is tempting to believe that environment plays a role in aging, and the research on dietary restriction in rodents indicates that it can. However, it is difficult to know in a specific case whether the environmental factor influences aging processes, or rather, simulates an effect on aging processes, but in fact acts by a different mechanism.

REFERENCES

1. **Finch, C. E.,** *Longevity, Senescence and the Genome,* University of Chicago Press, Chicago, 1990, chap. 1.
2. **Schneider, E. L.,** Theories of aging, a perspective, in *Modern Biological Theories of Aging,* Butler, R. N., Schneider, E. L., Sprott, R. L., and Warner, H. R., Eds., Raven Press, New York, 1987, 1.
3. **Rockstein, M., Chesky, J., and Sussman, M.,** Comparative biology and evolution of aging, in *Handbook of the Biology of Aging,* Finch, C. E. and Hayflick, L., Eds., Van Nostrand Reinhold, New York, 1977, chap. 1.
4. **Sacher, G. A.,** Life table modification and life prolongation, in *Handbook of the Biology of Aging,* Finch, C. E. and Hayflick, L., Eds., Van Nostrand Reinhold, New York, 1977, chap. 24.
5. **Pearl, R.,** *The Rate of Living,* Alfred Knopf, New York, 1928.
6. **Rubner, M.,** Das problem der Lebensdauer und seine Beziehungen zum *Wachstum und Ernäbrung,* Oldenbourg, Munich, 1908.
7. **Masoro, E. J.,** Biology of aging: facts, thoughts and experimental approaches, *Lab. Invest.,* 65, 500, 1991.
8. **Economos, A. C.,** Beyond the rate of living, *Gerontology,* 27, 258, 1981.
9. **Szilard, L.,** On the nature of the aging process, *Proc. Natl. Acad. Sci. U.S.A.,* 45, 30, 1959.
10. **Cristofalo, V. J.,** Overview of biological mechanism of aging, *Annu. Rev. Gerontol. Geriatr.,* 10, 1, 1991.
11. **Orgel, L. E.,** The maintenance of the accuracy of protein synthesis and its relevance to aging, *Proc. Natl. Acad. Sci. U.S.A.,* 49, 517, 1963.
12. **Rothstein, M.,** Age-related changes in enzyme levels and enzyme properties, *Rev. Biol. Res. Aging,* 1, 421, 1985.

13. **Bjorksten, J.**, The Crosslinking Theory of Aging, *J. Am. Geriatr. Soc.*, 16, 408, 1968.
14. **Hayflick, L.**, Human cells and aging, *Sci. Am.*, 218(3), 32, 1968.
15. **Finch, C. E. and Landfield, P. W.**, Neuroendocrine and autonomic functions in aging mammals, in *Handbook of the Biology of Aging*, Finch, C. E. and Schneider, E. L., Eds., Van Nostrand Reinhold, New York, 1985, chap 21.
16. **Sapolsky, R. M., Krey, L. C., and McEwen, B. S.**, The neuroendocrinology of stress and aging: the glucocorticoid cascade hypothesis, *Endocrine Res.*, 7, 284, 1986.
17. **Sabatino, F., Masoro, E. J., McMahan, C. A., and Kuhn, R. W.**, Assessment of the role of the glucocorticoid system in the aging processes and in the action of food restriction, *J. Gerontol.: Biol. Sci.*, 46, B171, 1991.
18. **Harman, J.**, Aging: a theory based on free radical and radiation biology, *J. Gerontol.*, 11, 98, 1956.
19. **Cadenas, E.**, Biochemistry for oxygen toxicity, *Annu. Rev. Biochem.*, 58, 79, 1989.
20. **Cerami, A.**, Hypothesis: glucose as a mediator of aging, *J. Am. Geriatr. Soc.*, 33, 626, 1985.
21. **Wolff, S. P., Bascal, Z. A., and Hunt, J. V.**, "Autooxidative glycosylation": free radicals and glycation, in *The Maillard Reaction in Aging, Diabetes, and Nutrition*, Baynes, J. W. and Monnier, V. M., Eds., Alan R. Liss, New York, 1989, 259.
22. **Kirkwood, T. B. L. and Cremer, T.**, Cytogerontology since 1881: a reappraisal of August Weisman and a review of modern progress, *Hum. Genet.*, 60, 101, 1982.
23. **Hayflick, L.**, Theories of biological aging, *Exp. Gerontol.*, 20, 145, 1985.
24. **Lack, D.**, *The Natural Regulation of Animal Numbers*, Clarendon Press, Oxford, 1954.
25. **Russell, R. L.**, Evidence for and against developmentally programmed aging, in *Modern Biological Theories of Aging*, Butler, R. N., Schneider, E. L., Sprott, R. L., and Warner, H. R., Eds., Raven Press, New York, 1987, 35.
26. **Rose, M. R.**, *Evolutionary Biology of Aging*, Oxford University Press, New York, 1991.
27. **Medawar, P. B.**, *An Unsolved Problem in Biology*, H. K. Lewis, London, 1952.
28. **Williams, G. C.**, Pleiotropy, natural selection and the evolution of senescence, *Evolution*, 11, 398, 1957.
29. **Kirkwood, T. B. L.**, The Disposable Soma Theory of Aging, in *Genetic Effects on Aging II*, Harrison, D. E., Ed., Telford Press, Caldwell, NJ, 1990, chap. 2.
30. **Masoro, E. J.**, Food restriction in rodents: an evaluation of its role in the study of aging, *J. Gerontol.: Biol. Sci.*, 43, B59, 1988.
31. **Holehan, A. M. and Merry, B. J.**, The experimental manipulation of ageing by diet, *Biol. Revs.*, 61, 329, 1986.
32. **Masoro, E. J.**, Assessment of nutritional components in prolongation of life and health by diet, *Proc. Soc. Exp. Biol. Med.*, 193, 31, 1990.
33. **Gilchrest, B. A.**, *Skin and Aging Processes*, CRC Press, Boca Raton, FL, 1984.
34. **Lavkin, R. M.**, Structural alterations in exposed and unexposed aged skin, *J. Invest. Dermatol.*, 73, 59, 1979.

Chapter 2

FREE RADICALS AND DIFFERENTIATION: THE INTERRELATIONSHIP OF DEVELOPMENT AND AGING

Robert G. Allen

TABLE OF CONTENTS

0-8493-4518-9/93/$0.00 + $.50

I. INTRODUCTION

Free radicals are believed to play a fundamental role in a wide variety of biological phenomena. Although the number of cellular reactions thought to be catalyzed by free radicals has steadily increased over several decades, virtually none of these reactions can be regarded as biologically beneficial. As discussed elsewhere in this volume, free radicals inactivate enzymes, break DNA, and initiate the chain reactions that peroxidize lipids. Indeed, most free radical involvement in cellular processes generally has been attributed to the destabilizing effects of structural damage.

It might be assumed that the potentially disastrous consequences of any large upsurge in the number of free radical reactions would effectively preclude the evolution of any cellular strategy that utilized these highly reactive substances as a biological stimulus. Paradoxically, a number of recent studies have demonstrated that bursts of oxidant production, as well as dramatic changes in the activities of various antioxidant defenses, are closely associated with alterations in gene expression in a variety of tissues from phylogenetically diverse organisms.[1,2] Furthermore, perturbations in the cellular equilibrium between oxidant generation and removal have been repeatedly observed to alter gene expression in a number of different types of cells.[2,3] Evidence has also accumulated that suggests that free radical-induced modulation of gene expression occurs in the absence of irreparable damage to DNA (for review, see Allen and Balin,[1] Allen,[2] and Sohal et al.[3,4]). Free radical reactions have been postulated to influence molecular and biochemical processes and to directly cause some of the changes observed in cells during differentiation, aging, and transformation.[3-5] In the discussion that follows, evidence is presented that supports a nondestructive role for free radical reactions in modulating molecular events, and the possible consequences of such mechanisms on the aging process are considered.

II. OXIDATIVE INFLUENCE ON THE METABOLIC CLOCK

A central question that underlies both the theories of aging and development is the nature of the mechanisms by which various events are initiated or terminated at critical times. For example, differentiation proceeds by the transcription of tissue-specific genes and the concomitant suspension of transcription of genes that are specific to pluripotent stem cells. Age-associated changes in gene expression that are both species and tissue specific also occur; however, in contrast to developmental changes in gene expression, age-associated changes neither completely halt the expression of a particular gene nor lead to the appearance of new genes. Instead, aging alters the rate of transcription for some, but not all genes.[6] It is, in fact, this apparent selectivity that leads to the conclusion that age-associated changes in gene expression are programmed and not random.[7,8]

Perhaps the strongest evidence for any influence of a metabolic clock on aging stems from the repeated observations that the life-span of poikilotherms (such as insects) can be predictably altered by experimentally varying their metabolic rate.[9-12] Poikilotherms also exhibit a metabolic potential, or maximum energy expenditure, that is species specific.[13-15] Although the metabolic potential of different phylogenetic groups is variable, within each group the rate of metabolism and life-span are inversely correlated.[15-18] For example, milkweed bugs, *Oncopeltus fasciatus,* raised at 18°C live fourfold longer and consume oxygen at only about one fourth the rate observed in insects reared at 30°C,[19] yet the total amount of oxygen consumed during life by both groups of insects is similar. Similar results have been found in other organisms.[15] Trout and Kaplan[20] observed that mutant *Drosophila,* which made characteristic twitching motions, exhibited a higher rate of metabolism and shorter life-span than normal controls. However, the total volume of oxygen consumed during life was similar in the "shaker" mutants and normal controls.

The existence of a specific metabolic potential for a given species supports the concept of a genetically controlled clock which runs in relation to energy expenditure rather than time. It might also be noted that the influence of the metabolic clock is not limited to biological senescence. The rate of development in poikilotherms is directly related to the rate of metabolism.[21] Since the duration of both development and aging phases of life can be varied by altering metabolic rate, it would seem reasonable to infer that any genetic mechanisms that control these biological events are directly influenced by the rate of metabolism.

A. THE FREE RADICAL THEORY OF AGING

One seemingly plausible explanation for the influence of metabolic rate on life-span was that oxygen radicals generated in metabolic pathways damaged cells and ultimately killed them. This hypothesis formed the basis of the "Free Radical Theory of Aging" as first presented by Harman in 1956.[22] Free radical reactions have been shown to promote a variety of deleterious reactions and probably account for the accumulation of lipofuscin pigment during the natural aging of untreated organisms,[23,24] as well as for certain aspects of age-associated diseases such as heart disease.[25] Furthermore, it has been demonstrated that species longevity is inversely correlated with the rate of free radical generation.[26,27] However, the postulate that damage alone was the basis for aging left many unresolved questions. One of the most troubling aspects of the theory has been the complete failure of most investigations to identify the target molecules that are damaged during aging.[28] Although it is relatively simple to damage molecules by free radical bombardment *in vitro,* the identification of *in vivo* damage that can account for any age-associated changes has remained elusive. An examination of age-associated changes reveals that neither gross structural damage to cellular components nor decreased repair capacity can account for cellular dysfunction and death.[7,28-30] A second inconsistency stems from the fact that antioxidant administration decreases the rate of accumulation of some types of cellular damage, such as lipofuscin pigment,[31] but fails to increase maximum life-span.[28,32] Several studies indicate that antioxidants can increase mean life-span,[33,34] but their failure to influence maximum life-span probably indicates that their effects are actually due to a decrease in vulnerability to aging-unrelated causes rather than an alteration of the rate of aging.[28,35]

Many experimental perturbations in antioxidant defenses have also failed to produce the result predicted by the free radical theory. Chemical oxidants and inhibition of various antioxidant enzymes often fail to decrease life-span in houseflies and can even increase mean longevity.[7,17,18] Whereas the growth of mammalian cell cultures is inhibited by oxygen partial pressures that exceed normoxic levels,[36] inhibition of either catalase or superoxide dismutase (SOD) activity stimulates their growth.[37] Furthermore, a comparison of the levels of various antioxidant defenses in different species reveals that some of them correlate inversely with longevity.[16,38]

One of the more puzzling aspects of free radical biology is the apparent existence of an equilibrium between oxidants and antioxidants. Organisms challenged by an oxidative stress often decrease their rate of metabolism, which presumably would lead to a corresponding decrease in their rate of free radical generation. This type of compensatory response has been implicated as the underlying cause of the radiation resistance observed in postmitotic organisms[39,40] and may also account for the fact that some chemical oxidants fail to decrease longevity in poikilothermic organisms.[17,18] Chemical oxidants also stimulate endogenous antioxidant defenses, which can prevent at least some damage.[41] A second aspect of the equilibrium is that administration of exogenous antioxidants tends to depress endogenous antioxidant levels.[18,42,43] This suggests that cells respond to either excessive oxidation or antioxidation. The net effect of these responses is to maintain a tightly controlled cellular balance between oxidizing and reducing equivalents. Thus, the relationship between oxidants and antioxidants is far more dynamic than originally predicted by the free radical theory. On the basis of these observations, it is evident that apparent conflicts with the free radical theory do not exclude free radical damage as a cause of aging; however, it would also seem probable that free radical-induced damage alone can not account for the relationship between metabolic rate and life-span. On the other hand, free radicals may influence life-span by mechanisms that are independent of structural damage.

B. GENE EXPRESSION AS A TARGET OF FREE RADICALS

Aside from inducing gross structural damage to cellular components, free radical reactions may also lead to specific but more subtle changes in homeostatic responses. Cutler[16,38] postulated that DNA regulatory mechanisms become altered by environmental factors, and that these alterations resulted in a gradual loss of cellular control over the genome. He termed this process "dysdifferentiation". Because dysdifferentiation changes occur randomly, only a small population of cells should exhibit a given set of alterations. Since dysdifferentiation loosens genetic control, it would be expected that new proteins would appear in aging cells. In fact, the expression of c-Ha-*ras*-1 increases in proliferatively aged cell cultures,[44] and several studies have revealed decreased repression of viral DNA in aging mammalian cells.[45-47] There is also evidence that conformational changes in controlling proteins may alter cellular responses to environmental stress as a function of age.[48] Additionally, changes such as the appearance of abnormal proteins[49] increased incidence of metaplasias,[50] and the appearance of biochemically distinct subpopulations of lymphocytes[51,52] are all examples of dysdifferentiation. However, it is not clear that any of these phenomena occur widely enough to be regarded as part of a general mechanism of aging.[6] For example, Parker et al.[53] and later Fleming et al.[54] used 2D gel electrophoresis to demonstrate that aging in insects is associated with some qualitative changes in the expression of proteins, but with the appearance of no new ones. It has also been argued that the randomness of the changes proposed by Cutler cannot account for the relatively specific time course of aging events.[7,8]

Recently, Sohal and Allen[7] proposed the ''Oxidative Stress'' hypothesis. It postulated that development and aging changes are both genetically controlled, and that the programs which govern these changes are driven to completion by incremental increases in cellular oxidation. They noted that developmental changes in gene expression cause both the disappearance of some proteins and the appearance of other new proteins, and that once development is completed, the appearance of new proteins would not be expected. Instead, age-associated changes in gene expression would largely result in variations in the cellular capacity to synthesize proteins, which is consistent with observations made in aging tissues.[6] According to the oxidative stress hypothesis,[7] aging is a continuation of differentiation rather than a loss of differentiation as postulated by the dysdifferentiation hypothesis. Although others have proposed similar hypotheses to explain aging,[55-57] the oxidative stress hypothesis encapsulated by Sohal and Allen is unique because it postulates that both aging and development are governed by a free radical-driven metabolic clock. A second difference between the oxidative stress hypothesis and its predecessors is that it offers a test for its validity: according to Sohal and Allen, ''the completion of the genetic program governing the sequence and duration of various ontogenetic phases is linked to the expenditure of a definite sum of energy.''[7] Accordingly, changes in the rate of energy expenditure should alter the course and/or the duration of development and aging. In fact, both development and life-span can be influenced by the rate of metabolism.[11,21,40,58-62]

The principle weakness of the oxidative stress hypothesis is that it remains largely untested. Nevertheless, several studies exist which support the hypothesis. Munkres[63] has demonstrated that the age gene modulates the antioxidant defenses, development, and life-span of *Neurospora*. Although increases in antioxidant enzymes are observed during their development, age⁻ mutants exhibit an impaired capacity to respond to oxidative stress and they are incapable of asexual differentiation[64-66] unless their medium is supplemented with antioxidants such as α-tocopherol.[65] These observations implicate a single locus in both development and aging. Furthermore, the locus implicated regulates cellular oxidative stress.

The oxidative stress hypothesis would also seem to be supported by studies conducted *in vitro*. It has recently been demonstrated that human fetal lung fibroblasts nearing the end of their proliferative life-span selectively repress the expression of *c-fos;* other oncogenes, such as *H-ras* and *c-myc*, were not repressed.[67] It has also been observed that the posttranscriptional processing of proliferating cell nuclear antigen (PCNA) is blocked in proliferatively senescent cells.[68] Interestingly, the age-associated decrease in avian ovalbumin also appears to result from a failure of oviduct cells to posttranscriptionally process hnRNA.[69] In this latter case, it was found that oxidizing treatments stimulated the release of unprocessed RNA (see discussion below). These observations indicate that the changes in gene expression associated with senescence are specific. It is also well established that the finite proliferative life-span of cultured cells is inversely related to the age of the cell donor. An analysis of proliferative life-span reveals that limited proliferative capacity may stem from changes in the state of differentiation of the cells.[70,71] The inverse relationship between donor age and proliferative life-span (before terminal differentiation) indicates that progressive changes in the state of differentiation may also occur during aging *in vivo*.

As seen later in this discussion, several mechanisms by which the environment influences gene expression have been determined. Most of the evidence supporting an oxidative influence on gene expression has been obtained from studies of developing organisms and differentiating cells. Some of these data are summarized in the discussion that follows.

C. OXYGEN, OXIDATIVE STRESS, AND DEVELOPMENT

Early in this century, developmentalists established that gradient effects were operative during early development, but the nature of these gradients could not be clearly defined.[72,73] In a series of elegant experiments using metabolic inhibitors and redox sensitive dyes, C. M. Child[58-62] demonstrated that both development and regeneration were influenced by regional variations in rate of metabolism, i.e., metabolic gradients. He observed that both the size of organs and the type of tissue which developed from precursor cells could be influenced by experimentally-induced alterations in the metabolic rate of developing sea urchins.[61] Similarly, on the basis of studies in the hydra and in amphibians, Chernavskii et al.[74,75] inferred that a high level of metabolism results in a "limitation of tissue potency" and thus promotes differentiation; whereas, the lowering of metabolic intensity "expands tissue potency" and leads to dedifferentiation (as in regeneration) and transformation.

Oxygen is an absolute requirement for differentiation, and only aerobic organisms have the capacity to establish physiological diversity via differentiation. Even very simple aerobes are often capable of a type of differentiation. Considerable evidence has accumulated to implicate oxygen as one of the primary regulatory factors that controls microbial differentiation.[76] For example, the syncitial slime mold, *Physarum polycephalum* essentially differentiates by forming cell walls. The ability of *Physarum* to differentiate is abolished when it is cultured anaerobically; however, admission of oxygen to the culture flasks permits the process to proceed.[77] Similarly, mycelial development in the fungus *Mucor racemosus* is oxygen dependent; conversely, anaerobic conditions promote only yeast-like morphogenesis.[78]

Oxygen is necessary for differentiation to proceed; however, it is more than an essential cofactor for aerobic metabolism. Variations in ambient oxygen concentration strongly modulate the developmental fate of embryonic tissues. In cultures of fetal chick-limb rudiments, bone development is supported only by hyperoxic conditions, whereas cells maintained at 5% O_2 differentiate into cartilage.[79] More striking are the observations of Caplan and Koutroupus,[80] who reported that chick mesenchymal cells exposed to low oxygen concentrations differentiated into cartilage, while those cultured at higher oxygen concentration formed muscle cells.

Paradoxically, the influence of oxygen on development is not mediated by any effects on respiration. Meal worms reared under 10.5% O_2 exhibit a high rate of abnormal metamorphosis. As many as one third of the pupae maintained under hypoxia develop into pupae-adult intermediates that exhibit features of both pupae and adults; however, due to the structure of the insect respiratory system and the relatively low K_M of their cytochrome oxidase, the actual rate of oxygen consumption is not altered by maintenance under hypoxia.[81] Similarly, hyperoxia induces differentiation in neuroblastoma, even in the presence of enough cyanide to abolish aerobic metabolism.[82] Thus, the effects of oxygen on differentiation are independent of aerobic metabolism. Many oxygen-mediated reactions occur via oxygen-free radical intermediates. Although respiratory inhibitors decrease the rate of oxygen utilization, they also promote cytochrome reduction and thereby stimulate free radical generation.[83] Furthermore, the rate of free radical generation in cells is strongly modulated by ambient oxygen concentration.[84] Oxygen radicals and their derivatives can react deleteriously with most of the organic components of cells; however, their extremely short half-life and their ability to mediate changes in the electrical charge of the cellular microenvironment suggest that they might also serve as subcellular messengers. As seen in the discussion that follows, several lines of evidence implicate them as the probable effectors of oxygen-mediated changes in gene expression.

D. OXIDANTS, ANTIOXIDANTS, AND DIFFERENTIATION
1. Superoxide Dismutase and Development

Large variations in the levels of antioxidant defenses have been observed during the development of an extremely wide variety of tissues in phylogenetically diverse organisms.[1,2] For example, total SOD activity increases dramatically during the differentiation of tissues in syncitial slime mold,[85] acellular slime mold,[86] fruit flies,[87] nematodes,[88] amphibians,[89] mice,[90] guinea pigs,[90] rabbits,[90,91] hamsters,[90] rats,[92] and humans.[93-95] SOD exists as two forms, a manganese-containing form (MnSOD) localized primarily in mitochondria and a copper/zinc form (Cu/Zn SOD) usually found in the cytosol. When the activity of these two forms has been determined, it has usually been changes in the MnSOD activity that were most strongly associated with differentiation.[2] Recently, it has been demonstrated that the increase in activity corresponds to increased transcription of the MnSOD gene.[95]

The underlying causes of the stimulation of SOD during development are not entirely clear. It has been suggested that the changes in ambient oxygen tension associated with birth contribute to differences observed in the SOD activity of pre- and postnatal tissues; however, only the Cu/Zn form of SOD appears to respond to the changes in ambient oxygen tension associated with birth.[96] Additionally, SOD activity increases markedly prior to birth,[91,94] and both forms of SOD exhibit distinctive developmental patterns, which would argue against induction by variations in ambient oxygen tension.[97]

Studies in cultured cells have also revealed that the developmental changes in SOD activity are independent of ambient oxygen tension. Oxygen tension presumably would not vary during *in vitro* differentiation, yet SOD activity triples in human monocytes induced to differentiate in culture,[98] and doubles during the *in vivo* differentiation of erythrocytes in rabbit bone marrow.[99] A study of confluent (nonmitotic) human skin fibroblast cultures, obtained from fetal (15 to 16-week gestational age) and postnatal donors (4 to 96-year old), that were maintained under six different oxygen tensions (0% to 95% O_2) for 1 week revealed no significant change in SOD activity at any concentration of oxygen examined.[100] At all of the oxygen tensions employed, the activity of the mangano form of SOD (MnSOD) was fivefold greater in the 14 postnatal lines than in the seven fetal lines examined. No developmental differences were observed in the Cu/Zn form of SOD. No sex-related differences were found in either form of SOD activity. These data indicate that development-associated differences in MnSOD activity are maintained in cultures of cutaneous fibroblasts and that these differences are not due to variations in ambient oxygen concentration. Since all of the cultures were confluent when transferred to different ambient oxygen tensions, the possibility of differences in activity associated with differences in mitotic activity could also be eliminated. As to this last point, it should be noted that MnSOD activity accumulates in growth-arrested cells.[101] Yet, MnSOD activity increases in regenerating liver tissue in which mitotic activity would presumably be stimulated.[102] Also, the very large increase in MnSOD activity associated with differentiation in *Physarum* is not maintained in the resulting quiescent cells; MnSOD activity declines sharply once the organism has differentiated into mitotically quiescent cells.[103]

2. Glutathione and Development

Three distinct patterns of change in glutathione (GSH) concentration have been reported during cellular differentiation. In cells that lose mitotic capacity during development, GSH concentration decreases. For example, GSH concentration declines by 60% in houseflies during metamorphosis[104] and by 50% in developing rat lung.[105] A loss of GSH has also been reported in preadipocytes[106] that were induced to differentiate in culture. A notable exception to the changes in GSH associated with differentiation into postmitotic cells is seen in muscle development. GSH concentration increases during much of the differentiation phase of avian skeletal muscle; the only decreases observed occur just prior to hatching.[107] It has been suggested that this unusual pattern results from an equilibrium between GSH and small histidine-containing peptides.[107] GSH levels remained high during a period when the dipeptides were low or absent from muscle tissue. Histidine-containing peptides reach their highest level prior to hatching, and GSH concentration drops to nearly zero.

The concentration of GSH- and ⁻SH-containing peptides increases during the mitotic phase of regeneration and decreases during redifferentiation of regenerating tissues in amphibians.[108] Regeneration also leads to an increased chemical reducing capacity in mammalian tissue.[1,109-111] Cells that differentiate into tissues which retain a high regenerative capacity, such as liver tissue, exhibit no loss of GSH during development.[2] GSH concentration increases sharply during the development of meiotic tissues.[112]

The changes in GSH concentration that occur during development may influence the developmental fate of cells. For example, the inductive capacity of postnodal pieces taken from chick embryos can be modified by soaking the tissue in a solution of GSH or cysteine.[113,114] Furthermore, the types of tissue that arise from induction are affected by sulfhydryl status.[113,114] Experimentally induced changes in GSH concentration stimulate the expression of heat shock proteins.[115]

3. Lipid Peroxidation and Development

Lipid peroxidation has been implicated in a large number of cellular processes and has been postulated to play an integral role in some synthetic pathways and in the controlling mechanisms that govern mitosis.[116,117] Many organisms exhibit a marked increase in lipid peroxidation or in the susceptibility of their tissues to peroxidation during development.[85,118-121] In contrast, lipid peroxidation decreases during periods of increased mitotic activity such as regeneration[122] or in transformed cells.[17,123] The addition of antioxidant enzymes to lung homogenates from young rats is reported to have no effect on the susceptibility to lipid peroxidation, and, while tocopherol inhibits peroxidation, the concentration required to achieve inhibition in neonatal tissue is far greater than would ever be found in fetal or adult tissue.[124] Strains of mice that exhibit higher SOD activity in early neonatal development are less vulnerable to peroxidation than strains which contain low SOD activity in early postpartum life.[119]

The greater susceptibility of mammalian neonatal lipids to peroxidation is largely due to differences in lipid composition between adults and newborns.[125] Although peroxidation is generally deleterious, unsaturated lipids may remove radicals and thus provide a type of antioxidant protection for other cellular components at a time when other enzymic defenses are low in neonates. Feeding mature rats diets rich in saturated fat will decrease their susceptibility to peroxidation, but it also proves fatal to them after 68-h hyperoxic exposure, whereas 46% of the rats fed a normal diet survive after 96-h hyperoxic exposure.[126] Neonatal animals that contain large amounts of polyunsaturated lipid in their lung tissues are known to be more resistant to oxygen than organisms with a low polyunsaturated lipid concentration.[1]

E. THE EFFECTS OF OXIDANTS AND ANTIOXIDANTS ON DIFFERENTIATION

The changes in oxidative metabolism that occur during differentiation appear to play a causal role in stimulation of at least some types of differentiation. The syncitial slime mold *Physarum polycephalum* has been used extensively as a model to examine the effects of oxidants and antioxidants on differentiation. *Physarum* exhibits a 46-fold increase in MnSOD activity and a 70 to 80% loss of GSH during its transition from mitotically active to mitotically quiescent cells.[85,127] A strain of *Physarum* that fails to differentiate under identical culture conditions exhibits neither a sustained increase in SOD activity nor any significant loss of GSH.[77,85,127] In differentiating strains of *Physarum*, the rate of cyanide-resistant respiration doubles, and there is also a sharp increase in the concentration of organic peroxides and H_2O_2 during spherulation; the nondifferentiating strain of *Physarum* exhibits none of these changes.[85]

Experimental perturbations of the antioxidant defenses of *Physarum* exert profound effects on its state of differentiation. Buthionine sulfoximine (BSO), an inhibitor of GSH synthesis, increases the rate of differentiation in organisms cultured in a nonnutrient medium; however, BSO fails to induce differentiation in growth medium. Treatments that increase GSH concentration strongly retard the rate of differentiation.[127] Treatment of a nondifferentiating strain of *Physarum* with paraquat, a free radical-generating herbicide, and BSO induces a type of incomplete differentiation.[128]

Introduction of bovine Cu/ZnSOD into cells of the nondifferentiating strain of *Physarum* via liposomes induced differentiation.[129] The effect could be significantly increased by pretreatment of the cells with BSO for 48 h prior to treatment with SOD-containing liposomes. Conversely, other antioxidants such as dithiothreitol, ascorbate, GSH, β-carotene, α-tocopherol, and butylated hydroxytoluene all failed to induce differentiation. Strong oxidants such as cumene hydroperoxide, plumbagin, and intracellular generation of H_2O_2 by liposomal addition of either D-amino acid oxidase or xanthine oxidase also stimulate spherulation in the nondifferentiating strain. SOD itself was observed to increase intracellular H_2O_2.[129]

In similar studies, Beckman et al.[130] observed that Friend erythroleukemia cells (FLC) treated with liposomally encapsulated SOD were stimulated to differentiate (produce hemoglobin). Treatments with other antioxidants failed to induce differentiation and, in fact, were found to inhibit differentiation of FLC induced by treatment with hexamethylene (bis)acetamide (HMBA). In contrast, oxidants such as plumbagin, potassium superoxide, cumene hydroperoxide, and liposomally encapsulated xanthine oxidase or D-amino acid oxidase were all found to stimulate the differentiation of FLC. As in the case of *Physarum*, decreasing GSH concentration with BSO prior to addition of oxidizing compounds or SOD-containing liposomes increased the effectiveness of these treatments.

SOD is an antioxidant enzyme; however, the large increases in its activity observed during differentiation or after treatment of the nondifferentiating strain with SOD-containing liposomes were both associated with a significant rise in parameters of oxidation.[85,129] Increased H_2O_2 production and stimulation of peroxidation in the presence of elevated SOD activity have been observed in tumor cell homogenates[131] and in HeLa cells that contained an inserted SOD gene.[132] It would also seem noteworthy that, in *Drosophila,* a threefold increase in SOD activity resulting from insertion of a bovine SOD gene exerted deleterious effects on development that were associated with a marked increase in peroxidation.[133] Since O_2^- spontaneously dismutates quite rapidly, it is improbable that high SOD activity alone stimulates production of H_2O_2. Some oxidation reactions as well as some oxidative enzymes are inhibited by O_2^-; its removal by SOD would be expected to accelerate oxidation in the case of these reactions.[1,2]

The capacity of cellular oxidation to induce differentiation is not unique to *Physarum* or FLC, but this effect is not universal. Antioxidants have repeatedly been observed to induce differentiation in other types of cells. Cu(II)(3,5-diisopropylsalicylate), a chemical that mimics SOD activity, has been used to induce differentiation in mouse neuroblastoma.[5] Numerous studies have indicated that treatment of tumor cells with lipid soluble antioxidants can induce a type of reversible differentiation.[134-136] Furthermore, p16, a protein that regulates growth in erythroid progenitor cells, was recently purified and identified as Cu/Zn SOD.[137] What is apparent from these studies is that changes in the rate of generation or the rate of removal of cellular oxidants can potentially stimulate alterations in gene expression in a wide variety of cell types. It is also apparent that the timing of oxidative changes must be tightly controlled for development to proceed normally. The mechanisms by which oxidants and reductants influence gene expression have only recently been investigated and remain poorly understood. It will probably not be possible to determine whether the genes that regulate the biological clock are themselves influenced by redox mechanisms until these genes have been identified.

F. OXIDANTS AND ANTIOXIDANTS IN AGING ORGANISMS

Changes in the antioxidant defenses have been observed during the aging of several organisms, but unlike the variations seen in developing organisms, the age-associated changes in antioxidant enzymes lack uniformity; most are species-specific and some are strain-specific.[18,123] Decreased SOD activity has been observed in several types of insects during aging.[87,138] In mammals, age-associated changes in SOD activity are highly variable. Total SOD appears to decrease slightly in the liver tissue of Sprague-Dawley rats, but not in their brain.[139] Conversely, total SOD activity decreases by roughly 36% in the brains of C57BL/6J mice.[140] Cu/Zn SOD activity decreases in the brains of Wistar rats, but MnSOD activity increases at a proportional rate.[141] A second point that should be raised is that the regulation of some genes (including the SODs) differs in adult and fetal animals.[142] Adult tissues appear to respond to an oxidative stress by increasing translation of existing mRNA; conversely, fetal tissues respond by increasing their rate of transcription.[142-144] Thus, if stochastic mechanisms are involved in any developmental or age-associated changes in antioxidant protection, then clearly the regulatory targets of these mechanisms differ in different phases of life.

Aside from SOD, most of the other antioxidant defenses such as catalase and GSH peroxidase decline during the aging of animal tissues.[138,145,146] However, changes in these enzymes are tissue-specific. For example, a significant decrease in catalase activity was observed in rat brain, but not in liver or heart tissues; GSH peroxidase increases in liver and heart, but declines in brain; and GSH reductase decreased in heart, but increased in liver and brain.[26] Cellular redox status tends to become consistently more prooxidizing with age. This loss of reducing equivalents stems from loss of GSH as well as other sources of reducing equivalents such as NAD(P)H.[104,147,148] Whether age-associated loss of antioxidant enzyme activities plays any role in this shift in redox state is presently unclear.

Evidence derived from a variety of methods clearly demonstrates that the rate of oxidant generation increases during the aging of many types of cells and tissues in diverse organisms. For example, the rate of alkane production increases with age in both insects[149] and mammals.[150] On the basis of age-associated changes in membrane structure and increases in the production of dienes, aldehydes, and ketones, Nohl and Hegner[151-153] inferred that the rate of free radical generation increased as a function of aging in the heart tissues of rats. The rate of O_2^- production from submitochondrial particles is higher in old houseflies as compared with young animals.[154] H_2O_2 has also been observed to increase in houseflies during aging.[155] A similar comparison of liver, heart, and brain tissues in aging rats revealed that both the rates of O_2^- and H_2O_2 generation were elevated in 18-month-old animals as compared with 3-month-old animals.[26] Similar observations have been reported by others in rat hearts.[156]

III. THE MECHANISMS OF OXIDATIVE INFLUENCE ON GENE EXPRESSION

The influence of oxidative stress on gene expression can be direct; however, it would be expected that these direct effects would chemically modify either the DNA or structural proteins of chromatin. In many instances, oxidants are reported to alter the expression of genes without physically interacting with the components of chromatin. Aside from transcriptional changes induced by oxidative stress, both posttranscriptional and translational effects are also observed. As might be expected, more than one mechanism is necessary to account for all of these effects. The effects of oxidant/antioxidant equilibrium on gene expression are mediated by both biophysical and genetic elements.

A. REDOX STATUS, METAL IONS, AND CYTOSKELETON

Several physical factors that are strongly influenced by the cellular generation of oxidants appear to exert general effects on gene expression. Thus, oxidative changes in redox state, cellular ion distribution, and the cytoskeleton and nuclear matrix may directly alter gene expression, or in some cases, make the cellular environment permissive to activation of preexisting, but inactive regulatory factors.

1. Redox Status

The activity of proteins is strongly influenced by their charge which is largely a product of microenvironmental factors such as pH, redox state, and surrounding metal ions.[157] Environmental effects on protein activities will have a far-reaching influence if the protein affected is involved in chromatin regulation. As discussed above, changes in GSH concentration associated with development are largely dependent on the cell type resulting from differentiation. Variations in redox state have been demonstrated to play a key role in the induction of some genes. For example, the production of adenylylated nucleotides, which function as regulatory molecules that signal the onset of oxidative stress,[158] is stimulated by a wide variety of oxidants. Sulfhydryl group oxidants appear to be particularly effective.[159] Furthermore, $^-$SH groups have been implicated as targets for several inducers of heat shock proteins in eukaryotic cells,[115,159,160] and sulfhydryl-containing compounds appear to modulate the expression of heat shock proteins.[161] It would seem noteworthy that heat shock has been observed to induce SOD activity in *Escherichia coli*.[162]

Aside from differentiation, cell mitosis presents a period of intense gene activity with highly controlled changes in gene expression. A very strong correlation exists between the phase of mitosis and the redox state of cells.[163] It has in fact been demonstrated that modulation of GSH concentration can be employed to control cell cycle in human T lymphocytes.[164] Although a comparison of cultures reveals a greater GSH content in proliferating cultures than in stationary growth arrested cultures, in individual cells (and in synchronous cultures) $^-$SH concentration decreases prior to metaphase and is lowest during cytokinesis.[1,163] This suggests that cells are more oxidized during mitosis. It has also been demonstrated that interference with oxidant production tends to inhibit cellular proliferation.[165,166] Redox status also appears to play a key role in the rate of proliferative aging. Chronic stimulation of GSH synthesis increases proliferative life-span by about 40%, while chronic inhibition of GSH synthesis decreases proliferative life-span.[167]

The effects of redox changes on gene expression are not limited to cell cycle. Roederer et al.[168] found that the expression of human immunodeficiency virus (HIV) could be controlled by modulation of the cellular GSH concentration.

2. Metal Ions

Cells maintain an extremely tight control over free metal ion concentrations. Since a rise in the concentration of any of several metal ions can stimulate a large number of biochemical pathways, any failure to effectively sequester metal ions can rapidly lead to cellular chaos and death. The mitochondria and endoplasmic reticula are the primary sites for storage of metal ions within cells. Physiological stimulation of various biochemical pathways by metal ions appears to proceed by their release from cellular stores followed by rapid resequestration.[169]

Sequestration of metal ions by cells is strongly modulated by a cellular redox state.[170-172] It has been postulated that an upsurge in the rate of free radical generation during development could stimulate a release of mitochondrial stores of metal ions, particularly calcium ions, and thereby initiate a cascade of biochemical events that ultimately change gene expression.[1] These effects appear to be selective since O_2^- decreases free Mg^{2+} ions.[172] Fluctuations in the intracellular ion concentration and particularly calcium ion concentration have been implicated as the physiological signal that initiates many cellular processes, including some biochemical and genetic phenomena associated with both mitosis and development.[169-171] Variations in the ionic strength of other metals such as (Mg^{2+}, Na^+, K^+) has been shown to induce puffing in insect salivary glands.[173,174] Oxidants stimulate calcium release from mitochondria and induce cytoskeletal contraction; in extreme cases of cellular oxidation, surface blebbing occurs due to contraction of the cytoskeleton.[175,176] The influence of oxidants on calcium sequestration appears to be mediated by changes in cellular redox state. Lotscher et al.[177] have implicated utilization of reduced nicotinamide-adenine dinucleotide (NADH) during ribosylation of proteins as a probable cause of calcium release from mitochondria. Although redox changes resulting from GSH oxidation do not directly stimulate calcium release, they do make the cellular environment permissive to reactions that will stimulate calcium release.[170,171] For example, loss of GSH and its effect on the cellular environment could, at some point, stimulate ADP-ribose transferase, an enzyme that consumes reduced nicotinamide-adenine dinucleotide phosphate (NAD(P)H) and that is sensitive to oxidation.

Calcium is required for differentiation in the syncytial slime mold, *Physarum polycephalum*. Citrate buffered calcium alone provides an environment sufficient for differentiation to occur, but the associated changes in MnSOD activity and GSH concentration are diminished in this environment.[103] Although the stimulus that causes increased SOD activity is apparently decreased when citrate buffered calcium is employed to induce differentiation, cellular peroxidation (as indicated by thiobarbituric [TBA] reactants) is both rapid and extensive in organisms cultured in this medium. Treatment of either differentiating or nondifferentiating strains with an extremely high calcium concentration (54 mM) induces differentiation even in nutrient medium, albeit, over a vastly increased time course (4 to 5 d).[103] Deletion of calcium from the medium completely inhibits differentiation; however, spherulation can proceed normally in the absence of any of the other cations usually present in the differentiation medium.[103]

Calcium ions, sequestered by mitochondria, usually react with inorganic phosphate to form small granules which are visible in electron micrographs. The mitochondria of *Physarum* cultured in nutrient medium contain relatively few granules. Within 6 h of transfer of cultures to differentiation medium, a marked increase in the number of mitochondrial granules is observed. The number of granules subsequently decreased and had virtually vanished after 30 h in differentiation medium. X-ray probe analysis of these granules revealed that they were composed primarily of calcium and phosphorus.[178] In contrast to the differentiating strain, the nondifferentiating strain accumulated no mitochondrial granules when transferred to differentiation medium; instead, the organism died after a few hours.

In *Physarum*, NADH concentration increases after transfer of the organism to differentiation medium, reaching its acme in about 6 h. During this same period, calcium is accumulated in granules by mitochondria. The concentration of NADH subsequently declines and by 30 h after transfer to differentiation medium it is 75% lower than the highest concentration observed at 6 h. It is during this same period that the mitochondrial calcium granules disappear.[178]

The development of multicellular organisms is closely associated with a selective uptake and release of calcium ions. The resulting orderly flow of positively charged calcium ions through tissues produces bioelectricity, which has been postulated to influence the course of development.[179] Transcellular currents of this type have been demonstrated in a wide variety of organisms.[169,180,181] Such currents have also been implicated in regeneration.[179,182,183] It is likely that the establishment of bioelectrical currents is augmented by metabolic gradients and the resulting redox gradients which they establish.[100]

3. Cytoskeleton

A physical factor that strongly modulates gene expression is the spatial arrangement of chromatin, i.e., chromatin configuration.[184-187] The redox status, as well as the ionic milieu of cells, affects chromatin configuration.[188-190] Changes in chromatin configuration arise partly from direct interactions with ions.[191,192] Thus, a change in redox status that stimulates the release of cellular stores of ions may indirectly alter chromatin configuration and gene activity.

It has been demonstrated repeatedly that cellular oxidation induces chromosomal puff formation in a variety of organisms.[115,159-161] The formation of chromosomal puffs is at least partly due to changes in the cellular electrolyte balance;[173,174] however, oxidants also influence nuclear matrix proteins and the karyoskeleton.[193] The cytoskeleton reciprocally transmits information between the cell membrane and chromatin.[194] Variations in membrane fluidity and polarity induced by free radicals can therefore alter chromatin configuration[190,194,195] and, presumably, gene expression. Both ionic and redox gradients are established at relatively early stages of development.[169,179] The influence of these gradients on chromatin configuration may partially account for the positional divergence of the developmental fates of cells. Age-associated changes in membranes have been postulated to result in broad changes in gene expression; albeit, these alterations are probably more quantitative than qualitative.[7]

B. TRANSCRIPTIONAL EFFECTS

Treatment of bacteria with small amounts of H_2O_2 induces the synthesis of more than 30 proteins. Nine of these are now known to be under the control of the *oxyR* gene.[196-198] The gene also appears to regulate its own transcription.[196,198] Activation of the *oxyR* gene product is not due to disulfide bond formation, conjugation with short chain sulfhydryl compounds such as GSH, or reduction of a metal ion core.[196] Storz et al.[196] have postulated that the *oxyR* protein may have an active site that captures oxidants directly with a concomitant conformational change. They further suggested that the change in conformation releases the protein from the *oxyR* gene and stimulates its binding to the other genes that it regulates. The mechanism by which the *oxyR* protein stimulates transcription of other genes is presently unknown.

Similar mechanisms may exist in mammalian cells.[199] NF-κ-B is a multisubunit transcriptional factor that activates the expression of genes associated with inflammatory and immune responses. Although a wide variety of chemicals have previously been observed to activate NF-κ-B, it was recently demonstrated that all of these agents act via active oxygen species. On the basis of this study, it has been postulated that oxidants act as subcellular messengers that, in this case, cause the release of an inhibitory subunit from the NF-κ-B complex.[199] Oxidation of cultured human fibroblasts has been observed to stimulate transcription of the collagen gene.[200] Inhibition of peroxidation with antioxidants such as α-tocopherol was found to also inhibit the transcription of the collagen gene. It was postulated that either a direct interaction of lipid peroxidation byproducts with a transactivating protein alters its binding properties and permits it to activate collagen transcription, or that peroxidation may act to make the collagen gene more accessible to transcription factors.[200]

C. RNA PROCESSING

Both microscopic[201] and biochemical evidence[202,203] has implicated the karyoskeleton in posttranscriptional RNA processing. Presently, the karyoskeleton is believed to provide anchor points for pre-mRNA.[201-203] Although anchoring pre-mRNA appears to be essential for processing to occur, the precise role of the anchoring is unknown. Experimentally induced disruption of the karyoskeleton by O_2^- stimulates the release of unprocessed RNA from nuclei.[69] This suggests that physiological levels of O_2^- may regulate or at least influence the anchoring of pre-mRNA to the karyoskeleton.

D. TRANSLATIONAL EFFECTS

Changes in cellular redox status exert a controlling influence on the translation of ferritin. A 28-nucleotide sequence at the 5' end of the ferritin transcript, called the iron responsive element (IRE), is the binding site for an iron-sensitive translational repressor or iron responsive element binding protein (IRE-BP).[204,205] In fact, the binding affinity of the IRE-BP to the IRE is redox sensitive. A prooxidizing environment inhibits binding of the inhibitor protein to ferritin mRNA and, thus, stimulates translation.[205]

The protein products of *c-fos* and *c-jun* act as transcriptional factors after forming either homodimeric or heterodimeric complexes via a leucine zipper domain. A redox mechanism has also been reported to control the post-translational activity of *fos* and *jun* proto-oncogene protein products.[206] The binding of the *fos-jun* complex to DNA is strongly modulated by redox status of a single conserved cysteine in the DNA-binding domains of the two proteins. It is noteworthy that the changes in the redox status of the protein complex appear to be catalyzed by a nuclear protein rather than through the more general mechanism of an alteration in cellular redox state.[206] Taken together, the studies of ferritin and *fos-jun* may be indicative of a widespread subcellular control mechanism, namely, redox sensitivity of DNA- and RNA-controlling proteins.

V. CONCLUSIONS

A probable link between metabolism and longevity is the ubiquitous generation of partially reduced oxygen species by the biochemical pathways of aerobic cells. Although free radicals may contribute to aging by directly inflicting structural damage, they may also decrease homeostatic control without causing massive structural damage, either by damaging nuclear control mechanisms or by causing cellular changes that influence gene expression. Studies conducted with developing organisms and tumor cells clearly demonstrate that oxidants stimulate changes in gene expression which can alter the state of differentiation. As techniques in molecular analysis improve, a more thorough understanding of oxidative mechanisms that contribute to cellular aging via effects on gene expression should become possible. Such an assessment of free radical influences on gene expression should also prove invaluable to a comprehensive understanding of the elements that control development and transformation.

REFERENCES

1. **Allen, R. G. and Balin, A. K.**, Oxidative influence on development and differentiation: an overview of a free radical theory of development, *J. Free Radical Biol. Med.*, 6, 631, 1989.
2. **Allen, R. G.**, Oxygen-reactive species and antioxidant responses during development: the metabolic paradox of cellular differentiation, *Proc. Soc. Exp. Biol. Med.*, 196, 117, 1991.
3. **Sohal, R. S., Allen, R. G., and Nations, C.**, Oxidative stress and cellular differentiation, in *Membrane in Cancer Cells*, Galeotti, T., Cittadini, A., Neri, G., and Scarpa, A., Eds., Ann. N.Y. Acad. Sci., New York, 1988, 59.
4. **Sohal, R. S., Allen, R. G., and Nations, C.**, Oxygen free radicals play a role in cellular differentiation: an hypothesis, *J. Free Radical Biol. Med.*, 2, 175, 1986.
5. **Oberley, L. W.**, Superoxide dismutases in cancer, in *Superoxide Dismutase*, Oberley, L. W., Ed., CRC Press, Boca Raton, FL, 1983, 127.
6. **Richardson, A. and Semsei, I.**, Effect of aging on translation and transcription, in *Review of Biological Research in Aging*, Rothstein, M., Ed., Alan R. Liss, New York, 1987, 467.
7. **Sohal, R. S. and Allen, R. G.**, Oxidative stress as a causal factor in differentiation and aging: a unifying hypothesis, *Exp. Gerontol.*, 25, 499, 1990.
8. **Allen, R. G.**, Role of free radicals in senescence, in *Annual Review of Gerontology and Geriatrics*, Cristofalo, V. J. and Lawton, M. P., Eds., Springer, New York, 1990, 198.
9. **Liu, R. K. and Walford, R. L.**, Mid-life temperature transfer effects on life-span of the annual fish, *J. Gerontol.*, 30, 129, 1975.
10. **Sacher, G. A.**, Life table modification and life prolongation, in *The Handbook of the Biology of Aging*, Finch, C. E. and Hayflick, L., Eds., Van Nostrand Reinhold, New York, 1977, 582.
11. **Ragland, S. S. and Sohal, R. S.**, Mating behavior, physical activity and aging in the housefly, *Musca domestica, Exp. Gerontol.*, 8, 135, 1973.
12. **Miquel, J., Lungren, P. R., Bensch, K. J., and Atlan, H.**, Effect of temperature on the life-span vitality and fine structure of *Drosophila melanogaster, Mech. Ageing Dev.*, 5, 347, 1976.
13. **Sohal, R. S.**, Metabolic rate and life-span, *Interdisciplinary Top. Gerontol.*, 9, 25, 1976.
14. **Sohal, R. S.**, Oxygen consumption and adult life-span in the adult housefly, *Musca domestica, Age*, 5, 21, 1982.
15. **Sohal, R. S.**, The Rate of Living Theory: a contemporary interpretation, in *Comparative Biology of Insect Aging: Strategies and Mechanisms*, Collatz, K. G. and Sohal, R. S., Eds., Springer-Verlag, Heidelberg, 1986, 23.
16. **Cutler, R. G.**, Antioxidants, aging and longevity, in *Free Radicals in Biology*, Pryor, W. A., Ed., Academic Press, New York, 1984, 371.

17. **Sohal, R. S. and Allen, R. G.**, Relationship between metabolic rate, free radicals, differentiation and aging: a unified theory, in *The Molecular Biology of Aging (Brookhaven Symposium)*, Woodhead, A., Blackett, A. D., and Hollaender, A., Eds., Plenum Press, New York, 1985, 75.

18. **Sohal, R. S. and Allen, R. G.**, Relationship between oxygen metabolism, aging and development, *Adv. Free Radical Biol. Med.*, 2, 117, 1986.

19. **McArthur, M. C. and Sohal, R. S.**, Relationship between metabolic rate, aging, lipid peroxidation and fluorescent age pigment in milkweed bug, *Oncopeltus fasciatus* (Hemiptera), *J. Gerontol.*, 37, 268, 1981.

20. **Trout, W. E. and Kaplan, W. D.**, A relationship between longevity and activity in shaker mutants of *Drosophila melanogaster*, *Exp. Gerontol.*, 5, 83, 1970.

21. **Loeb, J. and Northrop, J.**, On the influence of food and temperature upon the duration of life, *J. Biol. Chem.*, 32, 103, 1917.

22. **Harman, D.**, Aging: a theory based on free radical and radiation biology, *J. Gerontol.*, 11, 298, 1956.

23. **Sohal, R. S.**, Metabolic rate, aging, and lipofuscin accumulation, in *Age Pigments*, Sohal, R. S., Ed., Elsevier/NorthHolland, New York, 1981, 303.

24. **Donato, H.**, Lipid peroxidation, crosslinking reactions, and aging, in *Age Pigments*, Sohal, R. S., Ed., Elsevier/North-Holland, New York, 1981, 63.

25. **McCord, J. M.**, Oxygen-derived free radicals in postischemic tissue injury, *N. Engl. J. Med.*, 312, 159, 1985.

26. **Sohal, R. S., Arnold, L. A., and Sohal, B. H.**, Age-related changes in antioxidant enzymes and prooxidant generation in tissues of the rat with special reference to parameters in two insect species, *Free Radical Biol. Med.*, 9, 495, 1990.

27. **Sohal, R. S., Svensson, I., Sohal, B. H., and Brunk, U. T.**, Superoxide radical production in different animal species, *Mech. Ageing Dev.*, 49, 129, 1989.

28. **Mehlhorn, R. J. and Cole, G.**, The free radical theory of aging: a critical review, *Adv. Free Radical Biol. Med.*, 1, 165, 1985.

29. **Newton, R. K., Ducore, J. M., and Sohal, R. S.**, Effect of age on endogenous DNA single-strand breakage, strand break induction and repair in the adult housefly, *Musca domestica*, *Mutation Res.*, 219, 113, 1989.

30. **Newton, R. K., Ducore, J. M., and Sohal, R. S.**, Relationship between life expectancy and endogenous DNA single-strand breakage, strand break induction and DNA repair capacity in the adult housefly, *Musca domestica*, *Mech. Ageing Dev.*, 49, 259, 1989.

31. **Nandy, K.**, Effects of antioxidants on neuronal lipofuscin pigment, in *Free Radicals in Molecular Biology, Aging and Disease*, Armstrong, D., Sohal, R. S., Cutler, R. G., and Slater, T. F., Eds., Raven Press, New York, 1984, 223.

32. **Kohn, R. R.**, Effects of antioxidants on the life-span of C57BL mice, *J. Gerontol.*, 26, 378, 1971.

33. **Harmon, D.**, The free radical theory of aging, in *Free Radicals in Biology*, Pryor, W. A., Ed., Academic Press, New York, 1982, 255.

34. **Harman, D.**, Free radicals in aging, *Mol. Cell. Biol.*, 84, 155, 1984.

35. **Balin, A. K.**, Testing the free radical theory of aging, in *Testing the Theories of Aging*, Adelman, R. C. and Roth, G. C., Eds., CRC Press, Boca Raton, FL, 1982, 137.

36. **Balin, A. K., Goodman, D. G., Rassmussen, H., and Cristofalo, V. J.**, The effect of oxygen tension on the growth and metabolism of WI-38 cells, *J. Cell. Physiol.*, 89, 235, 1976.

37. **Oberley, T. D.**, The possible role of reactive oxygen metabolites in cell division, in *Superoxide Dismutase*, Oberley, L. W., Ed., CRC Press, Boca Raton, FL, 1985, 83.

38. **Cutler, R. G.**, Antioxidants and longevity in mammalian species, in *Molecular Biology of Aging*, Woodhead, A. D., Blackett, A. D., and Hollaender, A., Eds., Plenum Press, New York, 1985, 15.

39. **Allen, R. G. and Sohal, R. S.**, Life-lengthening effects of γ-radiation on the adult male housefly, *Musca domestica*, *Mech. Ageing Dev.*, 20, 369, 1982.

40. **Allen, R. G.**, Relationship between γ-irradiation, life-span, metabolic rate and accumulation of fluorescent age pigment in the adult male housefly *Musca domestica, Arch. Gerontol. Geriatrics*, 4, 169, 1985.

41. **Halliwell, B.**, Free radicals, oxygen toxicity and aging, in *Age Pigments*, Sohal, R. S., Ed., Elsevier/North Holland, Amsterdam, 1981, 1.

42. **Blakely, S. R., Slaughter, L., Adkins, J., and Knight, E. V.**, Effect of β-carotene and retinyl palmitate on corn oil-induced superoxide dismutase and catalase in rats, *J. Nutr.*, 118, 152, 1988.

43. **Sohal, R. S., Allen, R. G., Farmer, K. J., Newton, R. K., and Toy, P. L.**, Effects of exogenous antioxidants on the levels of endogenous antioxidants, lipidsoluble fluorescent material and life-span in the housefly, *Musca domestica, Mech. Ageing Dev.*, 31, 329, 1985.

44. **Goldstein, S., Srivastava, A., Riabowol, K. T., and Shmookler-Reis, R. J.**, Changes in genetic organization and expression in aging cells, in *Molecular Biology of Aging*, Woodhead, A. D., Blackett, A. D., and Hollaender, A., Eds., Plenum Press, New York, 1985, 255.

45. **Florine, D. L., Ono, T., Cutler, R. G., and Getz, M. J.**, Regulation of endogenous murine leukemia virus-related nuclear and cytoplasmic RNA complexity in C57BL/6J mice of increasing age, *Cancer Res.*, 40, 19, 1980.

46. **Ono, T. and Cutler, R. G.**, Age-dependent relaxation of gene repression: increase of endogenous murine leukemia virus-related and globin-related RNA in brain and liver of mice, *Proc. Natl. Acad. Sci. U.S.A.*, 75, 4431, 1978.

47. **Dean, R. G., Socher, S. H., and Cutler, R. G.**, Dysdifferentiation nature of aging: age-dependent expression of mouse mammary tumor virus and casein genes in the brain and liver tissues of the C57BL/6J mouse strain, *Arch. Gerontol. Geriatrics*, 4, 43, 1985.

48. **Niedzwiecki, A., Kongpachith, A. M., and Fleming, J. E.**, Aging affects expression of 70-kDa heat shock proteins in *Drosophila, J. Biol. Chem.*, 266, 9332, 1991.

49. **Wisniewski, H. M. and Terry, R. D.**, Neuropathology of the aging brain, in *Neurobiology of Aging*, Terry, R. D. and Gershon, S., Eds., Raven Press, New York, 1976, 265.

50. **Hartman, P.**, Putative mutagens and carcinogens in foods. I. Nitrate/nitrite ingestion and gastric cancer mortality, *Environ. Mutagenesis*, 5, 111, 1983.

51. **Hallgren, H. M., Jackola, D. R., and O'Leary, J. J.**, Unusual patterns of surface marker expression on peripheral lymphocytes from aged humans suggestive of a population of less differentiated cells, *J. Immunol.*, 131, 191, 1983.

52. **O'Leary, J. J., Jackola, D. R., Hallgren, H. M., Abbasnezhad, M., and Yasmineh, W. G.**, Evidence for a less differentiated subpopulation of lymphocytes in people of advanced age, *Mech. Ageing Dev.*, 21, 109, 1983.

53. **Parker, J., Flanagan, J., Murphy, J., and Gallant, J.**, On the accuracy of protein synthesis in *Drosophila melanogaster, Mech. Ageing Dev.*, 16, 127, 1981.

54. **Fleming, J. E., Quattrocki, E., Latter, G., Miquel, J., Marcuson, R., Zuckerkandl, E., and Bensch, G.**, Age-dependent changes in the proteins of *Drosophila melanogaster, Science*, 231, 1157, 1986.

55. **Cristofalo, V. J.**, Overview of biological mechanism of aging, in *Annual Review of Gerontology and Geriatrics*, Cristofalo, V. J. and Lawton, M. P., Eds., Springer, New York, 1990, 1.

56. **Krooth, R. G.**, A deterministic mechanism for cellular and organismic aging, *J. Theor. Biol.*, 46, 501, 1974.

57. **Russel, R. L.**, Evidence for and against the theory of developmentally programmed aging, in *Modern Biological Theories of Aging*, Warner, H. R., Butler, R. N., Sprott, R. L., and Schneider, E. L., Eds., Raven Press, New York, 1987, 35.

58. **Child, C. M.**, Axial gradients in the early development of the starfish, *Am. J. Physiol.*, 37, 203, 1915.

59. **Child, C. M.**, *Individuation and Reproduction in Organisms; Senescence and Rejuvenescence*, Chicago University Press, Chicago, 1915.

60. **Child, C. M.**, Axial susceptibility gradients in the early development of the sea urchin, *Biol. Bull.*, 30, 391, 1916.

61. **Child, C. M.**, Experimental control and modification of larval development in the sea urchin in relation to the axial gradients, *J. Morphol.*, 28, 65, 1916.

62. **Child, C. M.**, Physiological dominance and physiological isolation in development and reconstitution, *Wilhelm Roux's Arch. Entwicklungsmechanik Organismen*, 113, 556, 1929.

63. **Munkres, K. D.**, The role of genes, antioxidants, and antioxygenic enzymes in aging of Neurospora: a review, in *Superoxide Dismutase*, Oberley, L. W., Ed., CRC Press, Boca Raton, FL, 1985, 237.

64. **Munkres, K. D.**, Genetical, developmental, and thermal regulation of antioxidant enzymes in *Neurospora*, *Free Radical Biol. Med.*, 9, 23, 1990.

65. **Munkres, K. D. and Furtek, C. A.**, Selection of conidial longevity mutatants of *Neurospora crassa*, *Mechanisms Ageing Dev.*, 25, 47, 1984.

66. **Munkres, K. D. and Furtek, C. A.**, Linkage of conidial longevity determinant genes in *Neurospora crassa*, *Mech. Ageing Dev.*, 25, 63, 1984.

67. **Sushadri, T. and Campisi, J.**, Repression of c-*fos* transcription and an altered genetic program in senescent human fibroblasts, *Science*, 247, 205, 1990.

68. **Chang, C.-D., Phillips, P., Lipson, K. E., Cristofalo, V. J., and Baserga, R.**, Senescent human fibroblasts have a post-transcriptional block in the expression of the proliferating cell nuclear antigen gene, *J. Biol. Chem.*, 266, 8663, 1991.

69. **Schroder, H. C., Messer, R., Bachmann, M., Bernd, A., and Muller, W. E. G.**, Superoxide radical-induced loss of nuclear restriction of immature mRNA: a possible cause for ageing, *Mech. Ageing Dev.*, 41, 251, 1987.

70. **Kontermann, K. and Bayreuther, K.**, The cellular aging of rat fibroblasts *in vitro* is a differentiation process, *Gerontology*, 25, 261, 1979.

71. **Bell, E., Marek, L. F., Levinstone, D. S., Merril, C., Sher, S., and Eden, M.**, Loss of division potential *in vitro*: aging or differentiation?, *Science*, 202, 1158, 1980.

72. **Boveri, T.**, Ueber die polaritaet des seeigeleies, *Verh. Phys. Med. Ges. Wurz.*, 34, 145, 1901.

73. **Morgan, T. H.**, "Polarity" considered as a phenomenon of gradation of materials, *J. Exp. Zool.*, 2, 495, 1905.

74. **Chernavskii, D. S., Polezhaev, A. A., and Volkov, E. I.**, Cell surface and cell division, *Cell Biophys.*, 4, 143, 1982.

75. **Chernavskii, D. S., Solyanik, G. I., and Belousov, L. V.**, Relation of the intensity of metabolism with the process of determination in embryonic cell, *Biol. Cybern.*, 37, 9, 1980.

76. **Hansberg, W. and Aguirre, J.**, Hyperoxidant states cause microbial cell differentiation by cell isolation from dioxygen, *J. Theor. Biol.*, 142, 201, 1990.

77. **Nations, C., Allen, R. G., Farmer, K., Toy, P. L., and Sohal, R. S.**, Superoxide dismutase activity during the plasmodial life cycle of *Physarum polycephalum*, *Experientia*, 42, 64, 1986.

78. **Philips, G. J. and Borgia, P. T.**, Effects of oxygen on morphogenesis and polypeptide expression by *Mucor racemosus*, *J. Bacteriol.*, 164, 1039, 1985.

79. **Shaw, J. L. and Bassett, C. A.**, The effects of varying oxygen concentrations on osteogenesis and embryonic cartilage *in vitro*, *J. Bone Jt. Surg.*, 49-A, 73, 1967.

80. **Caplan, A. I. and Koutroupus, S.**, The control of muscle and cartilage development in the chick limb: the role of differential vascularization, *J. Embryol. Exp. Morphol.*, 29, 571, 1973.

81. **Loudon, C.**, Development of *Tenebrio molitor* in low oxygen levels, *J. Insect Physiol.*, 34, 97, 1988.

82. **Erkell, L. J.**, Differentiation of mouse neuroblastoma under increased oxygen tension, *Exp. Cell Biol.*, 48, 374, 1980.

83. **Foreman, H. J. and Boveris, A.**, Superoxide radical and hydrogen peroxide in mitochondria, in *Free Radicals in Biology,* Pryor, W. A., Ed., Academic Press, New York, 1982, 65.

84. **Turrens, J. F., Freeman, B. A., Levitt, J. G., and Crapo, J. D.**, The effect of hyperoxia on superoxide production by lung submitochondrial particles, *Arch. Biochem. Biophys.,* 217, 401, 1982.

85. **Allen, R. G., Newton, R. K., Sohal, R. S., Shipley, G. L., and Nations, C.**, Alterations in superoxide dismutase, glutathione, and peroxides in the plasmodial slime mold *Physarum polycephalum* during differentiation, *J. Cell. Physiol.,* 125, 413, 1985.

86. **Lott, T., Gorman, S., and Clark, J.**, Superoxide dismutase in *Didymium iridis:* characterization of changes in activity during senescence and sporulation, *Mech. Ageing Dev.,* 17, 119, 1981.

87. **Massie, H. R., Aiello, V. R., and Williams, T. R.**, Changes in superoxide dismutase activity and copper during development and ageing in the fruit fly *Drosophila melanogaster, Mech. Ageing Dev.,* 12, 279, 1980.

88. **Anderson, G. L.**, Superoxide dismutase activity in Dauerlarvae of *Caenorhabditis elegans* (Nematoda: Rhabditidae), *Can. J. Zool.,* 60, 288, 1982.

89. **Barja de Quiroga, G. and Gutierrez, P.**, Superoxide dismutase during the development of two amphibian species and its role in hyperoxia tolerance, *Mol. Physiol.,* 6, 221, 1984.

90. **Frank, L., Bucher, J. R., and Roberts, R. J.**, Oxygen toxicity in neonatal and adult animals of various species, *J. Appl. Physiol. Respir. Environ. Exercise Physiol.,* 45, 699, 1978.

91. **Frank, L. and Groseclose, E. E.**, Preparation for birth into an O_2-rich environment: the antioxidant enzymes in developing rabbit lung, *Pediatr. Res.* 18, 240, 1984.

92. **Mavelli, I., Mondovi, B., Federico, R., and Rotilio, G.**, Superoxide dismutase activity in developing rat brain, *J. Neurochem.,* 31, 363, 1978.

93. **Autor, A. P., Frank, L., and Roberts, R. J.**, Developmental characteristics of pulmonary superoxide dismutase: relationship to idiopathic respiratory distress syndrome, *Pediatr. Res.,* 10, 154, 1976.

94. **Hien, P. V., Kovacs, K., and Matkovics, B.**, Properties of enzymes. I. Study of superoxide dismutase activity changes in human placenta of different ages, *Enzyme,* 18, 341, 1974.

95. **Church, S. L., Farmer, D. R., and Nelson, D. M.**, Induction of manganese superoxide dismutase in cultured human trophoblast during *in vitro* differentiation, *Dev. Biol.,* 149, 177, 1992.

96. **Tanswell, A. K. and Freeman, B. A.**, Pulmonary antioxidant enzyme maturation in the fetal and neonatal rat. I. Development profiles, *Pediatr. Res.,* 18, 584, 1984.

97. **Mariucci, G., Ambrosini, M. V., Colarieti, L., and Bruschelli, G.**, Differential changes in Cu, Zn and Mn superoxide dismutase activity in developing rat brain and liver, *Experientia,* 46, 753, 1990.

98. **Nakagawara, A., Nathan, C. F., and Cohn, Z. A.**, Hydrogen peroxide metabolism in human monocytes during differentiation *in vitro, J. Clin. Invest.,* 68, 1243, 1981.

99. **Russanov, E. M., Kirkova, M. D., Setchenska, M. S., and Arnstein, H. R. V.**, Enzymes of oxygen metabolism during erythrocyte differentiation, *Biosci. Rep.,* 1, 927, 1981.

100. **Allen, R. G. and Balin, A. K.**, Developmental changes in the superoxide dismutase activity of human skin fibroblasts are maintained *in vitro* and are not caused by oxygen, *J. Clin. Invest.,* 82, 731, 1988.

101. **Yamanaka, N. and Deamer, D.**, Superoxide dismutase activity in WI-38 cell cultures: effect of age, trypsinization and SV-40 transformation, *Physiol. Chem. Phys.,* 6, 95, 1974.

102. **Oberley, L. W., Bize, I. B., Sahu, S. K., Leuthauser, S. W. H. C., and Gruber, H. E.**, Superoxide dismutase activity of normal murine liver, regenerating liver, and H6 hepatoma, *J. Natl. Cancer Inst.*, 61, 375, 1978.

103. **Nations, C., Allen, R. G., Balin, A. K., Reimer, R. J., and Sohal, R. S.**, Superoxide dismutase activity and glutathione concentration during the calcium-induced differentiation of *Physarum polycephalum* microplasmodia, *J. Cell. Physiol.*, 133, 181, 1987.

104. **Allen, R. G. and Sohal, R. S.**, Role of glutathione in aging and development of insects, in *Aging in Insects: Strategies and Mechanisms*, Collatz, K. G. and Sohal, R. S., Eds., Springer-Verlag, Heidelberg, 1986, 168.

105. **Warshaw, J. B., Wilson, C. W., Saito, K., and Prough, R. A.**, The response of glutathione and antioxidant enzymes to hyperoxia in developing lung, *Pediatr. Res.*, 19, 819, 1985.

106. **Takahashi, S. and Zeydel, M.**, γ-Glutamyl transpeptidase and glutathione in aging IMR-90 fibroblasts and in differentiating 3T3 L1 preadipocytes, *Arch. Biochem. Biophys.*, 214, 260, 1982.

107. **Boldyrev, A. A., Dupin, A. M., Siambela, M., and Stvolinsky, S. L.**, The level of natural antioxidant glutathione and histidine-containing dipeptides in skeletal muscles of developing chick embryos, *Comp. Biochem. Physiol.*, 89B, 197, 1988.

108. **Balinsky, B. I.**, *Embryology*, W. B. Saunders, Philadelphia, 1970.

109. **Fraser, L. B. and Carter, D. B.**, Variation of acid soluble sulfhydryl groups during liver regeneration, *Bri. J. Cancer*, 21, 235, 1967.

110. **Ferrari, V. and Harkness, R. D.**, Free amino-acids in liver and blood after partial hepatectomy in normal and adrenalectomized rats, *J. Physiol.*, 124, 443, 1954.

111. **Hopsu, V. K. and Harkonen, M.**, Protein-bound SH-groups in liver tissue after partial hepatectomy, *Acta Pathol. Microbiol. Scand.*, 48, 94, 1960.

112. **Calvin, H. I. and Turner, S. I.**, High levels of glutathione attained during postnatal development of rat testis, *J. Exp. Zool.*, 219, 389, 1982.

113. **Rao, K. V.**, A study of the role of sulfhydryl groups in morphogenesis of the chick embryo, *Wilhelm Roux's Arch. Entwicklungsmechanik Organismen*, 163, 161, 1969.

114. **Waheed, M. A. and Mulherkar, L.**, Studies on induction by substances containing sulfhydryl groups in post-nodal pieces of chick blastoderms, *J. Embryol. Exp. Morphol.*, 17, 161, 1967.

115. **Freeman, M. L., Scidmore, N. C., Malcolm, A. W., and Meredith, M. J.**, Diamide exposure, thermal resistance and synthesis of stress (heat shock) proteins, *Biochem. Pharmacol.*, 36, 21, 1987.

116. **Cornwell, D. G. and Morisaki, N.**, Fatty acid paradoxes in the control of cell proliferation: prostaglandins, lipid peroxides, and co-oxidation reactions, in *Free Radicals in Biology*, Pryor, W. A., Ed., Academic Press, New York, 1984, 95.

117. **Lands, W. E. M., Kulmacz, R. J., and Marshall, P. J.**, Lipid peroxide actions in regulation of prostaglandin biosynthesis, in *Free Radicals in Biology*, Pryor, W. A., Ed., Academic Press, New York, 1984, 39.

118. **Utsumi, K., Yoshioka, T., Yamanaka, N., and Nakazawa, T.**, Increase in superoxide dismutase activity concomitant with a decrease in lipid peroxidation during post partum development, *FEBS Lett.*, 79, 1, 1977.

119. **Novak, R., Matkovics, M., Marik, M., and Fachet, J.**, Changes in mouse liver superoxide dismutase activity and lipid peroxidation during embryonic and postpartum development, *Experientia*, 34, 1134, 1978.

120. **Yoshioka, T., Shimada, T., and Sekiba, K.** Lipid peroxidation and antioxidants in the rat lung during development, *Biol. Neonate*, 38, 161, 1980.

121. **Yoshioka, T., Utsumi, K., and Sekiba, K.**, Superoxide dismutase activity and lipid peroxidation of the rat liver during development, *Biol. Neonate*, 32, 147, 1977.

122. **Wolfson, N., Wilber, K. M., and Bernheim, F.**, Lipid peroxide formation in regenerating rat liver, *Exp. Cell Res.*, 10, 556, 1956.

123. **Sohal, R. S. and Allen, R. G.**, Oxygen radicals in cellular differentiation and the aging process, *Age,* 8, 91, 1985.
124. **Kehler, J. P. and Autor, A. P.**, Age-dependent lipid peroxidation in neonatal rat lung tissue, *Arch. Biochem. Biophys.,* 181, 73, 1977.
125. **Kehler, J. P. and Autor, A. P.**, Changes in the fatty acid composition of rat lung lipids during development and following age-dependent lipid peroxidation, *Lipids,* 12, 596, 1977.
126. **Kehler, J. P. and Autor, A. P.**, The effect of dietary fatty acids on the composition of adult rat lung lipids: relationship to oxygen toxicity, *Toxicol. Appl. Pharmacol.,* 44, 423, 1978.
127. **Allen, R. G., Farmer, K. J., Toy, P. L., Newton, R. K., Sohal, R. S., and Nations, C.**, Involvement of glutathione in the differentiation of the slime mold, *Physarum polycephalum, Dev. Growth Differentiation,* 27, 615, 1985.
128. **Allen, R. G., Newton, R. K., Farmer, K. J., and Nations, C.**, Effect of the free radical generator paraquat on differentiation, superoxide dismutase, glutathione and inorganic peroxides in microplasmodia of *Physarum polycephalum, Cell Tissue Kinet.,* 18, 623, 1985.
129. **Allen, R. G., Balin, A. K., Reimer, R. J., Sohal, R. S., and Nations, C.**, Superoxide dismutase induces differentiation in the slime mold, *Physarum polycephalum, Arch. Biochem. Biophys.,* 261, 205, 1988.
130. **Beckman, B. S., Balin, A. K., and Allen, R. G.**, Superoxide dismutase induces differentiation in Friend erythroleukemia cells, *J. Cell. Physiol.,* 139, 370, 1989.
131. **Dionisi, O., Galleotti, T., Terranova, T., and Azzi, A.**, Superoxide radicals and hydrogen peroxide formation in mitochondria from normal and neoplastic tissues, *Biochim. Biophys. Acta,* 403, 293, 1975.
132. **Elroy-Stein, O., Bernstein, Y., and Groner, Y.**, Overproduction of human Cu/Zn superoxide dismutase in transfected cells: extenuation of paraquat-mediated cytotoxicity and enhancement of lipid peroxidation, *EMBO J.* 5, 615, 1986.
133. **Reveillaud, I., Neidzwiecki, A., Bensch, K. G., and Fleming, J. E.**, Expression of bovine superoxide dismutase in *Drosophila melanogaster* augments resistance to oxidative stress, *Mol. Cell. Biol.,* 11, 632, 1991.
134. **Prasad, K. N. and Edwards-Prasad, J.**, Effects of tocopherol (vitamin E) acid succinate on morphological alterations and growth inhibition in melanoma cells in culture, *Cancer Res.,* 42, 550, 1982.
135. **Prasad, K. N., Edwards-Prasad, J., Ramanujam, S., and Sakamoto, A.**, Vitamin E increases the growth inhibitory and differentiating effects of tumor therapeutic agents on neuroblastoma and glioma cells in culture (40840), *Proc. Soc. Exp. Biol. Med.,* 164, 158, 1980.
136. **Prasad, K. N., Gaudreau, D., and Brown, J.**, Binding of vitamin E in mammalian tumor cell culture (41041), *Proc. Soc. Exp. Biol. Med.,* 166, 167, 1981.
137. **Pluthero, F. G., Shreeve, M., Eskinazi, D., van der Gaag, H., Huang, K.-S., Hulmes, J. D., Blum, M., and Axelrad, A. A.**, Purification of an inhibitor of erythroid progenitor cell cycling and antagonist to interleukin 3 from mouse marrow cell supernatants and its identification as cytosolic superoxide dismutase, *J. Cell Biol.,* 111, 1217, 1990.
138. **Sohal, R. S., Farmer, K. J., Allen, R. G., and Cohen, N. R.**, Effects of age on oxygen consumption, superoxide dismutase, catalase, glutathione, inorganic peroxides, and chloroform-soluble antioxidants in the adult male housefly, *Musca domestica, Mech. Ageing Dev.,* 24, 185, 1983.
139. **Kellog, E. W., III and Fridovich, I.**, Superoxide dismutase in the rat and mouse as a function of age and longevity, *J. Gerontol.,* 31, 405, 1976.
140. **Massie, H. R., Aiello, V. R., and Iodice, A. A.**, Changes with age in copper and superoxide dismutase levels in the brains of C57BL/6J mice, *Mech. Ageing Dev.,* 10, 93, 1979.

141. **Vanella, A., Geremia, E., D'Urso, G., Tiriolo, P., DiSilvestro, I., Germaldi, R., and Pinturo, R.,** Superoxide dismutase activities in the aging rat brain, *Gerontology,* 28, 108, 1982.

142. **Frank, L.,** Developmental aspects of experimental pulmonary oxygen toxicity, *Free Radical Biol. Med.,* 11, 463, 1991.

143. **Hass, M. A. and Massaro, D.,** Differences in CuZn superoxide dismutase induction in lungs of neonatal and adult rats, *Am. J. Physiol.,* 253, C66, 1987.

144. **Fleming, R. E. and Gitlin, J. D.,** Developmental regulation of Cu/Zn superoxide dismutase gene expression, *Pediatr. Res.,* 23, 242A, 1988.

145. **Nicolisi, R. J., Baird, M. B., Massie, H. R., and Samis, H. V.,** Senescence in *Drosophila*. II. Renewal of catalase activity in flies of different ages, *Exp. Gerontol.,* 8, 101, 1973.

146. **Stohs, S. J., El-Rashidy, F. H., Angle, C. R. L. T, Kabayashi, R. H., Wulf, B. G., and Patter, J. F.,** Changes in glutathione and glutathione metabolising enzymes in human erythrocytes and lymphocytes as a function of age of donor, *Age,* 7, 3, 1984.

147. **Noy, N., Schwartz, H., and Gafni, A.,** Age-related changes in the redox status of rat muscle cells and their role in enzyme aging, *Mech. Ageing Dev.,* 29, 63, 1985.

148. **Gandhi, C. R. and Chowdhury, D. R.,** Effects of Diabetes mellitus on sialic acid and glutathione content of human erythrocytes of different ages, *Indian J. Exp. Biol.,* 17, 585, 1977.

149. **Sohal, R. S., Muller, A., Koletzko, B., and Sies, H.,** Effect of age and ambient temperature on *n*-pentane production in the housefly, *Musca domestica, Mech. Ageing Dev.,* 29, 317, 1985.

150. **Sagai, M. and Ishinose, T.,** Agerelated changes in lipid peroxidation as measured by ethane, butane and pentane in respired gases of rats, *Life Sci.,* 27, 731, 1980.

151. **Nohl, H. and Hegner, D.,** Do mitochondria produce oxygen radicals *in vivo?*, *Eur. J. Biochem.,* 82, 563, 1978.

152. **Nohl, H. and Hegner, D.,** Responses of mitochondrial superoxide dismutase, catalase and glutathione peroxidase activities to aging, *Mech. Ageing Dev.,* 11, 145, 1979.

153. **Hegner, D.,** Age-dependence of molecular and functional changes in biological membranes, *Mech. Ageing Dev.,* 14, 101, 1980.

154. **Farmer, K. J. and Sohal, R. S.,** Relationship between superoxide anion generation and aging in the housefly, *Musca domestica, Free Radical Biol. Med.,* 7, 23, 1989.

155. **Sohal, R. S., Svensson, I., and Brunk, U. T.,** Hydrogen peroxide production by liver mitochondria in different species, *Mech. Ageing Dev.,* 53, 209, 1990.

156. **Nohl, H.,** Oxygen release in mitochondria: influence of age, in *Free Radicals, Aging, and Degenerative Disease,* Johnson, J. E., Walford, R., Harman, D., and Miquel, J., Eds., Alan R. Liss, New York, 1986, 79.

157. **Douzou, P. and Maurel, P.,** Ionic regulation in genetic translation systems, *Proc. Natl. Acad. Sci. U.S.A.,* 74, 1013, 1977.

158. **Lee, P. C., Bochner, B. R., and Ames, B. N.,** AppppA, heat-shock stress, and cell oxidation, *Proc. Natl. Acad. Sci. U.S.A.,* 80, 7496, 1983.

159. **Bochner, B. R., Lee, P. C., Wilson, S. W., Cutler, C. W., and Ames, B. N.,** AppppA and related adenylylated nucleotides are synthesized as a consequence of oxidative stress, *Cell,* 37, 225, 1984.

160. **Levenson, W., Oppermann, H., and Jackson, J.,** Transition series metals and sulfhydryl reagents induce the synthesis of four proteins in eukaryotic cells, *Biochim. Biophys. Acta,* 606, 170, 1980.

161. **Whelan, S. A. and Hightower, L. E.,** Differential induction of glucose-regulated and heat shock proteins: effects of pH and sulfhydral-reducing agents on chicken embryo cells, *J. Cell. Physiol.,* 125, 251, 1985.

162. **Privalle, C. T. and Fridovich, I.,** Induction of superoxide dismutase in *Escherichia coli* by heat shock, *Proc. Natl. Acad. Sci. U.S.A.,* 84, 2723, 1987.

163. **Smirnova, I. B.,** Thiols in mitosis and cleavage, *Sov. J. Dev. Biol.,* 4, 407, 1974.

164. **Suthanthiran, M., Anderson, M. A., Sharma, V. K., and Meister, A.,** Glutathione regulates activation-dependent DNA synthesis in highly purified normal T lymphocytes stimulated via CD2 and CD3 antigens, *Proc. Natl. Acad. Sci. U.S.A.,* 87, 3343, 1990.
165. **Amstad, P., Peskin, A., Shah, G., Mirault, M.-E., More, R., Zbinden, I., and Cerrutti, P.,** The balance between Cu,Zn-superoxide dismutase and catalase affects the sensitivity of mouse epidermal cells to oxidative stress, *Biochemistry,* 30, 9305, 1991.
166. **Oberley, T. D., Allen, R. G., Schultz, J. L., and Lauchner, L. J.,** Antioxidant enzymes and steroid-induced proliferation of kidney tubular cells, *Free Radical Biol. Med.,* 10, 79, 1991.
167. **Honda, S. and Matsuo, M.,** Relationships between the cellular glutathione level and *in vitro* life-span of human diploid fibroblasts, *Exp. Gerontol.,* 23, 81, 1988.
168. **Roederer, M., Staal, F. J. T., Raju, P. A., Ela, S. W., Herzenberg, L. A., and Herzenberg, L. A.,** Cytokine-stimulated human immunodeficiency virus replication is inhibited by *N*-acetyl-L-cysteine, *Proc. Natl. Acad. Sci. U.S.A.,* 87, 4884, 1990.
169. **Kretsinger, R. H.,** Mechanisms of selective signalling by calcium, *Neurosci. Res. Prog. Bull.,* 19, 211, 1980.
170. **Richter, C. and Kass, G. E. N.,** Oxidative stress in mitochondria: its relationship to cellular Ca^{2+} homeostasis, cell death, proliferation, and differentiation, *Chemico-Biol. Interactions,* 77, 1, 1991.
171. **Richter, C. and Frei, B.,** Ca^{2+} release from mitochondria induced by prooxidants, *Free Radical Biol. Med.,* 4, 365, 1988.
172. **Masumoto, N., Tasaka, K., Miyake, A., and Tanizawa, O.,** Regulation of intracellular Mg^{2+} by superoxide in amnion cells, *Biochem. Biophys. Res. Commun.,* 182, 906, 1992.
173. **Kroeger, H. and Muller, G.,** Control of puffing activity in three chromosomal segments of explanted salivary gland cells of *Chironomus thummi* by variations in extracellular Na^+, K^+, Mg^{2+}, *Exp. Cell Res.,* 82, 89, 1973.
174. **Kroeger, H., Trosch, W., and Muller, G.,** Changes in nuclear electrolytes of *Chironomus thummi* salivary gland cells during development, *Exp. Cell Res.,* 80, 329, 1973.
175. **Jewell, S. A., Bellomo, G., Thor, H., Orrenius, S., and Smith, M. T.,** Bleb formation in hepatocytes during drug metabolism is caused by disturbances in thiol and calcium ion homeostasis, *Science,* 217, 1257, 1982.
176. **Smith, M. T., Thor, H., Jewell, S. A., Bellomo, G., Sandy, M. S., and Orrenius, S.,** Free radical-induced changes in the surface morphology of isolated hepatocytes, in *Free Radicals in Molecular Biology, Aging and Disease,* Armstrong, D., Sohal, R. S., Cutler, R. G., and Slater, T. F., Eds., Raven Press, New York, 1984, 103.
177. **Lotscher, H. R., Winterhalter, K. H., Carfalo, E., and Richter, C.,** Hydroperoxides can modulate the redox state of pyridine nucleotides and calcium balance in rat liver mitochondria, *Proc. Natl. Acad. Sci. U.S.A.,* 76, 4340, 1979.
178. **Nations, C., Allison, V. F., Aldrich, H. C., and Allen, R. G.,** Superoxide dismutase and the mobilization of mitochondrial calcium during the differentiation of *Physarum polycephalum, J. Cell. Physiol.,* 140, 311, 1989.
179. **Borgens, R. B., Vanable, J. W., and Jaffe, L. F.,** Bioelectricity and regeneration, *Bioscience,* 29, 468, 1979.
180. **Nuccitelli, R. and Jaffe, L. F.,** The ionic component of the current pulses which cross growing tips of *Pelvetia* embryos, *Dev. Biol.,* 49, 518, 1975.
181. **Weisenseel, M. H., Nuccitelli, R., and Jaffe, L. F.,** Large electrical currents traverse growing pollen tubes, *J. Cell Biol.,* 66, 556, 1975.
182. **Borgens, R. B., Vanable, J. W., and Jaffe, L. F.,** Bioelectricity and regeneration: large currents leave the stump of regenerating newt limbs, *Proc. Natl. Acad. Sci. U.S.A.,* 74, 4528, 1977.
183. **Borgens, R. B., Vanable, J. W., and Jaffe, L. F.,** Bioelectricity and regeneration. I. Initiation of frog limb regeneration by minute currents, *J. Exp. Zool.,* 200, 451, 1977.
184. **Pruss, G. J. and Drlica, K.,** DNA supercoiling and suppression of the leu-500 promoter mutation, *J. Bacteriol.,* 164, 947, 1985.

185. **Stirdivant, S. M., Crossland, L. D., and Bogorad, L.,** DNA supercoiling affects *in vitro* transcription of two maize chloroplast genes differently, *Proc. Natl. Acad. Sci. U.S.A.,* 82, 4886, 1985.

186. **Weintraub, H. and Groudine, M.,** Chromosomal subunits in active genes have an altered conformation, *Science,* 193, 848, 1976.

187. **Wallace, R. B., Dube, S. K., and Bonner, J.,** Localization of the globin gene in the template active fraction of chromatin of Friend Leukemia cells, *Science,* 198, 1166, 1977.

188. **Aaronson, R. P. and Woo, E.,** Organization in the cell nucleus: divalent cations modulate the distribution of condensed and diffuse chromatin, *J. Cell. Physiol.,* 90, 181, 1981.

189. **Tas, S. and Walford, R. L.,** Increased dissulfide-mediated condensation of nuclear DNA-protein complex in lymphocytes during postnatal development and aging, *Mech. Ageing Dev.,* 19, 73, 1982.

190. **Means, A. R., Tash, J. S., Chafouleas, J. G., Lagace, L., and Guerriero, V.,** Regulation of the cytoskeleton by Ca^{2+} − calmodulin and cAMP, *Ann. New York Acad. Sci.,* 383, 69, 1982.

191. **Manning, G. S.,** Packaged DNA: an elastic model, *Cell Biophys.,* 7, 59, 1985.

192. **Laundon, C. H. and Griffith, J. D.,** Cationic metals promote sequence-directed DNA bending, *Biochemistry,* 26, 3759, 1987.

193. **McConnell, M., Whalan, A. M., Smith, D. E., and Fisher, P. A.,** Heat shock-induced changes in the structural stability of proteinaceous karyoskeletal elements *in vitro* and morphological effects *in situ, J. Cell Biol.,* 105, 1087, 1987.

194. **Scott, J. A.,** The role of cytoskeletal integrity in cellular transformation, *J. Theor. Biol.,* 106, 183, 1984.

195. **Scott, J. A., Kahn, B.-A., Homcy, C. J., and Rabito, C. A.,** Oxygen radicals alter the cell membrane potential in a renal cell line (LLC-PK1) with differentiated characteristics of proximal tubular cells, *Biochim. Biophys. Acta,* 897, 25, 1987.

196. **Storz, G., Tartaglia, L. A., and Ames, B. N.,** Transcriptional regulator of oxidative stress-inducible genes: direct activation by oxidation, *Science,* 248, 189, 1990.

197. **Tartaglia, L. A., Storz, G., and Ames, B. N.,** Identification and molecular analysis of *oxyR*-regulated promoters important for the bacterial adaptation to oxidative stress, *J. Mol. Biol.,* 210, 709, 1989.

198. **Storz, G., Tartaglia, L. A., and Ames, B. N.,** The *oxyR* regulon, *Antonie van Leeuwenhoek,* 58, 157, 1990.

199. **Schreck, R., Rieber, P., and Baeuerle, P. A.,** Reactive oxygen intermediates as apparently widely used messengers in the activation of the NFκ-B transcription factor and HIV-1, *EMBO J.,* 10, 2247, 1991.

200. **Chojkier, M., Houglum, K., Solis-Herruzo, J., and Brenner, D. A.,** Stimulation of collagen gene expression by ascorbic acid in cultured human fibroblasts, *J. Biol. Chem.,* 264, 16957, 1989.

201. **Herman, R., Weymouth, L., and Penman, S.,** Heterogenous nuclear protein fibers in chromatin depleted nuclei, *J. Cell Biol.,* 78, 663, 1978.

202. **Ciejek, E. M., Nordstrom, J. N., and O'Malley, B. W.,** Ribonucleic acid precursors are associated with the chick oviduct nuclear matrix, *Biochemistry,* 21, 4945, 1982.

203. **Schroder, H. C., Trolltsch, D., Wenger, R., Bachmann, M., Diehl-Siefert, B., and Muller, W. E. G.,** Cytochalasin B selectively releases ovalbumin mRNA precursors but not the mature ovalbumin mRNA from hen oviduct nuclear matrix, *Eur. J. Biochem.,* 167, 239, 1987.

204. **Walden, W. E., Patino, M. M., and Gaffield, L.,** Purification of specific repressor of ferritin mRNA translation from rabbit liver, *J. Biol. Chem.,* 264, 13765, 1989.

205. **Hentze, M. W., Rouault, T. A., Harford, J. B., and Klausner, R. D.,** Oxidative-reduction and the molecular mechanism of a regulatory RNA-protein interaction, *Science,* 244, 357, 1989.

206. **Abate, C., Patel, L., Rauscher, F. J., and Curran, T.,** Redox regulation of FOS and JUN DNA-binding activity *in vitro, Science,* 249, 1157, 1990.

Chapter 3

BASIC FREE RADICAL BIOCHEMISTRY

Robert A. Floyd

TABLE OF CONTENTS

0-8493-4518-9/93/$0.00 + $.50

I. INTRODUCTION

Free radicals have been considered important to aging processes for many years, but only lately has it become an area of intense research effort. Significant advances are being made in this area, and thus more understanding is needed regarding the fundamental aspects of free radicals. This brief chapter will review the basic concepts of free radicals with an emphasis on aspects that are of importance to help understand the aging process. Oxidative damage is an important aspect of aging, and the mechanisms involved have as their basis oxygen free radical intermediates. Therefore, oxygen free radical chemistry will be treated in greater detail. The involvement of the trace metals Fe and/or Cu in oxidative damage and the mechanisms which nature has evolved to protect from oxidative damage will be detailed as well as newer methods now used to assess oxygen free radical flux *in vivo*. Finally, recently collected data from our own research effort on oxidative damage in the brain will be summarized. Novel developments indicate that certain spin-trapping compounds, chemicals that react with and stabilize free radicals, appear to reverse certain age-associated oxidative damage in gerbil brain. The lessons learned from these experiments will be viewed in the light of what they reveal about oxidative events and the processes involved in aging.

II. WHAT IS A FREE RADICAL?

Understanding the characteristics of a free radial ultimately rests upon an understanding of the Pauli Exclusion Principal, which in very general terms states that no two electrons in an atom can have the same four quantum numbers n, 1, m, and s. The quantum number s, designating spin, describes the two possible orientations of the magnetic moment generated by an electron resulting from rotation on its own axis; i.e., it acts as if it is a tiny bar magnet. The spin quantum numbers have values of $s = \frac{1}{2}$ and $s = -\frac{1}{2}$. Nature builds atoms and molecules such that they have matched or paired electrons, in terms of spin. That is, the outer orbital will have two electrons, one with spin $s = \frac{1}{2}$ and the other with spin $s = -\frac{1}{2}$. Therefore, if a free (i.e., unpaired electron) resides in a molecule and is not matched in terms of spin state, it is therefore called a free radical. Free radicals are present at very low levels in biological systems.

Free radicals are in general very reactive chemically, due mainly to the fact that they are not in a stable spin state. That is, free radicals in general readily give up or accept an electron to stabilize their unpaired electron. Since a free radical reacts to either accept or donate a free electron, this causes the production of another free radical; i.e.,

$$\dot{R} + X \rightarrow R + \dot{X} \tag{1}$$

The newly produced free radical is unstable in most cases and thus it can also react with another molecule to produce another free radical; i.e.,

$$\dot{X} + Y \rightarrow X + \dot{Y} \tag{2}$$

Thus, a chain of radical reactions can occur, leading to many damaging unstabilizing reactions. The reaction of one free radical with another free radical will, in general, terminate the chain of free radical reactions; i.e.,

$$\dot{R} + \dot{R} \rightarrow R\text{--}R \tag{3}$$

It is also possible to quench or stabilize free radical intermediates by reaction with a compound that is not a free radical, but which becomes a very stable free radical once the free radical has added to it; i.e.,

$$\dot{R}_{(reactive)} + ST \rightarrow \dot{S}A_{(stable)} \tag{4}$$

Some chemicals known as spin traps (ST) react with free radicals to yield relatively stable, i.e., unreactive products, called spin adducts ($\dot{S}A$). Spin traps are not the only compounds that will react with and stabilize free radicals.

III. OXYGEN: AN INSULT TO EARLY EVOLUTIONARY LIFE FORMS

The best available knowledge clearly indicates that life on earth began about four billion years ago under conditions where oxygen was completely absent. About one billion years later, photosynthetic processes appeared, and in a relatively short time (geologically), caused an increase in oxygen content from zero to much higher levels, perhaps nearly to the 21% now present in our atmosphere. Life forms adapted to the presence of oxygen which, no doubt, caused a massive oxidative insult to their normal anaerobic life styles. They adapted well; in fact they evolved to take advantage of the omnipresent oxygen molecules and used them as electron sinks for reductants, whereby during respiration the free energy loss from reductant to oxygen is conserved in high energy molecules (ATP), and in the process, oxygen is reduced to form water. Thus, through adaptation, oxygen, (which at first was an oxidative insult) was made to serve in a process whereby more energy is captured from the reductants available.

IV. FUNDAMENTAL PROPERTIES OF OXYGEN

There is one fundamental property of oxygen that prevents it from reacting rapidly with and completely oxidizing all biological material. That property is the fact that its two "outer" electrons are in a triplet spin state. The orbitals

ORBITALS

	$^3\Sigma g^- \; O_2$		$O_2^{\cdot -}$		O_2^{2-}		$^1\Delta gO_2$	
π^*2p	↑	↑	↑↓	↑	↑↓	↑↓	↑↓	
$\pi 2p$	↑↓	↑↓	↑↓	↑↓	↑↓	↑↓	↑↓	↑↓
$\sigma 2p$	↑↓		↑↓		↑↓		↑↓	
σ^*2S	↑↓		↑↓		↑↓		↑↓	
$\sigma 2S$	↑↓		↑↓		↑↓		↑↓	
σ^*1S	↑↓		↑↓		↑↓		↑↓	
$\sigma 1S$	↑↓		↑↓		↑↓		↑↓	

FIGURE 1. Molecular orbital occupation for ground state molecular oxygen, $(^3\Sigma\,g - O_2)$, superoxide $(O_2^{\cdot -})$, hydrogen peroxide (O_2^{2-}) and singlet oxygen $(^1\Delta gO_2)$.

of several oxidative states of oxygen are shown in Figure 1. Thus, molecular oxygen is a free radical in a technical sense. That is, the two "outer" electrons are unpaired but exist in two separate orbitals, π^*2p. This is fortunate because molecules having triplet state electrons do not react with molecules having singlet state electrons. Almost all biological molecules are in a singlet state, and thus, molecular ground state oxygen will not readily react with (oxidize) biological molecules. If, however, molecular oxygen is energized (addition of 23 kcal) to form singlet oxygen (both electrons exist in one π^*2p orbital), which allows it to readily react with biological molecules; it thus causes oxidative damage. These principles are illustrated in the following relationships:

$$
\begin{array}{ccc}
\underset{\substack{\text{triplet state} \\ \text{(molecular oxygen)}}}{\uparrow\,\uparrow} & + & \underset{\substack{\text{singlet state} \\ \text{(biological molecules)}}}{\uparrow\,\downarrow} = \text{no reaction}
\end{array} \qquad (5)
$$

$$
\underset{\substack{\text{triplet state} \\ \text{(molecular oxygen)}}}{\uparrow\,\uparrow} + \text{Energy (23 kcal)} \rightarrow \underset{\substack{\text{singlet oxygen}}}{\uparrow\,\downarrow} \qquad (6)
$$

$$
\underset{\substack{\text{singlet oxygen}}}{\uparrow\,\downarrow} + \underset{\substack{\text{biological molecules}}}{\uparrow\,\downarrow} \rightarrow \text{oxidation} \qquad (7)
$$

V. OXYGEN FREE RADICALS OF IMPORTANCE IN LIFE PROCESSES

If molecular oxygen in its ground state does not readily react with (oxidize) biological molecules, then how does oxygen mediate oxidative damage? The answer to this puzzle resides in the fact that reactive species of oxygen having reduction states between the two extremes, i.e., molecular oxygen and water, are formed at very low levels in biological systems and mediate oxidative damage. These "semi-reduced" toxic species of oxygen are superoxide, hydrogen peroxide, and hydroxyl free radical.[1,2] Superoxide, formed by the addition of one electron to oxygen, is negatively charged at the pH of physiological solutions, i.e., it has a pK of 4.8 and can readily pass through membranes on the anion channel.[2] Hydrogen peroxide is formed by several biological reactions and can readily pass through membranes.[1]

Superoxide is a good reductant, readily donating its extra electron to electron acceptors. Thus, superoxide will reduce Fe(III) to form Fe(II); i.e.,

$$O_2^- + Fe(III) \rightarrow O_2 + Fe(II) \tag{8}$$

Hydrogen peroxide will readily react with Fe(II) to form hydroxyl free radical; i.e.,

$$Fe(II) + H_2O_2 \rightarrow OH^- + \dot{O}H + Fe(III) \tag{9}$$

Thus the summation of reactions 8 and 9 is as such:

$$O_2^- + H_2O_2 \xrightarrow{Fe} OH^- + \dot{O}H + O_2 \tag{10}$$

It should be noted that even though Fe is involved in the reactions, it acts catalytically and is, therefore, needed only in very small amounts and as an "available" low molecular weight complex having redox properties which allow it to readily participate in the redox reactions.

Iron is present in biological systems mostly as an essential part of proteins such as hemoglobin, ferritin, cytochromes, Fe-S proteins, etc. and is present only at very low levels as an "available" low molecular weight complex.

Hydroxyl free radicals are formed and react rapidly and indiscriminately with almost any available molecule that is nearby their site of formation. Thus, hydroxyl free radicals will react at nearly diffusion mediated rates by either adding to or abstracting a hydrogen atom from molecules and forming another free radical; i.e.,

$$RH + \dot{O}H \rightarrow H\dot{R}OH \tag{11}$$

$$RH + \dot{O}H \rightarrow \dot{R} + HOH \tag{12}$$

In either case, a free radical chain reaction is set in motion, thus leading to the formation of more free radicals, etc. This is especially important when oxygen is present, for it will add to certain free radicals, forming alkoxy free radicals which then will subsequently react to form other free radicals, leading to chain reactions; i.e.,

$$\dot{R} + O_2 \rightarrow R\dot{O}O \qquad (13)$$

$$R\dot{O}O + R'H \rightarrow ROOH + \dot{R}' \qquad (14)$$

$$\dot{R}' + O_2 \rightarrow R'\dot{O}O \qquad (15)$$

$$R'\dot{O}O + R''H \rightarrow \dot{R}'' + R'OOH \qquad (16)$$

Thus, as illustrated above, the chain is propagated on and on. Each hydroperoxide that is formed can react in the presence of Fe and/or Cu to produce other free radicals, thus leading to further oxidative damage. The reactions noted above are particularly pertinent to the reactions which occur during lipid peroxidation, whereby the polyunsaturated fatty acids of membrane phospholipids are oxidized.

The reaction of H_2O_2 with Fe localized on a protein, or as an essential part of the active center of certain proteins such as glutamine synthetase, will produce oxidants that damage the protein by attacking specific amino acids, especially histidine, lysine, proline, and arginine, that may be located either very near to or participate as a part of the iron-binding site.[3] Thus, site specificity is an important aspect of oxidative damage to the biological macromolecules DNA, RNA, and proteins and is dictated, in large part, by the site specificity of the binding of the trace metals Fe and/or Cu to the macromolecule.

VI. ANTIOXIDANT PROTECTIVE MECHANISMS

Nature has evolved several enzymes and antioxidants which act in a combined fashion to help protect biological systems against oxidative damage. Their primary function is to lower the amount of oxygen free radicals or their precursors in the cell.

Superoxide dismutase (SOD), an enzyme discovered by McCord and Fridovich,[4] acts to dismutate superoxide to form hydrogen peroxide and oxygen; i.e.,

$$O_2^- + O_2^- + \xrightarrow[2H^+]{SOD} H_2O_2 + O_2 \qquad (17)$$

Several forms of SOD exist in the cell, including manganese-containing SOD (Mn-SOD) present in mitochondria and copper/zinc-SOD (Cu/Zn-SOD) present in the cytosol.[2] There also is a small amount of extracellular SOD apparently existing in the extra cellular matrix. Catalase (CAT) acts upon hydrogen peroxide to form molecular oxygen and water; i.e.,

$$2H_2O_2 \xrightarrow{\text{CAT}} O_2 + 2H_2O \tag{18}$$

Glutathione peroxidase (GSH-Px) acts to reduce hydrogen peroxide to water, utilizing reduced glutathione (GSH) as a source of reducing equivalents; i.e.,

$$H_2O_2 + 2GSH \xrightarrow{\text{GSH-Px}} 2H_2O + GSSG \tag{19}$$

In addition to the three enzymes illustrated above, glutathione, vitamin E, ascorbate, and uric acid also help to protect from oxidative damage. Glutathione acts not only as a reductant for GSH-Px, but most likely in other ways not fully understood at the present time. Vitamin E (α-tocopherol) is a lipid soluble antioxidant which resides within the membrane bilayer present at a level of about one α-tocopherol molecule per 1000 phospholipid molecules. α-tocopherol acts to scavenge lipid free radicals formed during the process of lipid peroxidation. The α-tocopherol free radical, formed as a result of its reaction with lipid free radicals, itself becomes reduced back to its original state by ascorbate which resides in the aqueous phase. The fate of the ascorbyl free radical is not known, but it will dismutate rapidly (6.3 to $10.0 \times 10^7 M^{-1}\text{sec}^{-1}$) to form ascorbate and dehydro-ascorbate.[5] In addition to ascorbate, uric acid also acts as an aqueous antioxidant.[6]

VII. OXIDATIVE STRESS

Oxidative stress is an important concept that helps not only formulate but critically evaluate the importance of oxidative damage in the aging process. The fact that a biological system is exposed to oxygen, even though it is absolutely necessary for aerobic life, also means that it experiences oxidative stress. That is, exposure to and use of oxygen in metabolic processes results in the formation of toxic "semireduced" oxygen by-products which causes oxidative stress to the organism. The imposed oxidative stress can be referred to as the oxidative damage potential, P_o. In the previous section, it was seen that nature has evolved several antioxidant systems capable of preventing the buildup of toxic oxygen by-products. Thus, the imposed oxidative damage potential is opposed by the antioxidant defense capacity, A_c, of the system. Thus, these two opposing processes are in dynamic equilibrium with each other, as expressed in Equation 20:

$$P_o \rightleftharpoons A_c \tag{20}$$

In reality, oxidative damage potential is greater than the antioxidant defense capacity, and thus there is a small amount of toxic oxygen by-products which escapes the defenses of the cells. This fact is expressed in Equation 21, where P'_o represents the fraction of toxic oxygen byproducts that escapes the defenses; i.e.,

$$P_o - A_c = P'_o \tag{21}$$

One may question the validity of this notion and ask why nature would allow a small amount of oxidation damage to occur at all times. In defense of the validity of the statement, it can be pointed out that a certain amount of, for instance, oxidized proteins and nucleic acids exist in cells at all times. The fact that these macromolecules are oxidized certainly reflects oxidative events that have occurred. Also, one of the most consistent observations in aging research is the almost universal presence of lipofuscin, aging pigment, in cells. Although debate exists about the exact nature of lipofuscin, there is very little doubt that it is formed by oxidative mechanisms, being most likely the product of oxidized lipids and oxidized proteins. With regard to the question of why nature allows oxidative damage to occur, it is due perhaps to the fact that: (1) it would require too much energy to build enough defenses to prevent *all* oxidative damage and, therefore, (2) nature probably uses the small amount of oxidative flux as triggering or signaling events in the process of development or differentiation. The latter notion is speculative, but certain observations support the concept.

As noted above, a small but significant fraction of the cellular proteins and nucleic acids are oxidized at any specific time. Their presence reflects not only the fact that they are formed by oxidative mechanisms, but also that they are not completely removed at any specific time. Thus, the amount present at any specific time reflects the equilibrium levels which is the sum of the rate of formation less the rate of repair and/or degradation processes responsible for removing or repairing the damaged products. This principle is presented in Equation 22, where B represents a biological molecule, B_{ox} is an oxidized molecule, and A represents the degradation products such as amino acids in the case of proteins; i.e.,

$$B \underset{R}{\overset{P'_o}{\rightleftharpoons}} B_{OX} \xrightarrow{D_{OX}} A \tag{22}$$

Thus, the rate of B_{ox} formation is governed by the amount of toxic "oxygen byproducts", P'_o, which have avoided the defense systems, R represents the repair of oxidized macromolecules, and D_{ox} represents the rate of degradation to individual components. Repair processes are probably of more importance in DNA damage, and degradation processes are important in the proteolytic decomposition of oxidized protein. It therefore follows that if the amount of oxidized protein is constant as a function of time at any specific age, then the rate of its formation is equal to its rate of decay.

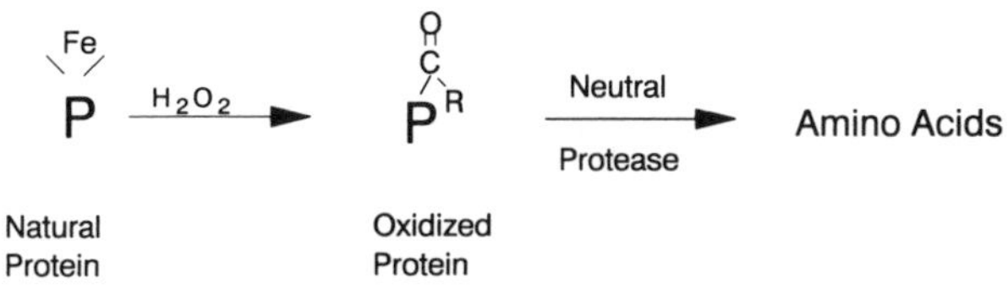

FIGURE 2. Scheme illustrating oxidation of protein (P) which involves binding of Fe to the protein, the reaction of hydrogen peroxide to oxidize amino acids on the protein and form carbonyl residues. The oxidized proteins acts a substrate for a neutral protease which degrades the protein into individual amino acids. (Summarized by Floyd, R. A. and Carney, J. M., *Ann. Neurol.,* 32, S22, 1992. With permission.)

The enzyme system responsible for catalyzing the decomposition of oxidized protein is a neutral protease which was discovered by Rivett in 1985.[7] It is probably a complex protease having several individual peptides similar if not identical to the macro-oxy protease (MOP) described by Davies and isolated from the red blood cell.[8] Formation of oxidized protein depends upon the presence of either Fe and/or Cu and is mediated by H_2O_2.[3] The formation and enzymatic decomposition of oxidized protein is illustrated in Figure 2. Oxidized proteins have an increased carbonyl content due to the oxidation of specific residues (i.e., histidine, proline, lysine, and arginine are the most sensitive) and are quantitated using a variety of methods.[9]

VIII. METHODS USED TO QUANTITATE OXYGEN FREE RADICALS *IN VIVO*

It is extremely difficult to determine the flux of oxygen free radicals in a living system. This is because, in general, oxygen free radicals are normally present at extremely low levels, i.e., perhaps at $10^{-11} M$ or less. One reason for this is because they react almost immediately as they are formed, depending upon the particular oxygen free radical under question. There are two general approaches that have been used to ascertain the *in vivo* flux of oxygen free radicals and/or the amount of oxidative damage which has occurred. The two general approaches are: (1) use of exogenous traps and (2) assay of oxidative damage to biological molecules. Both general approaches used in conjunction with each other yield the most critical information.

With regard to the use of exogenous traps, it is desired that a trap react rapidly with the oxygen free radicals under question, and that the product formed be unique and in addition stable, such that, even though the rate of free radical formation is small, the product will, with time, build up to where it can be quantitated. Figure 3 shows examples of two exogenous traps that have been used.

Salicylate reacts at diffusion limited rates with hydroxyl free radicals to form the 2,3- and 2,5-dihydroxybenzoic acid (DHBA) products.[10] The ratio of DHBA to salicylate present in tissue can be quantitated using high

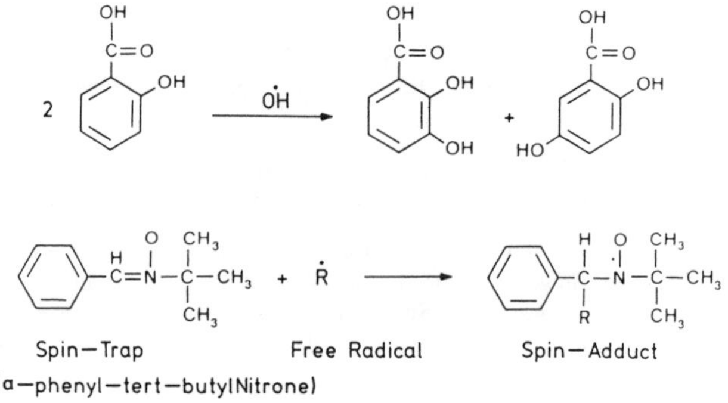

FIGURE 3. Equation showing the reaction of salicylate to form 2,3- and 2,5-dihydroxybenzoic acid product and the reaction of a free radical with the spin trap, PBN. (Summarized by Floyd, R. A. and Carney, J. M., *Ann. Neurol.*, 32, S22, 1992. With permission.)

performance liquid chromatography (HPLC) in combination with a fluorescence detector positioned in line with but before an electrochemical detector.[11] The salicylate content can be determined using 300-mm excitation and 412-mm emission, and the DHBA content determined using an electrochemical detector set at 0.8 V in the oxidation mode. The amount of DHBA present is usually about 0.1% of the salicylate present if the salicylate has been given intraperitoneal (i.p.) in saline at the level of 50 mg/kg 20 min prior to induction of the oxidative insult. Salicylate appears to permeate all tissues, perhaps transported by an organic acid transport system.

Phenyl-α-*tert*butyl nitrone (PBN) is only one of several so-called spin-trapping compounds available. Certain free radicals add to the carbon-nitrogen double bond, yielding a nitroxide product, termed a spin-adduct. The nitroxide is usually fairly stable, thus permitting characterization of the free radical which has been spin-trapped. The electron spin resonance spectrum of the spin-adduct is, in theory, unique for each free radical that adds to the spin-trap. PBN is both water soluble and lipid soluble and readily, within 20 min, permeates all tissues essentially equivalently.[12] It remains in the tissue as the parent compound with a half-life of about 3 to 4 h and is eliminated as one polar product, apparently metabolized by the liver, in the urine.[12]

Proteins and nucleic acids, two major cellular compounds, are damaged by oxidative events, and there are methods available to quantitate the amount of oxidized product formed. One particularly sensitive method which has been utilized to ascertain oxidative damage to nucleic acids is to determine the amount of 8-hydroxyguanine present. The modified nucleoside is measured using HPLC with electrochemical detection.[11] Amounts of 8-hydroxy-2'-deoxyguanosine (8-OHdG) as small as 20 fmol can be quantitated.[13] Tissue DNA normally has about 1 to 3 8-OHdG present for each 10^5 normal deoxyguanosines present. Therefore, the 8-OHdG content of as little as 10 μg of DNA can be assessed with this methodology.[11]

As noted earlier, oxidative damage to proteins produces an increase in the carbonyl content of the protein due to oxidation of the amino acids histidine, proline, arginine, and lysine.[3] These residues are very sensitive to oxidative damage, and in certain enzymes, for instance glutamine synthetase, histidine -269 is readily oxidized and causes loss of enzymatic activity. The essential metal cofactor of this enzyme is Fe and it is localized near the histidine -269 residue.[14] Thus, it is clear that hydrogen peroxide reacts with Fe in the active center and causes oxidative damage to the nearby histidine. This is a clear example of site-specificity in the oxidative damage of a protein.

IX. OXIDATIVE STRESS IN A MODEL AGING SYSTEM

The brain, the proper functioning of which is of prime importance to the quality of life, has certain properties that make it an important system for aging studies. The brain is highly organized and processes complex information. Therefore, small modifications may have drastic effects. Neurons are postmitotic; thus, death to a neuron is permanent. The brain consumes a significant fraction (20%), on the basis of its weight, of the total oxygen demand. The brain is prone to oxidative damage, apparently because: (1) it contains high amounts of the easily peroxidizable 20:4 and 22:6 fatty acids; (2) it is not particularly enriched in the antioxidant protective defense enzymes or vitamin E; and (3) certain regions of the brain, especially the human brain, contain significant levels of iron. We have shown that if the brain is disrupted, the homogenate readily peroxidizes in phosphate buffer at 37°.[15] Peroxidation of the homogenate is prevented by compounds that ligate Fe and that specific brain regions peroxidize at different rates, depending on the total Fe content of that region.[15] Addition of dopamine prevents brain homogenate peroxidation.[15]

Our *in vitro* research with the brain was extended into the live animal where an ischemia/reperfusion insult (IRI) was used to investigate oxidative damage in the brain. The animal model chosen was the mongolian gerbil, due mostly to the fact that the forebrain of this animal is entirely perfused by the two common carotids.[16] Thus, ligation and the subsequent release of the two common carotids shut down and then allow resumption of blood flow into the forebrain. Ligation of the carotids has no effect on blood flow into the brain stem or cerebellum region. Therefore, brain stem and cerebellum can be used as internal controls to ascertain the region specific modifications induced by an IRI.

We have used salicylate hydroxylation as well as protein oxidation and loss of glutamine synthetase (GS) activity, an enzyme, the activity of which is destroyed by oxidative damage, to monitor oxidative events in gerbil brain given an IRI.[17-19] A summary of the results of several studies is presented in Figure 4. The results show that salicylate hydroxylation in the cerebral cortex, but not in the brain stem, is dependent upon whether the animals have had

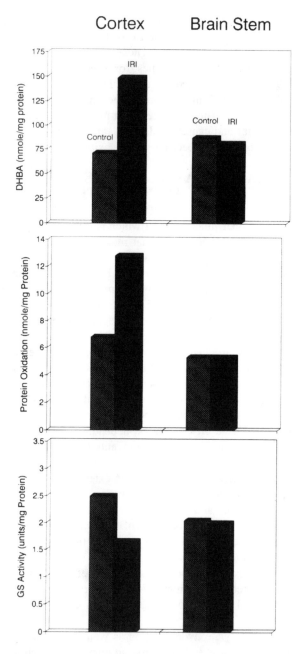

FIGURE 4. Summary of research results showing that salicylate hydroxylation increased in the cortex, but not in the brain stem,[19] and that an increase in protein oxidation as well as a decrease in glutamine synthetase (GS) activity was found in the cortex, but not in the brain stem of ischemia (10 min)/reperfusion (60 min)-treated gerbils. (Summarized by Floyd, R. A. and Carney, J. M., *Ann. Neurol.*, 32, S22, 1992. With permission.)

an IRI. In addition, the amount of protein oxidation and loss of GS activity in the cerebral cortex but not in the brain stem is also dependent upon whether the animals have had an IRI. This data strikingly demonstrates that oxidative events occur in the region of gerbil brain that has undergone an IRI, but not in the region that did not experience an IRI.

In the same model, we made a surprise observation, namely that administration of PBN protected the gerbils from an IRI-induced lethality, and that the spin-trap also diminished an IRI-dependent increase in the amount of protein oxidation or loss of GS activity in the cerebral cortex. This data is shown in Figure 5. It should also be noted that older gerbils are more sensitive to an IRI than are the younger animals. That is, 10-min ischemia eventually (7 d) killed all of the older gerbils, but only half of the younger gerbils were killed by 15-min ischemia.

X. PROTECTION AGAINST OXIDATIVE STRESS IN A MODEL AGING SYSTEM

The protective action which PBN provided in the gerbil brain ischemia/ reperfusion model and the age-associated lethality brought about by brain ischemia prompted us to test the notion that PBN may alter age-associated changes in the brain. Aging in the brain brings about a significant increase in oxidized protein and a significant decrease in the activity of glutamine synthetase as well as of neutral protease.[20] Comparing the brains of younger (3 to 4 month) gerbils with older (18 month) gerbils, we found that oxidized proteins were nearly double in older gerbils compared to young animals, and that GS activity had dropped to 65% in old animals, whereas the neutral protease activity had dropped to a value of only 33% of that found in the young animals.

With this background data, we administered PBN chronically (32 mg/kg twice daily) for 14 d, then after 1 d off PBN, determined the changes in brain-oxidized proteins and GS as well as in neutral protease activity. The results are presented in summary form in Figure 6. Chronic PBN administration caused a decrease in oxidized protein back down to levels noted in young gerbils. In addition to a change in oxidized proteins, PBN brought about an increase in GS activity and neutral protease activity. The activity of these two enzymes rebounded back nearly to levels noted in young animals. Chronic PBN administration to young gerbils (3 to 4 month) did not significantly alter the amount of oxidized protein or the GS or neutral protease activities.[20]

Cessation of PBN administration caused a rebound in the amount of oxidized protein in gerbil brain back to the normal levels after 14 d without PBN.[20] Figure 6 also shows that the activities of GS and neutral protease in the PBN-treated animals returned back down to their normal low levels. The return back to normal values was gradual, occurring in a monotonic fashion.[20]

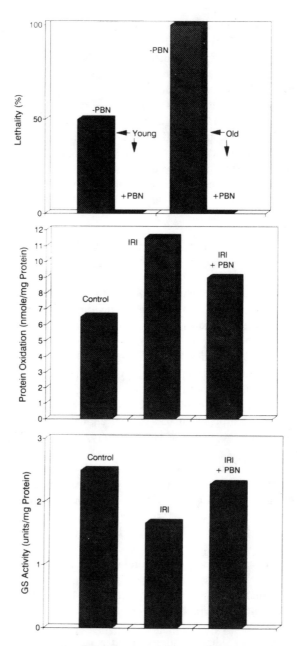

FIGURE 5. Summary of research results showing that lethality, assessed at 7 d was 50% for young (3 to 4 month) gerbils given 15-min brain ischemia, but was 100% for older (18 month) gerbils given 15-min ischemia; but 300 mg/kg PBN given ip. before the ischemia protected both young and old animals.[1] PBN given prior to an ischemia (10 min)/reperfusion (60 min)-insult helped to prevent protein oxidation and loss in GS activity in the cerebral cortex.[18] (Data summarized from Floyd, R. A. and Carney, J. M., *Ann. Neurol.*, 32, S22, 1992. With permission.)

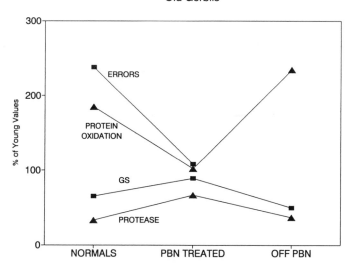

Old Gerbils

FIGURE 6. Summary of the research results demonstrating that chronic PBN administration to older gerbils caused a decrease in oxidized proteins in the brain and an increase in both glutamine synthetase and neutral protein activity, as well as a decrease in errors committed in a radial-arm maze designed to test short-term/spatial memory.[20] The cessation of PBN administration caused a reversion back to the older brain values observed prior to spin-trap administration. (From Floyd, R. A., *Science*, 254, 1597, 1991. With permission of ©AAAS.)

In addition to the brain chemistry data, we also tested the effect of PBN administration on one behavioral parameter.[20] The gerbils were tested for patrolling behavior in an eight-arm radial arm device which yields an index of short-term/spatial memory. Older gerbils consistently made about two times the amount of errors as younger gerbils in this test, as the data in Figure 6 show. Chronic PBN administration for 14 d did not alter the errors committed in the young gerbils, but significantly decreased the errors committed by older gerbils, back down to the levels found in younger animals.

Thus, the data we have collected so far has shown that PBN administered chronically causes a decrease in the age-associated increase in brain protein oxidation and loss of specific enzyme activities. There is also an associated decrease in a behavioral parameter which is an index of short-term/spatial memory.

The mechanism of how PBN brings about these changes is not known at the present time, but the most simple explanation is that it is trapping very crucial free radicals in an early phase, thus preventing oxidative damage. This remains to be proven, but the fact that all of the parameters tested change as would be expected if an interference in oxidative damage had occurred certainly adds credence to the notion that oxidative damage is an important parameter in aging-associated processes. The most remarkable feature of this set of experiments is the resiliency of the system. That is, PBN is able to alter the system such that it returns to the younger state, but cessation of PBN administration allows it to come back to its original state. This implies that there is an age-associated oxidative damage set-point which is fairly rigidly determined at any specific age. This may be determined by development-dictated gene-mediated events brought about by oxidative damage. Clearly this area of research is ripe for further investigation.

ACKNOWLEDGMENTS

The research results presented were made possible by the excellent collaborative efforts of Drs. John M. Carney, Cynthia N. Oliver, Pamella Starke-Reed, and Earl R. Stadtman. This research was supported in part by National Institutes of Health (NIH) Grants NS23307 and AG09690.

REFERENCES

1. **Floyd, R. A.**, Role of oxygen free radicals in carcinogenesis and brain ischemia, *FASEB J.*, 4, 2587, 1990.
2. **Fridovich, I.**, The Biology of oxygen radicals, *Science*, 201, 875, 1978.
3. **Stadtman, E. R.**, Metal ion catalyzed oxidation of proteins: biochemical mechanism and biological consequences, *Free Radical Biol. Med.*, 9, 315, 1990.
4. **McCord, J. M. and Fridovich, I.**, Superoxide dismutase: an enzymic function for erythrocuperin (Hemocuprein), *J. Biol. Chem.*, 244, 6049, 1969.
5. **Yamazaki, I. and Piette, L. H.**, Mechanism of free radical formation and disappearance during the ascorbic acid oxidase and peroxidase reactions, *Biochim. Biophys. Acta*, 50, 62, 1961.
6. **Ames, B. N., Cathcart, R., Schwiers, E., and Hochstein, P.**, Uric acid provides an antioxidant defense in humans against oxidant- and radical-caused aging and cancer: a hypothesis, *Proc. Natl. Acad. Sci. U.S.A.*, 78, 6858, 1981.
7. **Rivett, A. J.**, Preferential degradation of the oxidatively modified form of glutamine synthetase by intracellular mammalian proteases, *J. Biol. Chem.*, 260, 300, 1985.
8. **Pacifici, R. E., Salo, D. C., and Davies, K. J. A.**, Macroxyproteinase (M. O. P.): a 670 kDa proteinase complex that degrades oxidatively denatured proteins in red blood cells, *J. Free Radical Biol. Med.*, 7, 521, 1989.
9. **Levine, R. L., Garland, D., Oliver, C. N., Amici, A., Climent, I., Lenz, A.-G., Ahn, B.-W., Shaltiel, S., and Stadtman, E. R.**, Determination of carbonyl content in oxidatively modified proteins, *Methods Enzymol.*, 186, 464, 1990.
10. **Floyd, R. A., Henderson, R., Watson, J. J., and Wong, P. K.**, Use of salicylate with high pressure liquid chromatography and electrochemical detection (LCED) as a sensitive measure of hydroxyl free radicals in adriamycin treated rats, *J. Free Radical Biol. Med.*, 2, 13, 1986.
11. **Floyd, R. A., West, M. S., Eneff, K. L., Schneider, J. E., Wong, P. K., Tingey, D. T., and Hogsett, W. E.**, Conditions influencing yield and analysis of 8-hydroxy-2'deoxyguanosine in oxidatively damaged DNA, *Anal. Biochem.*, 188, 155, 1990.
12. **Chen, G., Bray, T. M., Janzen, E. G., and McCay, P. B.**, Excretion, metabolism and tissue distribution of a spin trapping agent, α-phenyl-N-*tert*-butyl-nitrone (PBN) in rats, *Free Radical Res. Commun.*, 9, 317, 1990.

13. **Floyd, R. A., Watson, J. J., Harris, J., West, M., and Wong, P. K.,** Formation of 8-hydroxydeoxyguanosine, hydroxyl free radical adduct of DNA in granulocytes exposed to the tumor promoter, tetradeconylphorbolacetate, *Biochem. Biophys. Res. Commun.,* 137(2), 841, 1986.

14. **Levine, R. L.,** Oxidative modification of glutamine synthetase. I. Inactivation is due to loss of one histidine residue, *J. Biol. Chem.,* 258, 11823, 1983.

15. **Zaleska, M. M. and Floyd, R. A.,** Regional lipid peroxidation in rat brain *in vitro:* possible role of endogenous iron, *Neurochem. Res.,* 10, 397, 1985.

16. **Chandler, M. J., DeLeo, J., and Carney, J. M.,** An Unanesthetized-gerbil model of cerebral ischemia-induced behavioral changes, *J. Pharmacol. Methods,* 14, 137, 1985.

17. **Cao, W., Carney, J. M., Duchon, A., Floyd, R. A., and Chevion, M.,** Oxygen free radical involvement in ischemia and reperfusion injury to brain, *Neurosci. Lett.,* 68, 233, 1988.

18. **Oliver, C. N., Starke-Reed, P. E., Stadtman, E. R., Liu, G. J., Carney, J. M., and Floyd, R. A.,** Oxidative damage to brain proteins, loss of glutamine synthetase activity, and production of free radicals during ischemia/reperfusion-induced injury to gerbil brain, *Proc. Natl. Acad. Sci. U.S.A.,* 87, 5144, 1990.

19. **Floyd, R. A. and Carney, J. M.,** Age influence on oxidative events during brain ischemia/reperfusion, *Arch. Gerontol. Geriatr.,* 12, 155, 1991.

20. **Carney, J. M., Starke-Reed, P. E., Oliver, C. N., Landrum, R. W., Cheng, M. S., Wu, J. F., and Floyd, R. A.,** Reversal of age-related increase in brain protein oxidation, decrease in enzyme activity, and loss in temporal and spatial memory by chronic administration of the spin-trapping compound *N*-tert-butyl-α-phenylnitrone, *Proc. Natl. Acad. Sci. U.S.A.,* 88, 3633, 1991.

21. **Floyd, R. A.,** Oxidative damage to behavior during aging, *Science,* 254, 1597, 1991.

22. **Floyd, R. A. and Carney, J. M.,** Free radical damage to protein and DNA; mechanisms involved and relevant observations on brain undergoing oxidative stress, *Ann. Neurol.,* 32, S22, 1992.

Chapter 4

OXIDATIVE DAMAGE BY FREE RADICALS AND LIPID PEROXIDATION IN AGING

Byung Pal Yu

TABLE OF CONTENTS

I. INTRODUCTION

The idea that oxygen might have adverse effects on normal biological functions is not new. In fact, the deleterious effect of oxygen was first noted before the turn of the century.[1] However, the mechanistic explanation for the deleterious actions of oxygen molecules was unknown until the identification of the reactive chemical intermediates known as free radicals.[1] Advances in radiation biology in the 1950s provided evidence of widespread radiation-induced damage through free radical reactions in biological systems. The implications of the havoc that could be produced by free radicals and the cumulative results that lead to many age-related disease processes were collected together and formulated, in 1956, into a hypothesis — the Free Radical Theory of Aging.[2] Data acquired during the last two decades on free radicals have led many modern gerontologists to adopt this view that time-dependent, functional deterioration may be causally related to the oxidative stress of the organism due to deleterious actions of free radicals.[3-8] The basic premise making this hypothesis so attractive is the fact that free radicals are generated endogenously from respiring oxygen. As a consequence, the chronic exposure to oxidative stress due to the unusually high reactivity of free radicals (Table 1) could impose serious threats to the organism.[9-11]

To survive under such threats, organisms have developed intricate defense mechanisms against free radicals. Indeed, the existence of such defense systems (in all aerobic organisms examined) may be one of the strongest supports, attesting to the presence of an oxidative threat in living biological systems. Furthermore, the existence of these adaptive processes has provided strong biological evidence, albeit circumstantial, linking free radical involvement to aging processes. A very strong positive correlation exists between maximum life-span potential of a species and its antioxidant capacity (Figure 1); the biological significance of this correlation has been discussed by Cutler.[9] If free radicals are in fact the causative factors responsible for senescence, it would be of prime importance for organisms to maintain efficient defense systems throughout their life to minimize damage. An unfortunate consequence of aging is that these protective defense components themselves become targets of free radical attack and deteriorate during senescence.[11] Thus, the net balance between free radical production and protection shifts towards greater damage with advancing age.[12] As depicted in Figure 2, the assessment of the overall oxidative status requires consideration of several interrelated but distinct aspects of free radical metabolism — free radical generation, antioxidant protection, free radical damage, damage repair, and detoxification/elimination of potentially harmful free radical by-products. In this chapter, discussion of these topics is a major focus. Particular attention is given to membrane-related events because membranes house the major production apparatus of free radicals and because membranes suffer the greatest damage from free radicals. Finally, the importance of nutritional intervention in modulating these processes is discussed in some detail.

TABLE 1
Half-Life of Some Free Radicals

Chemical Species	Symbol	Half-life (sec) at 37°C
Superoxide	O_2^-	1×10^{-6}
Singlet oxygen	$^1O_2$	1×10^{-6}
Hydroxyl	$\cdot OH$	1×10^{-9}
Lipid peroxide	ROOH	$>10^2$
Alkoxyl	RO·	1×10^{-6}
Peroxyl	ROO·	1×10^{-2}
Molecular oxygen	O_2	$>10^2$

Adapted from Florence, T. M., *Proc. Nutr. Aust.*, 15, 88, 1990.

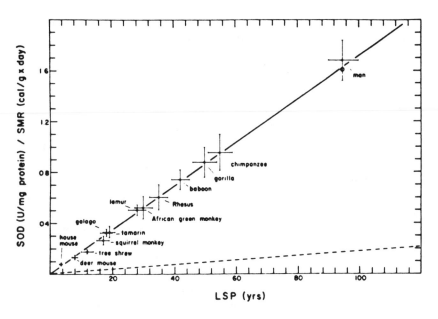

FIGURE 1. Correlation between maximum life-span potential and superoxide dismutase. (From Cutler, R. G., Antioxidants and longevity of mammalian species, in *Molecular Biology of Aging*, Woodhead, A. D., Blackett, A. D., and Hollaender, A., Eds., Plenum Press, New York, 1985, 15. With permission.)

II. MEMBRANE INVOLVEMENT IN FREE RADICALS AND LIPID PEROXIDATION

It is generally accepted that the biological membrane and its structural lipids are vulnerable to oxidation,[13-15] particularly to the free radical-mediated peroxidation catalyzed by transition metals such as Fe and Cu.[16-18] The

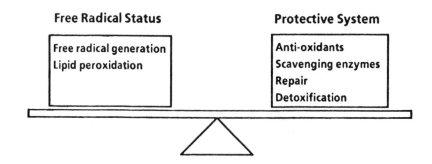

FIGURE 2. Schematic view depicting overall balance in cellular oxidative stress by the interaction between free radical status and protective defense systems.

susceptibility of membrane lipids to oxidative alterations is related to at least two inherent properties, the chemical nature of the lipids composing the membrane bilayer and the functional activities of membranes.[19-21] The first property is the peroxidizability of membrane lipids due to the degree of unsaturation of the fatty acid moieties. The second is related to the fact that most intracellular sites of free radical production are localized within biological membranes. The combination of these two properties makes membranes the likeliest candidates for oxidative injury.[23-25]

A. MEMBRANES AS SITES OF FREE RADICAL GENERATION

The activities related to free radical generation are mainly associated with membrane function and occur at various levels of cellular organization.[24] Biological sources of free radical production are widely distributed throughout the cell, as indicated in Table 2.[24] Quantitatively, however, mitochondria and microsomes are responsible for the bulk of the free radicals produced and have attracted the attention of many investigators in both the fields of free radicals and aging.[15,25-35]

The mitochondria,[25-32] being the respiratory powerhouse of the cell, is the major cellular site where substantial amounts of free radicals are formed. Loschen et al.[26] first supplied evidence for the mitochondrial generation of superoxide radicals and showed that superoxide is the precursor of mitochondrial H_2O_2. Subsequent studies identified two loci of superoxide generation, both localized in the inner membrane of the mitochondrial respiratory chain.[31] Suggested sites are the ubiquinone-cytochrome b region, probably by autoxidation of ubisemiquinone. Superoxide production rate is expected to be higher in state 4 with low ADP when respiratory chains are in reduced conditions.[36] The rate is low in state 3 or in the presence of uncouplers when oxygen consumption is high and the components of the respiratory component are oxidized. The amount of free radicals produced by mitochondria has been estimated to range anywhere from 1% to as much as 4% of oxygen respired by the organism under physiological conditions. Approximately 80% of superoxide radicals produced by the mitochondria become H_2O_2, which is de-

TABLE 2
Biological Sources of Free Radicals

Plasma membrane
  Lipooxgenase
  Cyclooxygenase
  NADPH oxidase
Mitochondria
  Electron transport
  Ubiquinone
  NADH dehydrogenase
Microsomes
  Electron transport
  Cytochrome P_{450}
  Cytochrome b_5
Peroxisomes
  Oxidases
  Flavoproteins
Others
  Hemoglobin
  Xanthine oxidase
  Flavins

Adapted from Freeman, B. D., *Free Radicals in Molecular Biology, Aging and Disease,* Armstrong, D., Sohal, R. S., Cutler, R. G., and Slater, T. F., Eds., Raven Press, New York, 1984, 43.

rived from dismutation of superoxide by mitochondrial superoxide dismutase.[31] Mitochondrial catalase converts the H_2O_2 to more reactive hydroxyl radical.[37] Hydroxyl radicals can also be generated nonenzymatically through the Haber-Weiss reaction in which H_2O_2 reacts with superoxide in the presence of transition metals.[15] To counteract endogenous oxidative stress, mitochondria are equipped with their own defense line, Mn/Zn superoxide dismutase, catalase, and peroxidase.

The second major membrane-associated source of free radicals and H_2O_2 is the endoplasmic reticulum (i.e., the microsomal membrane) which is involved in nicotinamide-adenine dinucleotide (reduced) (NADH)- or nicotinamide-adenine dinucleotide phosphate (reduced) (NADPH)-dependent oxidation of both endogenous and exogenous substrates.[38] Several studies[33-35] have shown that microsomes can generate superoxide and H_2O_2 during oxidation processes in which cytochrome P-450 and NADPH-cytochrome c reductase are involved. Although the exact site of superoxide formation has yet to be established, evidence suggests that cytochrome P-450, but not NADPH-dependent reductase itself, may be the source of the oxygen-derived free radicals. A proposed scheme for the involvement of various components and reaction steps in microsomal electron transport system is illustrated in Figure 3. According to the scheme,[39] binding of oxygen to the reduced heme Fe^{2+} leads to the formation of oxyferrous complex (IV), which in turn leads to the formation of either ferric peroxyl or ferrous-superoxide complex (V). When

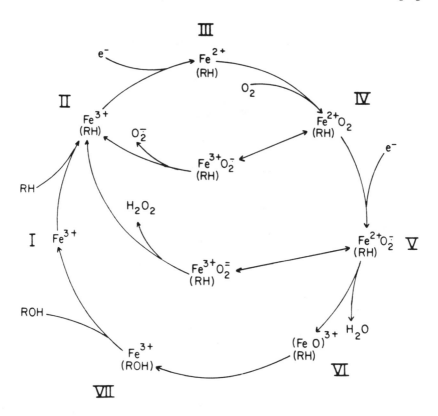

FIGURE 3. Schematic diagram for cytochrome P_{450} oxidation cycle. (From Morehouse, L. A. and Aust, S. D., *Cellular Antioxidant Defense Mechanisms,* Vol. 1, Chow, C. K., Ed., CRC Press, Boca Raton, FL 1988, 1. With permission.)

electron transport is tightly coupled, very little superoxide or H_2O_2 is generated during these reactions. However, if the systems are uncoupled, an increased generation of superoxide from oxyferrous and/or H_2O_2 from ferric peroxyl complexes occurs. Several factors may be involved in the uncoupling process. A change in the spin state of cytochrome P-450 may be one of the factors. Because the cytochrome P-450 isozymes present in the membrane exist in equilibrium between high and low spin states,[39] a shift in equilibrium to the high spin state would lead to the more reduced cytochrome P-450 and a decrease in production of superoxide or H_2O_2. Recent findings[40-42] on the selective modification of cytochrome isozymes by *in vitro* peroxidation suggest that damage to microsomal membranes might effect shifts in the spin state and lead to the potential uncoupling process.

B. LIPID PEROXIDATION REACTIONS OF MEMBRANES
Lipid peroxidation is an oxidative process in which lipid molecules undergo a series of chemical alterations initiated by free radicals and

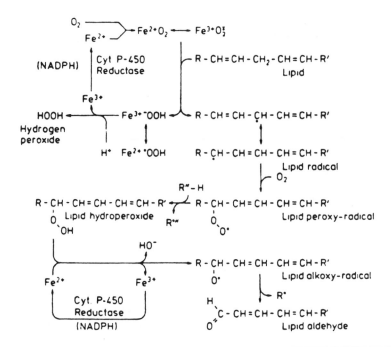

FIGURE 4. Diagram for iron-induced lipid peroxidation process. (From Kappus, H., Biochemical mechanisms of chemical-induced lipid peroxidation, in *Membrane Lipid Oxidation,* Vol. II, Vigo-Pelfrey, C., Ed., CRC Press, Boca Raton, FL, 1991, 104. With permission.)

oxygen.[18,24,29,43-45] In this process, molecular oxygen interacts with unsaturated membrane lipids through a series of complex multistage reactions. Under normal physiological conditions, oxygen, superoxide radicals, and H_2O_2 are not reactive enough to spontaneously interact with lipids. For lipid peroxidation to occur, activation of lipid molecules and pro-oxidants are both necessary. For instance, the activation of oxygen requiring transition metal-catalysis (Figure 4)[45] can be achieved by exciting one of the unpaired electrons to the singlet state by reducing oxygen to superoxide and hydroxyl radicals. Lipid peroxidation may occur under two different settings: (1) initiation by metal-oxygen interaction and (2) initiation by a hydroxyl radicals derived from superoxide on H_2O_2 through metal catalysis. The metal-oxygen interaction requires NADPH, ADP, Fe^{3+}, and reductase of the microsomal electron transport to reduce ADP-Fe^{3+} to a perferryl ion. Once initiation is started, the sequential propagative events follow. The reactive perferryl ion now can remove hydrogen atom (i.e., reduction) from the allylic bonds of lipid molecules, making conditions more unstable and more susceptible to further free radical attack (Figure 4). When reactive free radicals (e.g., · OH) break the allylic bonding, the lipid molecule itself becomes an alkyl radical through the loss of hydrogen. This activated lipid free radical itself can now interact with molecular oxygen to form lipid peroxyl radicals (LOO ·). Physiologically,

TABLE 3
Age-Related Changes in Membrane Structure

Membrane structure	Age	Dietary restriction	Ref.
Lipids			60
Hydroperoxide	↑	↓	
Fatty acids	↑	↓	
18:2	↓	↑	
20:4; 22:5; 22:6	↑	↓	
Peroxidizability index	↑	↓	
MDA Production	↑	↓	
Protein			13
Cytochrome P_{450}	↓	↑	
Cytochrome b_5	—	↑	
Membrane fluidity	↓	↑	13, 69
Membrane transition temperature	↑	—	13

Note: — , No change.

the process is even more complex since the overall *in vivo* oxidation of lipids involves transition metals. Because of this complexity, the "peroxidizability index of lipids" was proposed to quantitatively assess the potential peroxidizability (i.e., susceptibility) of total membrane lipids towards oxidation.[48] Since most polyunsaturated long-chained fatty acids in the cell are incorporated into membrane phospholipids, the index provides a useful means of evaluating how the change in fatty acid composition affects the overall membrane susceptibility to peroxidation (Table 3).

C. LIPOFUSCIN: EARLY HISTORICAL EVIDENCE FOR AGE-RELATED LIPID PEROXIDATION

Intracellular accumulation of fluorescent age-pigments[49-53] has been frequently used as an index of lipid peroxidation of most aged cells. Morphological observation of lipofuscin accumulation in aged human nerve cells was first reported before the turn of the century. Although the exact chemical composition of lipofuscin has yet to be determined, it is generally believed that oxidized lipid residues are the major constituents of fluorescent lipofuscin materials, and some of the physicochemical characteristics of these fluorescent materials have been partially identified.[49,50] The progressive increase and deposit of autofluorescent materials with age occurs in most tissues, particularly those tissues composed of postmitotic cells. Porta[55] reported that the accumulation of lipofuscin is most consistently detected in neurons and cardiac cells, while regenerative cells, like hepatocytes, exhibit only little accumulation. Subsequently, lipofuscin accumulation was considered an age-related event. Initially, evidence linking lipofuscin to lipid peroxidation was derived from nutritional intervention. For example, vitamin E deficiency results in greater lipofuscin accumulation.[53] In other studies, lipofuscin deposits were reduced by dietary supplementation of antioxidants.[49,51] Tappel et al.[49] showed that dietary supplementations of vitamin E and butylhydroxytuluol (BHT) suppressed the accumulation of fluorescent products in the testes and the heart. These studies further linked *in vivo* lipid peroxidation with the accumulation of lipofuscin.

III. HYPOTHESES FOR MEMBRANE ALTERATIONS IN AGING

In an attempt to establish a more direct relationship between free radical damage and aging, current interest has been directed toward membrane-related areas. The result has been the articulation of three aging hypotheses, all involving membrane-related alterations induced by free radical damage. These authors have implicated free radicals and other related reactive species, as well, as possible causative factors responsible for the age-related deterioration of structural and functional integrity leading to pathogenesis of many diseases associated with aging.

Zs-Nagy[56] proposed that the cell membrane structure undergoes physicochemical changes during aging, which ultimately causes an increased rigidity of the cell membrane. Specifically, this theory is based on observations of an increased intracellular potassium concentration during age, as detected by X-ray microanalysis, and relates the age-associated membrane changes with a decrease of membrane-potassium conductance. As the author speculated, the ramifications of this serious cellular deviation could lead to an increased intracellular ionic strength, causing major alterations of many important cellular activities, including increased chromatin condensation, instability of DNA-RNA, and decreased RNA-polymerase interactions. Although the evidence for increased membrane rigidity and decreased permeability was not definitive, Zs-Nagy speculated that free radicals lead to membrane damage during aging.

An earlier membrane hypothesis proposed by Hochschild[57] was the "lysosomal membrane hypothesis" which held that aging and many age-related pathologies were causally related to the increase in lysosomal activity due to destabilized lysosomal membranes. He suggested that the free radicals and lipid peroxidation caused the destabilized lysosomal membrane structure. A third membrane-related theory of aging was proposed by von Zglinicki.[58] This theory focused on the increase in the mitochondrial membrane permeability due to free radical damage seen during aging. The interesting point of the theory was that the mitochondrial membrane was proposed as the major target site of free radical injury. The deleterious action of free radicals in the mitochondria results in sequential changes in many essential cellular homeostatic regulatory processes, a predicament similar to that described by Zs-Nagy.[56] All three hypotheses emphasized the importance of cellular membrane integrity in aging, and implied that free radicals and lipid peroxidation were the underlying causes of membrane deterioration.

A. AGE-RELATED MEMBRANE CHANGES

If the aging process is characterized as a time-dependent, progressive modification of biological systems, it is highly unlikely that the complex structures, such as cell membranes, would escape from the age-related change. Consequently, the relevant question is: "What is changing, and what are the factors involved in the progression of alteration?"; not: "Why do membranes change with age?"

Biological membranes are superstructures consisting of phospholipids, cholesterol, proteins, and carbohydrates, all of which are intricately arranged in a thermodynamically stable state.[59] Since phospholipids are the major membrane constituents acting as the structural framework, the types of phospholipid in the membrane play an important role[58] in determining the membrane's physical characteristics, such as membrane fluidity. At present, the regulation of the membrane phospholipid biosynthesis in aging is poorly understood. However, as indicated by studies on the analysis of membrane phospholipids, substantial changes occur in phospholipid profiles[31,58-60] with age. Examples include the total amount, the composition of phospholipid subclasses,[61] and the asymmetrical distribution of phospholipids across the lipid bilayer of membranes.[62] The reduction in the total amount of phospholipid in membranes is one of the earliest signs of membrane-related alterations,[63] and such age-related changes are frequently observed, as reported by Grinna.[64] Although there is reason to believe that age-related decreases occur uniformly in all membranes, at present most of the documentation of these changes has been supplied for microsomal, mitochondrial, and plasma membrane preparations. In rat-liver microsomes, total phospholipid content decreased progressively from 3 to 22 months of age.[65] Similarly, Hegner[66] reported that phospholipid content of rat-plasma membranes was lower (by approximately 20%) in 780-d- than in 80-d- old male rats. These age-related changes are often associated with changing patterns of phospholipid subclasses, as shown in Figure 5.[63] Similar results were reported more recently in rat-liver microsomes and mitochondria by Laganiere and Yu.[60]

Cholesterol (Chol) is another major membrane constituent whose regulation in the aged membrane has not been extensively studied.[67] However, it is known that membrane cholesterol content increases with age.[32,46,63,68] The major function of cholesterol in the membrane lipid bilayer is to act as a stabilizer of membrane structure via its ability to promote hydrophobic interactions among fatty acid chains.[67] Under abnormally elevated levels, cholesterol was considered a membrane lipid solidifier which enhanced the overall lipid order and microviscosity of membranes. Since cholesterol molecules are thought to distribute evenly in the lipid bilayer, the molar ratio of Chol to phospholipid (PL) is often used as a marker for the membrane physical properties; e.g., a higher ratio suggests a more rigid membrane. Table 4 lists Chol:PL ratios in the cell membranes in relation to age.[68] A trend is evident which knows that membranes have increased Chol:PL ratio with age. The increase in the ratio is often considered a molecular explanation for the

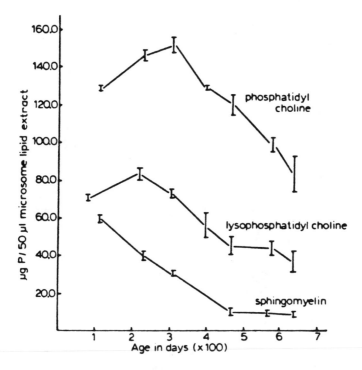

FIGURE 5. The effect of age on microsomal membrane phospholipids. (From Hawcroft, D. W. and Martin, P. A., *Mech. Ageing Dev.*, 3, 121, 1974. With permission.)

TABLE 4
Changes in Cholesterol: Phospholipid Ratios in Age

Tissue	Age	Chol	PL	Ratio
Red blood cells (human)	y (<30 years)	2.79 nmol/mg	363 nmol/mg	0:77
	o (>70 years)	2.79 nmol/mg	297 nmol/mg	0:94
Red blood cells (rat)	y (1.5 months)	0.334 (% total lipid)	0.077 (% total lipid)	4:34
	o (1–2 years)	0.598 (% total lipid)	0.077 (% total lipid)	7:72
Plasma membrane	y (80 d)	6.6 (% total lipid)	50 (% total lipid)	0:13
(rat liver)	o (780 d)	9.7 (% total lipid)	40 (% total lipid)	0:24
Microsomal membrane	y (6 months)	—	—	0:22
(rat liver)	o (24 months)	—	—	0:39
Mitochondrial membrane	y (6 months)	—	—	0:082
(rat liver)	o (24 months)	—	—	0:130

Note: — , No data available.

Adapted from Naeim, F. and Walford, R. L., *Handbook of the Biology of Aging*, 2nd ed., Finch, C. E. and Schneider, E. L., Eds., Von Nostrand Reinhold, New York, 1985, 272.

increased membrane rigidity of aging. However, as will be discussed in Section B, the age-related changes in the Chol:PL ratio may not be the sole factor contributing to membrane fluidity. Recent studies from our laboratory[69] show that age-related increases in lipid hydroperoxides and membrane lipid peroxidation can be membrane-rigidifying factors which influence the fluidity of aged membranes.[70,71]

Fatty acid composition represents another major alteration in membrane lipids. Increased hydroperoxides[60] and malondialdehyde (MDA) accumulation have been observed in aged tissues.[72,73] MDA is a major metabolite of arachidonic acid,[74] and the extent of MDA production has been used to measure lipid peroxidation. Numerous studies demonstrate that MDA content and production increase in aged tissues,[75-78] implying fatty acid alterations with age. Recent investigations show that fatty acid compositional changes in aging rat membranes[65,66,79] exhibit a distinct pattern: while the amounts of linoleic (18:2) and linolenic (18:3) acids decrease, the highly peroxidizable long-chained polyunsaturated acids, such as arachidonic (20:4) and docosapentaenoic (22:5) or docosahexaenoic (22:6) (Table 3), increase.[61] Therefore, it appears that a reduction in unsaturated 18 carbon fatty acids is accompanied by an elevation in polyunsaturated long-chained fatty acids. The mechanistic explanation for these changes is not known, but cellular adaptive responses may compensate for the age-related increase in membrane rigidity by elevating the polyunsaturation of fatty acids in the aged membranes. Such an adaptive response is unfortunate because it increases the peroxidizability index of the age membranes.[60,61] These age-related trends in fatty acid changes of membrane lipids have been reported by several other laboratories.[64,65,79] The molecular basis for the regulation of the membrane peroxidizability has yet to be defined; however, the regulation of the Δ^6-desaturase, a rate-limiting reaction converting 18:2 to 18:3, may be involved. A preliminary study from our laboratory[80] demonstrates an increased Δ^6-desaturase activity in the liver microsomes of aged rats. Further support comes from Choi et al.,[81] who observed an increased ratio of arachidonate to linoleate in aged rats, suggesting that changes in the regulation of the desaturation system of fatty acids occurred with aging in membranes.

B. MEMBRANE FLUIDITY CHANGES BY LIPID PEROXIDATION

Changes in membrane fluidity affect a variety of cellular functions.[62] Membrane fluidity, which is inversely related to the physical rigidity of membranes, represents the dynamic membrane property.[62,67] Fluidity depends on the physicochemical properties of membrane lipid constituents.[57,63,67,82,83] Major properties include: (1) the length of the fatty acid chain, (2) the degree of unsaturation, (3) the distribution of phospholipids in the membrane bilayer, and (4) the cholesterol content. Although it is generally accepted that aging causes a decline in membrane fluidity, the mechanistic nature of the decline has not been well characterized. To date, two membrane properties have received the most attention: (1) changes in fatty acid composition and (2) changes in cholesterol content with age.

The bulk of the evidence shows that both plasma and membrane cholesterol increase with age. Traditionally, the effect of cholesterol on membrane fluidity has been evaluated by the Chol:PL ratio because the amounts of both cholesterol and phospholipids in membranes vary with age. As shown in Table 4, the ratio increases with age.[68,69] The change in the ratio is caused either by an increased cholesterol and/or a decreased phospholipid content in membranes. As mentioned earlier, a rise in the ratio indicates that membrane rigidity has increased. However, recent examination of the fluidity of membranes from both aged *ad libitum*-fed and calorie-restricted rats revealed that fluidity is influenced by another age-modulated factor, namely, lipid peroxidation.[69] Utilizing membranes from dietary-restricted rats, which are known to be more resistant to peroxidation, we concluded that fatty acids from peroxidized membranes may contribute to the age-related increase in membrane rigidity.[69] This conclusion rests on the observations that the ratios of membrane Chol:PL of restricted and *ad libitum*-fed rats are very similar, yet the age-related increase in membrane rigidity did not occur in restricted rats.[69] Several other reports have shown that the loss in membrane fluidity with age correlates well with peroxidation of membranes from aged rats.[70,84] In addition, other work[71] demonstrated that the rigidity of liposomal membranes increased with *in vitro* peroxidation in the absence of cholesterol.

IV. FREE RADICAL GENERATION IN AGING

In the gerontological literature, it is often stated that overall oxidative stress of the organism increases with age.[7] This generalization is based mainly on evidence showing that free radical-induced damage or oxidatively modified cellular constituents accumulate with age. The commonly accepted underlying assumption is that there is a corresponding increase in the free radical production during senescence. Nohl and Hegner[31] first reported an increased production of superoxide by submitochondria particles (SMP) isolated from old rats. They showed that the superoxide production of SMP from 19-month-old rats was substantially higher than SMP from 6-month-old rats. These data of Nohl and Hegner form the basis for the general belief that free radical production increases with aging. The recent findings by Sawada et al.[85] on the superoxide formation by the plasma membrane of the brain, the heart, and the liver support the findings of Nohl and Hegner[31] in regard to the age-related increase of superoxide production. Moreover, these authors also showed that the age-related production of superoxide was organ-dependent, highest in the brain, followed by the heart, and lowest in the liver. However, a careful survey of the literature suggests that this generalization, that free radical generation increases with age, may not be tenable.[29,30,55,84]

The positive correlation between age and free radical production has not been a universal cathartic finding. For instance, a report by Zhan et al.,[84] utilizing electron spin resonance (ESR) in frozen tissue samples, showed, not only an absence of an age-related increase in superoxide production, but, in fact, a decrease with age. In their study, free radical generation in the liver, the testes, and the ovary of male and female Wistar rats significantly declined from ages 3 to 24 months. The authors speculated that the age-related reduction in superoxide production they observed could be secondary to the age-related decline of mixed functional oxidase activity in the liver and to cell loss in the ovary. Sawada and Carlson[86] quantitated mitochondrial superoxide generation by ESR measurement and showed that free radical production in mitochondria is also organ-dependent. They found a significant age-related increase in brain production of mitochondria followed by the heart, while only slight increases were found in liver mitochondria with age. This pattern was similar to that found in plasma membranes by Nohl and Hegner.[31] Additional proof that free radical production is not necessarily age-dependent was also obtained by other investigators. Floyd et al.[30] measured the free radical generation in aged brain by following the production of superoxide from intact synaptic and nonsynaptic mitochondria. Using oxygen electrode techniques, they found that brain mitochondria, especially the synaptic fraction from young rats, generated significantly higher amounts of superoxide compared to old rats, indicating an age-related decline in superoxide generation.

Our recent work[87] on the free radical production in liver microsomes utilizing dichlorofluorescin diacetate (DCFH-DA) dye is consistent with the data of Floyd et al.[30] This dye has been successfully used in the quantitation of oxygen-derived reactive species of superoxide, $\cdot$ OH, and H_2O_2 production in brain synaptosomes[88,89] and phagocytic cells.[90] The use of the lipophilic DCFH-DA dye has the distinct advantage of allowing measurement of reactive species without disruption of organelle membranes, due to its ability to permeate and incorporate into membrane hydrophobic regions. In addition, the fluorescence is emitted only when the dye is oxidized by oxygen reactive species, thereby permitting quantitative measurements. Data obtained with the fluorescent dye (Figure 6) indicate that free radical production does not increase with age. In agreement with this finding, our earlier studies[33] reported that the production of superoxide, hydroxyl radical, and H_2O_2 by liver microsomes isolated from rats at ages of 6, 12, 18, and 24 months also showed no age-related increases. In summary, the age-related increases in free radicals reported earlier are an inconsistent finding, as emphasized in Porta's review.[55] Because available data are inconsistent, further systematic investigation is warranted to define the precise quantitative significance of free radical production pertaining to the overall oxidative stress.

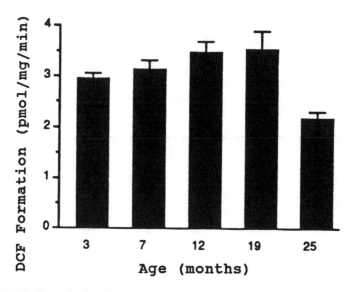

FIGURE 6. Determination of production of oxygen reactive species (O_2, $\cdot OH$, H_2O_2) by 2,7-dichlorofluorescence (DCF) dye method.[88] Mitochondria suspension was incubated with DCF ($5\mu M$), followed by centrifugation at $12,500 \times g$ for 8 min to pelletize. Induction of lipid peroxidation of dye-loaded mitochondria was carried out in the presence of NADPH (0.1 mM), ADP (1.7 mM), and FeCl$_3$ (0.1 mM). Fluorescence intensity was measured at wavelengths of 488 nm for excitation and 525 nm for emission.

V. MODULATION OF FREE RADICALS AND LIPID PEROXIDES

A. THE EFFECT OF DIETARY ANTIOXIDANTS

The existence of anti-radical defense systems in all aerobic organisms tested so far is probably the strongest evidence supporting the concept of a free radical threat to the organism. One experimental approach for validating this notion of an antioxidant defense against free radicals is to attenuate the threat or damage by administering exogenous antioxidants, as, for example, by adding antioxidants to food as dietary supplements. Feeding antioxidants to animals has attracted considerable interest from both nutritionists and gerontologists because of the capacity of antioxidants to neutralize or scavenge free radicals. Several investigators[8,91-95] have attempted to attenuate free radical injury by dietary antioxidants and have used the life-span as the index of antioxidant effectiveness (Table 5). Several well-known antioxidants, including 2-mercaptoethylamine (2-MEA)[92] and 2-mercaptoethanol (2-ME)[93] have been tested in the mouse,[5,94] *Drosophila*,[8] the nematode,[95] and the rotifer[96] (Table 5). It is clear from the results that dietary antioxidant supplementation improves survival by extending the average (median) life-span of rodents and the maximum life-spans of fruit flies and nematodes. Interpretation of life-span extension as a marker for the retardation of aging requires

TABLE 5
Antioxidant Effect on Life-Span

Compound	Increase in life-span (%)		Organisms	Sex	Ref.
	Median	Maximum			
2-Mercaptoethylamine (2-MEA)					
0.5% W	12.8	—	Mice, LAF	M	92
1.0% W	29.2	—	Mice, LAF	M	92
2-Mercaptoethanol (2-ME)					
0.25%	13.2	12.0	Mice, BCF	M	93
Santoquin					
0.5% W	18.1	—	Mice, C3H	M	94
	20.0	—	Mice, C3H	F	94
2-Ethyl-6-methyl-3hydroxypyridine	—	—	Mice, SHK	—	4
Tocopherol-*p*-chlorophen oxyacetate	13.0	13.0	*Drosophila*	—	7
Nordihydroguaiaretic acid	20.0	20.0	*Drosophila*	—	7
Magnesium thiazolidin carboxylate	20.0	20.0	*Drosophila*	—	7
α-Tocopherol	31.4	23.2	Nematode	—	95
Vitamin E	16.8	15.4	Rotifer	—	96
Sulfhydryl agent	28.0	—	Rotifer	—	9

Adapted from Harman, O., *Age,* 1, 143, 1978.

both theoretical and practical considerations. Average life-span extension without the maximum life-span extension, for instance as seen in rodents, is generally taken to indicate that the intervention exerts only a longevity hormesis without retarding the aging process per se. According to Neafsey,[97] hormesis is the beneficial effect of a toxicant seen at low-dose levels of the toxic substance. In practice, the extension of the median life-span generally occurs when genetically predisposed diseases are altered by particular treatments. Unfortunately, these potentially interesting experimental trials utilizing antioxidant paradigms suffer further from the fact that no other age-related functional changes were monitored to assess the efficacy of antioxidant treatment.

The work of Heidrick et al.[93] with 2-mercaptoethanol (2-ME) represents the most successfully executed study to date. Their study carefully monitored food intake, life-span, body weight, lipid peroxidation, and age-related changes in immune parameters. As shown in Table 5, the 2-ME treatment extended both the mean and maximum life-span. However, analysis of the survival data of these mice by Gompertz function revealed that 2-ME did not affect the mortality rate (i.e., aging) of the animals but merely postponed the onset of exponential death with age, i.e., longevity hormesis. These results imply that antioxidants exert very little effect on the rate of aging. With regard to the efficacy of 2-ME on lipid peroxidation, the study demonstrated a reduced accumulation of fluorescent lipid peroxidation products in spleen lymphocytes. A very interesting finding in this study was that 2-ME supplementation prevented the age-related deterioration of lymphocyte function. Considering the antioxidant action of 2-ME and the reduced lipid peroxidation, it is conceivable that the deterioration in lymphocyte function may be related to free radicals. Finally, it is noteworthy that the dietary antioxidant supplementation exerted its beneficial effects without reduced food intake. Reduction in calorie intake is a serious practical problem in most studies utilizing antioxidant supplementation.

Although antioxidant feeding promises to be a viable experimental paradigm in future studies, several theoretical and practical problems associated with dietary antioxidant supplementation need to be kept in mind. The first consideration is the proper selection of antioxidants because no antioxidant is capable of scavenging all free radical species. The second problem relates to the intestinal absorption and plasma levels of the antioxidant. The third consideration is the transport of antioxidants across the membrane barriers and the intracellular distribution of the antioxidant. Although the work of Schinitzky et al.[98] was not directly aimed at the antioxidant problem, their successful attempts to restore age-related membrane dysfunction by manipulating membrane fluidity with a diet supplemented with a membrane fluidizer may be applicable to anti-oxidant transport and distribution. In addition to these practical problems, a serious theoretical problem must be considered, namely, the disturbance of normal cellular redox balance by exogenous antioxidant and the possible undermining of the overall antioxidant defense competence. There are indications that overall antioxidant components are coordinated in such a way that increasing the concentration of one antioxidant would cause a compensatory reduction in another.

B. THE EFFECT OF DIETARY RESTRICTION

Dietary restriction is a term often used interchangeably with calorie restriction, food restriction, or undernutrition without malnutrition. In practice, restricted animals are given a reduced amount of chow (usually between 20% to 40% less than an *ad libitum*-fed cohort) for an extended period of time. The validity and utility of dietary restriction in the study of aging have been firmly established by numerous experiments on its antiaging actions.[99-105] Although the precise mechanisms underlying its diverse actions on the retardation of aging have not been established, dietary restriction has proven to be the most effective, interventive measure currently available for the retardation of aging in experimental gerontology.[106] Three characteristics of the actions of dietary restriction distinguish it from any other putative antiaging interventions: (1) retardation of physiological decline with age,[99] (2) postponement of the onset and/or progression of many age-related diseases,[107] and (3) extension of both the mean and maximum life-span.[102] In addition, the results of dietary restriction are experimentally highly consistent and reproducible, making it the most useful noninvasive intervention in aging animals.

TABLE 6
Age-Related Changes in Free
Radical Metabolism

Free radical metabolism	Age	Restriction	Ref.
Free radical and H_2O_2 production[a]			33
Superoxide	—	↓	
Hydroxyl	—	↓	
H_2O_2	—	↓	
Cytosolic antioxidant defense[b]			11
Superoxide dismutase	—	↑	
Catalase	↓	↑	
Reduced glutathione	↓	↑	
GSH Reductase	↓	↑	
GSH Peroxidase	↓	↑	
MDA Elimination[c]	↓	↑	154

Note: —, No change.

An earlier report by Enesco and Krurk[52] describing nutritional intervention on free radical damage showed that the reduction of dietary protein influenced the extent of lipid peroxidation. Restricting dietary protein to 4%, of the diet reduced the accumulation of lipofuscin in the heart and brain of mice. Although the oldest age of mice tested was only 12 months, a significant reduction of lipofuscin accumulation was observed in protein-restricted mice as compared with the control mice fed a 26% protein diet. The authors concluded that the consumption of a diet low in protein might modulate the level of free radical damage. The first report on the antiperoxidative action of calorie restriction was made by Chipalkatti et al.[108] Restriction of food intake to about one half that of the control group reduced lipofuscin in the brain and suppressed lipid peroxidation in liver homogenates as measured by malondialdehyde production. Koizumi et al.[109] found antioxidant effects of dietary restriction in liver homogenates from 12- and 24-month-old mice. The agerelated increase in lipid peroxidation as measured by the malondialdehyde formation was effectively suppressed by dietary restriction. These authors[109] extended their investigation to include the free radical scavenger enzymes, superoxide dismutase, catalase, and glutathione (GSH) peroxidase. While no diet-related modulation of superoxide dismutase or GSH peroxidase was seen, the age-related change in catalase was, interestingly, selectively up-regulated by dietary restriction. Further insights of antiradical actions of dietary restriction were obtained from studies on both soluble and membranous components of the cell. Laganiere and Yu[11] examined the effects of age and diet on cytosolic antioxidants, including catalase, GSH transferase, GSH peroxidase, GSH reductase, GSH, ascorbic acid, and vitamin E. They found that the age-mediated decrements in GSH, GSH reductase, and catalase were all strongly up-regulated by dietary restriction during senescence (Table 6), though GSH peroxidase and ascorbic acid were only slightly upregulated. Concerning membrane alterations, these same investigators[60] measured membrane peroxidation of liver microsomes and mitochondria from *ad libitum*-fed and dietary-restricted rats, aged 3, 6, 12, and 24 months. Lipid hydroperoxide content and MDA formation were significantly higher in the membranes from the *ad libitum*-fed rats, as was the membrane vitamin E content.

Additional evidence for the modulation of the free radical reactions by dietary restriction is found in studies which have measured the rate of free radical generation. Lee and Yu,[33] utilizing microsomes isolated from livers of *ad libitum*-fed and dietary-restricted rats aged 3, 6, 12, 18, and 24 months, investigated the formation of the superoxide, hydroxyl radicals, and hydrogen peroxide. Two points are especially noteworthy. First, no significant age-related increases in the production of these reactive species were observed. Second, throughout the life-span, the production of superoxide and hydroxyl radicals in *ad libitum*-fed rats were consistently higher than that of the dietary-restricted rats. In the same study, although no age-related decrease in superoxide dismutase was noted, dietary restriction elevated the activities of both cytosolic and mitochondrial superoxide dismutase relative to those observed in *ad libitum*-fed (Figure 7) rats, thus confirming the earlier work reported by Koizumi et al.[109]

VI. OTHER CELLULAR OXIDATIVE MODIFICATIONS WITH AGE

A. DNA DAMAGE AND MODULATION BY DIETARY RESTRICTION

Free radical-induced modifications are not limited to membrane lipids.[109,110] Because of their extreme reactivity, free radicals are capable of modifying most biological molecules, including DNA.[105,111-120] Alterations in DNA molecules induced by UV irradiation and free radicals has long been suspected of being a causal factor responsible for many age-related neoplastic diseases. As early as 1959, Szilard[121] proposed that the accumulation of DNA damage in the cell may be the major factor underlying the cellular aging process. The important consequences of oxidative DNA damage in relation to aging were further noted by Gensler and Bernstein,[122] who proposed that oxidative DNA damage is the primary cause of aging. Details of their discussion are presented in Chapter 5 of this volume. Their hypothesis is based on two major premises, namely, (1) DNA molecules represent the master code for cellular messages and (2) only a limited number of copies exist in diploid cells. Whether DNA molecules are more susceptible to oxidative attack under physiological conditions as compared to other macromolecules is not known at the present, but several lines of experimental data support the possibility that increased *in vivo* oxidative DNA damage occurs with age. A case in point is the work from Ames' laboratory.[111,112,120] This group showed that evidence of oxidatively modified DNA, such as thymine glycol, thimidine glycol, and hydroxymethyluracil, can be detected in the urine of both rats

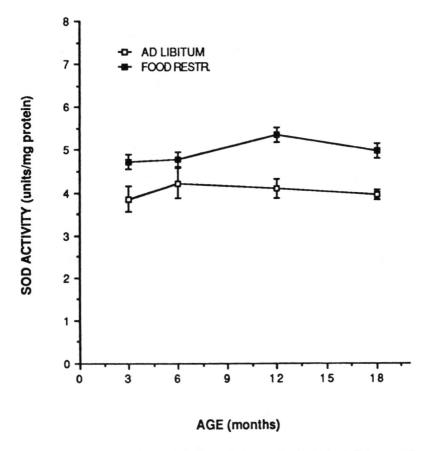

FIGURE 7.   The effects of age and dietary restriction on mitochondrial (Mn/Zn) superoxide dismutase.

and humans. Subsequently, these investigators also presented evidence indicating that *in vivo* DNA damage increases with advancing age.[116]

Recent findings suggest the possibility that oxidative damage of DNA can be lessened by the protective action of dietary restriction. Chung et al.[118] showed that a 40% dietary restriction reduced DNA damage significantly in both liver nuclear and mitochondrial DNA isolated from male Fischer 344 rats at the ages of 3 and 24 months. Dietary restriction reduced the amounts of 8-hydroxydeoxyguanosine (8-OH-dG) in oxidatively altered DNA molecules by about 20% in the liver and 35% in the mitochondria, respectively. It is noteworthy that in their study, the 3-month-old rats were restricted only for a period of $1 \frac{1}{2}$ months, indicating a rapid onset of the dietary effect. In addition, a significant difference was evident in the extent of DNA damage between nuclear and mitochondrial fractions. The amount of 8-OH-dG in mitochondrial DNA was about 15 times higher than that in nuclear DNA. This finding confirmed the previous results of Richter et al.,[112] who detected much higher 8-OH-dG in the mitochondrial than in the nuclear DNA fraction when damage was induced by UV irradiation. Protection of DNA from oxidative injury is considered significant in the overall action of dietary restriction because then the protection of DNA from oxidative damage by dietary restriction could effectively retard the onset and the progression of age-related diseases, such as tumorigenesis.[107] As proposed by Gensler and Bernstein,[122] oxidatively damaged DNA may be the underlying cause of many age-related diseases and could be a very important part of the mechanism by which diet extends life-span.

B. OXIDATIVELY ALTERED PROTEINS

Since proteins are major cellular structural and functional constituents, they also are targets of oxidative modification by free radicals.[110,123-126] It has been known for some time that *in vitro* oxidation of proteins is usually accompanied by structural modification, resulting in several physicochemical changes. For instance, fragmentation, aggregation, and increased susceptibility to proteolysis are the typical and dramatic changes seen in proteins when oxidized. Available experimental data suggest that modification of many proteins takes place *in vivo* with aging.[127-130] As far as membrane-associated proteins are concerned, only limited information is available on an aging effect. Starke-Reed and Oliver[131] showed that oxidation of proteins, specifically the histidine moieties, leads to increased carbonyl values. Oliver et al.[127] used this carbonyl value as an index of protein oxidation to assess the age-related increase in oxidatively altered proteins. They reported an increased concentration of oxidized proteins of red blood cell with the age of the cell. They also noted that the protein oxidation of cultured fibroblasts from normal individuals was lower than that observed in patients with progeria or Werner's Syndrome. The extent of the age-related increase in protein oxidation as estimated from carbonyl content of normal individuals was about two-fold between the ages of 10 and 80. Substantial oxidative modifications were also detected in the cytosolic proteins. Starke-Reed and Oliver[131] showed that the amount of oxidized hepatic protein increases in rats over the range of 3 to 24 months. The oxidative modification of proteins by various enzymatic and nonenzymatic mixed-function oxidation (MFO) was recently reviewed.[132]

Since oxidatively damaged proteins serve no apparent function[133,134] and are products[135] deleterious to the maintenance of cellular homeostasis, their removal is essential. A substantial body of evidence supports this position. The degradation of altered proteins by proteolytic digestion[136,137] is an extremely efficient process. In recognizing the importance of the proteolytic process, Davies[138] recently proposed that the proteolytic process represents a secondary free radical defense system (Table 7). An interesting feature of proteolytic degradation is the fact that, like digestion of oxidized lipids by phospholipase A_2,[69] oxidatively altered proteins become more susceptible to proteolysis, thereby making them preferred substrates for proteolytic enzymes.[139,140] For instance, when H_2O_2 inactivated superoxide dismutase is

TABLE 7
Proposed Scheme of Primary and Secondary Antioxidant Defenses

Primary defenses (to prevent damage)
    Antioxidant compounds   Vitamin E, β-carotene, ascorbic acid, uric acid, etc.
    Antioxidant enzymes   Superoxide dismutase, glutathione, peroxidase/reductase,
                                     DT-diaphorase, catalase, etc.
Secondary defenses (to remove or repair damaged products)
    Lipolytic enzymes   Phospholipase A_2
    Proteolytic systems   Proteinases, peptidases
    DNA, RNA repair systems   Endonucleases, exonucleases, etc.

From Davies, K. J. A., *Cellular Antioxidant Defense Mechanisms,* Vol. 2, Chow, C. K., Ed.,
CRC Press, Boca Raton, FL, 1988, 25.

incubated with cell-free RBC extracts, the damaged enzyme is digested several times faster than is the intact enzyme. This represents a cellular protective mechanism in which regeneration and repair of proteins is accelerated as efficiently as possible by the removal of nonfunctioning protein. This repair process is considered part of a well-coordinated, overall cellular defense mechanism in which oxidatively modified proteins are capable of activating the proteolytic system.[124] The preferential degradation of these oxidized molecules due to increased susceptibility to enzymatic degradation has been shown to relate to the extent of modification in the secondary and tertiary structures of proteins rather than in the primary structures, as seen with changes in hydrophobicity and denaturation.[141] Based on these data, Pacifici et al.[130] hypothesized that the enhanced susceptibility of the modified protein for degradation may, in part, be due to exposure and unfolding of the hydrophobic regions of proteins. The recent discovery of "proteosomes", a multicatalytic superstructure composed of 10 to 20 subunits with 600 to 700 kDa, was a significant advance in the understanding of cellular mechanisms for the proteolytic processing of many oxidatively modified proteins.[130]

VII. ELIMINATION OF OXIDATIVELY DAMAGED LIPID PRODUCTS

In order for degradation mechanisms to serve as secondary defense systems, they should encompass a broader range of oxidatively altered substances, including lipids. One such protective process is the degradation of by-products of lipid peroxidation.[142,143] The evidence for the existence of such an efficient elimination process arises from the detection of pentane and ethane in the expired gas of organisms.[144-147] The sources of pentane and ethane are the metabolites of lipid peroxidation. However, not all lipid moieties are metabolized, and if some nonmetabolizable lipid moieties accumulate, their deleterious effects may interfere with normal cellular functions.[74,148] Well-known examples of such by-product substances are malondialdehyde (MDA) and 4-hydroxynonenal (4-HNE), which have been studied previously.[72,149]

MDA has long been considered cytotoxic, mutagenic, and tumorigenic,[150-152] and has also been strongly implicated in the formation of age-pigments. In spite of all these putative actions, surprisingly little work has been done on the metabolic processes involved in MDA or 4-HNE elimination.

A brief description of MDA metabolism may help in understanding its fate. As indicated earlier, MDA is not an end-product of the lipid peroxidation process.[73,143] Rather, it is one of the intermediate metabolites which, under normal conditions, undergoes further metabolism to yield CO_2 and acetoacetate via a series of oxidation processes catalyzed by several enzymes, including aldehyde dehydrogenases.[73,153] However, during aging, the efficiency of MDA oxidation declines, leading to the accumulation of MDA in cells and tissues.[152] This situation could be aggravated with advanced age by increased lipid peroxidation. Evidence supporting an age-related decrease in the capacity to oxidize MDA was recently reported by our laboratory.[154] We found that the capacity to metabolize MDA by mitochondria (a major site of MDA oxidation) in aged *ad libitum*-fed rats decreased progressively with age, and, at 24 months, it was only 30% of the capacity of that of 3-month-old rats. On the other hand, dietary restriction with an enhanced antioxidant efficacy was able to partially prevent this mitochondrial functional decline. Although the precise mechanism responsible for this age-dependent decline remains to be explored, the deterioration of mitochondrial membranes and their membrane-associated aldehyde dehydrogenases by free radicals and lipid peroxidation may contribute to the decline. Our findings, therefore, provide a mechanistic explanation for the accumulated age-pigments seen in the aged cells and tissue, namely, the inability of mitochondria to oxidize MDA with age. Another reactive lipid metabolite which has only recently received attention is 4-hydroxynonenal (4-HNE).[72,155] Esterbauer,[72] who has done substantial amounts of work on aldehydic lipid peroxidation products, reports that 4-HNE reacts with cellular components much more strongly than does MDA.[156] Like MDA, 4-HNE, is a major by-product of 20:4 fatty acid autoxidation and should be processed to a less toxic compound under normal conditions. At present, little is known about the metabolic fate of 4-HNE. However, a preliminary observation showed that 4-HNE is preferentially bound to the mitochondria of *ad libitum*-fed rats, as compared with those from dietary-restricted rats.[157] It would be interesting to know how the metabolism of 4-HNE is compromised by age, and whether or not the age effect can be modulated by dietary restriction.

VIII. CONCLUDING REMARKS

Nearly 40 years have passed since the free radical theory of aging was proposed. During this period, numerous studies from both free radical and gerontological fields have attempted to validate the theory by generating experimental evidence. As a result, substantial advances have been made in the understanding of biological implications of free radicals and their potential

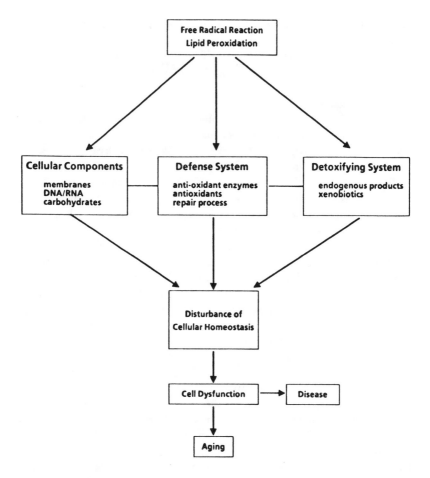

FIGURE 8. A proposed scheme showing the disruption of cellular homeostasis by free radicals and lipid peroxidation as a major cause of aging.

impact on the aging process. The interrelation of free radical metabolism with the aging process is schematically depicted in Figure 8. The main thrust of this scheme is that free radical and lipid peroxidation represent potential factors responsible for the disruption of cellular integrated system of homeostasis, leading to aging and age-related disease. In this chapter, emphasis was given to the changes occurring with age, which are the most likely impact sites of free radical actions and lipid peroxidation. Discussion centered around lipid peroxidation, membrane fluidity, and the modulatory action of dietary restriction. Although definite evidence linking free radicals to the cause of aging is lacking, the available evidence strongly suggests that the observed membrane alterations with age in terms of composition, physicochemical characteristics, and damage can be explained on the basis of free radical reactions. Advances in the field await technical and methodological breakthroughs which will allow the *in vivo* quantitative assessment of overall free radical metabolism.

ACKNOWLEDGMENTS

I should like to thank Drs. Helen Bertrand and Jeremiah Herlihy for their critical comments and editorial assistance this chapter. I should also like to thank Mrs. Kim Kennedy for helping in the preparation of the manuscript. This work was supported in part by Grant AGO-1188 from the National Institutes of Health.

REFERENCES

1. **Levine, J. S.,** The origin and evolution of atmospheric oxygen, in *Oxidases and Related Redox System,* King, T. E., Mason, H. S., and Morrison, M., Eds., Alan R. Liss, New York, 1988, 111.
2. **Harman, D.,** Aging: a theory based on free radical and radiation chemistry, *J. Gerontol.,* 11, 298, 1956.
3. **Ames, B. N.,** Endogenous DNA damage as related to cancer and aging, *Mutat. Res.,* 214, 41, 1989.
4. **Cutler, R. G.,** Antioxidants and longevity of mammalian species, in *Molecular Biology of Aging,* Woodhead, A. D., Blackett, A. D., and Hollaender, A., Eds., Plenum Press, New York, 1985, 15.
5. **Emanuel, N. M.,** Free radical and the action of inhibitor of radical processes under pathological states and aging in living organisms and in man, *Q. Rev. Biophys.,* 9, 283, 1976.
6. **Fleming, J. E., Miquel, J., Cottress, S. F., Yengoyan, L. S., and Economos, A. C.,** Is cell aging caused by respiration-dependent injury to the mitochondrial genome?, *Gerontology,* 28, 44, 1982.
7. **Sohal, R. S. and Allen, R. G.,** Oxidative stress as a causal factor in differentiation and aging: a unifying hypothesis, *Exp. Gerontol.,* 25, 499, 1990.
8. **Miquel, J. and Johnson, J. E.,** Effects of various antioxidants and radiation protectants on the life span and lipofuscin of drosophila and C57BL/6J mice, *Gerontologist,* 15, 11, 1975.
9. **Cutler, R. G.,** Antioxidants and longevity, in *Free Radicals in Molecular Biology, Aging and Disease,* Armstrong, D., Sohal, R. S., Cutler, R. G., and Slater, T. F., Eds., Raven Press, New York, 1984, 235.
10. **Bozovic, V. and Enesco, H. E.,** Effect of antioxidants on rotifer life-span and activity, *Age,* 9, 41, 1986.
11. **Laganiere, S. and Yu, B. P.,** Effect of chronic food restriction in aging rats. II. Liver cytosolic antioxidants and related enzymes, *Mech. Ageing Dev.,* 48, 221, 1989.
12. **Cutler, R. G.,** Antioxidants and aging, *Am. J. Clin. Nutr.,* 53, 373S, 1991.
13. **Lee, D. W. and Yu, B. P.,** The age-related alterations in liver microsomal membranes: the effect of lipid peroxidation and dietary restriction, in *Liver and Aging,* Kitani, K., Ed., Excerpta Medica, New York, 1991, 17.
14. **Agaronoff, B. W.,** Lipid peroxidation and membrane aging, *Neurobiol. Aging,* 5, 337, 1984.
15. **Cadenas, E.,** Biochemistry of oxygen toxicity, *Annu. Rev. Biochem.,* 58, 79, 1989.

16. **Halliwell, B. and Gutteridge, J. M. C.,** Oxygen toxicity, oxygen radicals, transition metals and disease, *Biochem. J.,* 219, 1, 1984.
17. **Winyard, P. G., Lunec, J., Brailsford, S. B., and Blake, D. R.,** Action of free radical generation systems upon the biological and immunological properties of ceruloplasmin, *Int. J. Biochem.,* 16, 1273, 1984.
18. **Minotti, G.,** Metal and membrane damage by oxy-radicals, in *Membrane in Cancer Cells,* Vol. 551, Galeotti, T., Cittadini, A., Neri, G., and Scarpa, A., Eds., Ann. N.Y. Acad. Sci., New York, 1988, 34.
19. **Porter, N. A. and Wagner, C. R.,** Phospholipid autoxidation, *Adv. Free Radical Biol. Med.,* 2, 283, 1986.
20. **Heinecke, J. W.,** Free radical modification of low-density lipoprotein: mechanisms and biological consequences, *Free Radical Biol. Med.,* 3, 65, 1987.
21. **Giacobini, E.,** Cellular and molecular mechanisms of aging of the nervous system: toward a unified theory of neuronal aging, in *The Aging Brain: Cellular and Molecular Mechanisms of Aging in the Nervous System,* Giacobini, E., Ed., Raven Press, New York, 1982, 271.
22. **Florence, T. M.,** Free radicals, antioxidants and cancer prevention, *Proc. Nutr. Aust.,* 15, 88, 1990.
23. **Bast, A.,** Is formation of reactive oxygen by cytochrome P-450 perilous and predictable?, *Trends Pharmacol. Sci.,* 7, 266, 1986.
24. **Freeman, B. D.,** Biological sites and mechanisms of free radical production, in *Free Radicals in Molecular Biology, Aging and Disease,* Armstrong, D., Sohal, R. S., Cutler, R. G., and Slater, T. F., Eds., Raven Press, New York, 1984, 43.
25. **Nohl, H.,** Formation of reactive oxygen species associated with mitochondrial respiration, in *Oxidative Damage and Repair,* Davies, K. J. A., Ed., Pergamon, New York, 1991, 105.
26. **Loschen, G., Azzi, A., Richter, C., and Flohe, L.,** Superoxide radicals as precursors of mitochondrial hydrogen peroxide, *FEBS Lett.,* 42, 68, 1974.
27. **Brandy, B. and Davison, A. J.,** Mitochondrial mutations may increase oxidative stress: implications for carcinogenesis and aging?, *Free Radical Biol. Med.,* 8, 523, 1990.
28. **Forman, H. J. and Boveries, A.,** Superoxide radical and hydrogen peroxide in mitochondria, in *Free Radicals in Biology,* Vol. V, Pryor, W. A., Ed., Academic Press, Orlando, FL, 1982, 65.
29. **Vladimirov, Y. A., Olievev, V. I., Suslova, T. B., and Cheremisina, Z. P.,** Lipid peroxidation in mitochondrial membrane, in *Advances in Lipid Research,* Vol. 17, Paoletti, R. and Kritchevsky, D., Eds., Academic Press, New York, 1980, 173.
30. **Floyd, R. A., Zaleska, M. M., and Harman, H. J.,** Possible involvement of iron and oxygen free radicals in aspects of aging brain, in *Free Radicals in Molecular Biology, Aging and Disease,* Armstrong, D., Sohal, R. S., Cutler, R. G., and Slater, T. F., Eds., Raven Press, New York, 1984, 143.
31. **Nohl, H. and Hegner, D.,** Do mitochondria produce oxygen radicals *in vivo?, Eur. J. Biochem.,* 82, 563, 1978.
32. **Paradies, G., Ruggiero, F. M., and Dinoi, P.,** Decreased activity of the phosphate carrier and modification of lipids in cardiac mitochondria from senescent rats, *Int. J. Biochem.,* 24, 783, 1992.
33. **Lee, D. W. and Yu, B. P.,** Modulation of free radicals and superoxide dismutase by age and dietary restriction, *Aging,* 2, 357, 1991.
34. **Cohen, G. and Cederbaum, A. I.,** Chemical evidence for production of hydroxyl radicals during microsomal electron transfer, *Science,* 204, 66, 1979.
35. **Tien, M. and Aust, S. D.,** Rabbit liver microsomal lipid peroxidation. The effect of lipid on the rate of peroxidation, *Biochim. Biophys. Acta,* 712, 1, 1982.
36. **Nohl, H., Breuninger, V., and Hegner, D.,** Influence of mitochondrial radical formation on energy-linked respiration, *Eur. J. Biochem.,* 90, 385, 1978.

37. **Fridovich, I. and Freeman, B.**, Antioxidant defenses in the lung, *Annu. Rev. Physiol.*, 48, 693, 1986.

38. **Svingen, B. A., Buege, J. A., O'Neal, F. O., and Aust, S. D.**, The mechanism of NADPH-dependent lipid peroxidation, *J. Biol. Chem.*, 254, 5892, 1979.

39. **Morehouse, L. A. and Aust, S. D.**, Microsomal oxygen radical generation-relationship to the initiation of lipid peroxidation, in *Cellular Antioxidant Defense Mechanisms*, Vol. 1, Chow, C. K., Ed., CRC Press, Boca Raton, FL, 1988, 1.

40. **Kitada, M., Komori, M., Ohi, H., Imaoka, S., Funae, Y., and Kamatako, T.**, Form-specific degradation of cytochrome P-450 by lipid peroxidation in rat liver microsomes, *Res. Commun. Chem.: Pathol. Pharmacol.*, 63, 175, 1989.

41. **Horbach, G. J. M. J., Asten, J. G., and van Bezoonjen, C. F. A.**, The influence of ageing on the induction of the mRNA of rat liver cytochromes P-450IIB1 and P-450IIB2, *Biochem. Pharmacol.*, 40, 529, 1990.

42. **Koizumi, A., Walford, R. L., Imamura, T.**, Treatment with poly I. C. enhances lipid peroxidation and the activity of xanthine oxidase, and decreases hepatic P-450 content and activities in mice and rats, *Biochem. Biophys. Res. Commun.*, 134, 632, 1986.

43. **Ivanov, I. I.**, A relay model of lipid peroxidation in biological membranes, *J. Free Radical Biol. Med.*, 1, 247, 1985.

44. **Girotti, A. W.**, Mechanisms of lipid peroxidation, *J. Free Rad. Biol. Med.*, 1, 87, 1985.

45. **Kappus, H.**, Biochemical mechanisms of chemical-induced lipid peroxidation, in *Membrane Lipid Oxidation*, Vol. II, Vigo-Pelfrey, C., Ed., CRC Press, Boca Raton, FL, 1991, 104.

46. **Hegner, D., Platt, D., Heckers, H., Schloeder, U., and Breuninger, V.**, Age-dependent physiological and biochemical studies of human red cell membranes, *Mech. Ageing Dev.*, 10, 117, 1979.

47. **Aust, S. D.**, Metal ions, oxygen radicals and tissue damage, in *Nutritional Impact of Food Processing*, Somogyi, J. C. and Müller, H. R., Eds., Bibl. Nutr. Dieta, Basel, Karger, 1989, 266.

48. **Witting, L. A. and Horwitt, M. K.**, Effect of degree of fatty acid unsaturation in tocopherol deficiency-induced creatinuria, *J. Nutr.*, 82, 19, 1964.

49. **Tappel, A., Fletcher, B., and Deamer, D.**, Effect of antioxidants and nutrients on lipid peroxidation fluorescent products and aging parameters in the mouse, *J. Gerontol.*, 28, 415, 1973.

50. **Tsuchida, M., Miura, T., and Aibara, K.**, Lipofuscin and lipofuscin-like substances, *Chem. Phys. Lipids*, 44, 297, 1987.

51. **Comporti, M.**, Biology of disease, lipid peroxidation and cellular damage in toxic liver injury, *Lab. Invest.*, 53, 599, 1985.

52. **Enesco, H. and Krurk, P.**, Dietary restriction reduces fluorescent age-pigment accumulation in mice, *Exp. Gerontol.*, 16, 357, 1981.

53. **Katz, M. L. and Robison, W. G., Jr.**, Nutritional influences on autoxidation, lipofuscin accumulation, and aging, in *Free Radicals, Aging and Degenerative Diseases*, Johnson, J. E., Walford, R., Harmon, D., and Miquel, J., Eds., Alan R. Liss, New York, 1986, 221.

54. **Nakano, M., Mizuno, T., Katoh, H., and Gotoh, S.**, Age-related accumulation of lipofuscin in myocardium of Japanese monkey (Macaca fusata), *Mech. Ageing Dev.*, 49, 41, 1989.

55. **Porta, E. A.**, Role of oxidative damage in the aging process, in *Cellular Antioxidant Defense Mechanisms*, Vol. 3, Chow, C. K., Ed., CRC Press, Boca Raton, FL, 1986, 1.

56. **Zs-Nagy, I.**, A membrane hypothesis of aging, *J. Theor. Biol.*, 75, 189, 1978.

57. **Hochschild, R.**, Lysosomes, membranes and aging, *Exp. Gerontol.*, 6, 153, 1971.

58. **von Zglinicki, T.**, A mitochondrial membrane hypothesis of aging, *J. Theor. Biol.*, 127, 127, 1987.

59. **Grinna, L. S.**, Changes in cell membrane during aging, *Gerontology*, 23, 452, 1977.

60. **Laganiere, S. and Yu, B. P.**, Effect of chronic food restriction in aging rats. I. Liver subcellular membranes, *Mech. Ageing Dev.*, 48, 207, 1989.
61. **Laganiere, S. and Yu, B. P.**, Modulation of membrane phospholipid fatty acid composition by age and food restriction, *Gerontology*, in press.
62. **Schroeder, F.**, Role of membrane lipid asymmetry in aging, *Neurobiol. Aging*, 5, 323, 1984.
63. **Hawcroft, D. W. and Martin, P. A.**, Studies on age-related changes in the lipids of mouse liver microsomes, *Mech. Ageing Dev.*, 3, 121, 1974.
64. **Grinna, L. S. and Barber, A. A.**, Lipid changes in the microsomal and mitochondrial membranes of rat liver during aging, *Fed. Proc.*, 35, 1525, 1976.
65. **Schmucker, D. R., Vessey, D. A., Wang, R. K., James, J. L., and Maloney, A.**, Age-dependent alterations in the physicochemical properties of rat liver microsomes, *Mech. Ageing Dev.*, 27, 207, 1984.
66. **Hegner, D.**, Age-dependence of molecular and functional changes in biological membrane properties, *Mech. Ageing Dev.*, 14, 101, 1980.
67. **Yeagle, P. L.**, Cholesterol and the cell membrane, *Biochim. Biophys. Acta*, 822, 267, 1985.
68. **Naeim, F. and Walford, R. L.**, Aging and cell membrane complexes: the lipid bilayer, integral proteins, and cytoskeleton, in *Handbook of the Biology of Aging*, 2nd ed., Finch, C. E. and Schneider, E. L., Eds., Von Nostrand Reinhold, New York, 1985, 272.
69. **Yu, B. P., Suescun, E. A., and Yang, S. Y.**, Effect of age-related lipid peroxidation on membrane fluidity and phospholipase A_2: modulation by dietary restriction, *Mech. Ageing Dev.*, 65, 17, 1992.
70. **Vorbeck, M. L., Martin, A. P., Long, J. W., Jr., Smith, J. M., and Orr, R. R.**, Aging-dependent modification of lipid composition and lipid structural order parameter of hepatic mitochondria, *Arch. Biochem. Biophys.*, 217, 351, 1982.
71. **Dobretsov, G. E., Borschevskaya, T. B., Petrov, V. A., and Vladimirov, Y. A.**, The increase of phospholipid bilayer rigidity after lipid peroxidation, *FEBS Lett.*, 84, 125, 1977.
72. **Esterbauer, H. and Chesseman, K. H.**, Determination of aldehydic lipid peroxidation products: malondialdehyde and 4-hydroxynonenal, *Meth. Enzymol.*, 186, 407, 199.
73. **Ikeda, H., Tauchi, H., Shimasaki, H., Ueta, N., and Sato, T.**, Age and organ difference in amount and distribution of autofluorescent granules in rats, *Mech. Ageing Dev.*, 31, 139, 1985.
74. **Marnett, L. J., Buck, J., Tuttle, M. A., Basu, A. K., and Bull, A. W.**, Distribution and oxidation of malondialdehyde in mice, *Prostaglandins*, 30, 241, 1985.
75. **Laganiere, S. and Yu, B. P.**, Anti-lipoperoxidation action of food restriction, *Biochem. Biophys. Res. Comm.*, 145, 1185, 1987.
76. **Hjelle, J. J. and Petersen, D. R.**, Metabolism of malondialdehyde by rat liver aldehyde dehydrogenase, *Toxicol. Appl. Pharmacol.*, 70, 57, 1983.
77. **Michiels, C. and Remacle, J.**, Cytotoxicity of linoleic acid peroxide, malondialdehyde and 4-hydroxynonenal towards human fibroblasts, *Toxicology*, 66, 225, 1991.
78. **Jozwiak, Z. and Jasnowska, B.**, Changes in oxygen-metabolizing enzymes and lipid peroxidation in human erythrocytes as a function of age of donor, *Mech. Ageing Dev.*, 32, 7, 1985.
79. **Laganiere, S. and Fernandes, G.**, Study on the lipid composition of aging Fischer 344 rat lymphoid cells: effect of long-term calorie restriction, *Lipids*, 26, 472, 1991.
80. **Yang, S. Y., Lee, D. W., and Yu, B. P.**, Enzymatic regulation of the age-related peroxidizability of membranes: the modulation of desaturases by dietary restriction, *Gerontology*, 30, 3214, 1990.
81. **Choi, Y. S., Goto, S., Ikeda, I., and Sugano, M.**, Age-related changes in lipid metabolism in rats: the consequence of moderate food restriction, *Biochim. Biophys. Acta*, 963, 237, 1988.

82. **Shinitzky, M. and Henkart, P.**, Fluidity of cell membranes: current concepts and trends, *Int. Rev. Cytol.*, 60, 121, 1979.

83. **Wahnon, R., Mokady, S., and Cogan, U.**, Age and membrane fluidity, *Mech. Age Dev.*, 50, 249, 1989.

84. **Zhan, H., Sun, C. P., Liu, C. G., and Zhou, J. H.**, Age-related change of free radical generation in liver and sex glands of rats, *Mech. Ageing Dev.*, 62, 111, 1992.

85. **Sawada, M., Sester, U., and Carlson, J. C.**, Superoxide radical formation and associated biochemical alterations in the plasma membrane of brain, heart and liver during the lifetime of the rat, *J. Cell. Biochem.*, 48, 296, 1992.

86. **Sawada, M. and Carlson, J. C.**, Changes in superoxide radicals and lipid peroxide formation in the brain, heart and liver during the lifetime of the rat, *Mech. Ageing Dev.*, 41, 125, 1987.

87. **Choi, J. H. and Yu, B. P.**, Free radical generation and membrane fluidity of aging brain synaptosomes: modulation by dietary restriction, *Gerontologist*, 32, 30 (Abstr.), 1992.

88. **Lebel, C. P. and Bondy, S. C.**, Persistent protein damage despite reduced oxygen radical formation in the aging rat brain, *Int. J. Dev. Neurosci.*, 9, 139, 1991.

89. **Lebel, C. P. and Bondy, S. C.**, Sensitive and rapid quantitation of oxygen reactive species formation in rat synaptosomes, *Neurochem. Int.*, 17, 435, 1990.

90. **Bass, D. A., Parce, J. W., Dechatelet, L. R., Szejda, P., Seeds, M. C., and Thomas, M.**, Flow cytometric studies of oxidative product formation by neutrophils: a graded response to membrane stimulation, *J. Immunol.*, 130, 1910, 1983.

91. **Harman, D.**, Free radical theory of aging: nutritional implications, *Age*, 1, 145, 1978.

92. **Harman, D.**, Free radical theory of aging: effect of free radical reaction inhibitors on mortality rate of mice, LAF_1 mice, *J. Gerontol.*, 23, 476, 1968.

93. **Heidrick, M. L., Hendricks, L. C., and Cook, D. E.**, Effect of dietary 2-mercapto-ethanol on the life-span, immune system, tumor incidence and lipid peroxidation damage in spleen lymphocytes of aging $BC3F_1$ mice, *Mech. Ageing Dev.*, 27, 341, 1984.

94. **Comfort, A.**, Effect of ethoxyquin on the longevity of C3H mice, *Nature*, 229, 254, 1971.

95. **Epstein, J. and Gershon, D.**, Studies on aging in nematodes. IV. The effect of antioxidants on cellular damage and life-span, *Mech. Ageing Dev.*, 1, 257, 1972.

96. **Sawada, M. and Enesco, H. E.**, Vitamin E extends life-span in the short-lived rotifer Asplanchna brightwella, *Exp. Gerontol.*, 19, 179, 1984.

97. **Neafsey, J. J.**, Longevity hormesis. A review, *Mech. Ageing Dev.*, 51, 1, 1990.

98. **Shinitzky, M., Lyte, M., Heron, D. S. and Samuel, D.**, Intervention in membrane aging — the development and application of active lipid, in *Intervention in the Aging Process*, Regelson, W. and Sinex, F. M., Eds., Alan R. Liss, New York, 1983, 175.

99. **Weindruch, R. and Walford, R. L.**, The retardation of aging and disease by dietary restriction, Charles C. Thomas, Springfield, IL, 1988.

100. **Weindruch, R. H., Cheung, M. K., Verity, A., and Walford, R. L.**, Modification of mitochondrial respiration by aging and dietary restriction, *Mech. Ageing Dev.*, 12, 375, 1980.

101. **Yu, B. P., Lee, D. W., and Choi, J. H.**, Prevention of free radical damage by food restriction, in *Biological Effects of Dietary Restriction*, Fishbein, L., Ed., Springer-Verlag, New York 1991, 191.

102. **Yu, B. P.**, Food restriction: past and present status, in *Review of Biological Research in Aging*, Vol. 4, Rothstein, M., Ed., Wiley-Liss, New York, 1990, 349.

103. **Yu, B. P. and Chen, J. J.**, Modification of mitochondrial aging by calorie restriction, *Age*, 13, 104, 1990.

104. **Weindruch, R.**, How does restriction retard disease and aging?, in *Dietary Restriction and Aging* Snyder, D. L., Ed., Alan R. Liss, New York, 1989, 97.

105. **Simic, G. M. and Bergtold, D. S.**, Dietary modulation of DNA damage in human, *Mutat. Res.*, 250, 17, 1991.

106. **Masoro, E. J., Shimokawa, I., and Yu, B. P.**, Retardation of the aging processes in rats by food restriction, in *Physiological Senescence and Its Postponement: Theoretical Approaches and Rational Intervention, 621,* Piepaoli, W. and Fabris, N., Eds., Ann. N.Y. Acad. Sci., New York, 1991, 337.

107. **Shimokawa, I., Yu, B. P., and Masoro, E. J.**, Influence of diet on fatal neoplastic disease in male Fischer rats, *J. Gerontol.,* 46, B228, 1991.

108. **Chipalkatti, S., De, A. K., and Aiyar, A. S.**, Effect of diet restriction on some biochemical parameters related to aging in mice, *J. Nutr.,* 113, 944, 1983.

109. **Koizumi, A., Weindruch, R., and Walford, R. L.**, Influences of dietary restriction and age on liver enzyme activities and lipid peroxidation in mice, *J. Nutr.,* 117, 361, 1987.

110. **Davies, K. J. A.**, Protein damage and degradation by oxygen radicals. I. General aspects, *J. Biol. Chem.,* 262, 9895, 1987.

111. **Ames, B. N., Saul, R. L., Schwiers, E., Adelman, R., and Cathcart, R.**, Oxidative DNA damage as related to cancer and aging: assay of thymine glycol, thymidine glycol and hydroxymethyluracil in human and rat urine, in *Molecular Biology of Aging: Gene Stability and Gene Expression,* Sohal, R. S., Birnbaum, L. S., and Cutler, R. G., Eds., Raven Press, New York, 1985, 137.

112. **Richter, C., Park, J. W., and Ames, B. N.**, Normal oxidative damage to mitochondrial and nuclear DNA is extensive, *Proc. Natl. Acad. Sci. U.S.A.,* 85, 6465, 1988.

113. **Hruszkewycz, A. M.**, Evidence for mitochondrial DNA damage by lipid peroxidation, *Biochem. Biophys. Res. Comm.,* 153, 191, 1988.

114. **Hruszkewycz, A. M. and Bergtold, D. S.**, The 8-hydroxyguanine content of isolated mitochondria increases with lipid peroxidation, *Mutat. Res.,* 244, 123, 1990.

115. **Halliwell, B. and Aruoma, O. I.**, DNA damage by oxygen-derived species, *FEBS Lett.,* 281, 9, 1991.

116. **Fraga, C. G., Shigenaga, M. K., Park, J. W., Degan, P., and Ames, B. N.**, Oxidative damage to DNA during aging: 8-hydroxy-2-deoxyguanosine in rat organ DNA and urine, *Proc. Natl. Acad. Sci. U.S.A.,* 87, 4533, 1990.

117. **Saul, R. L., Gee, P., and Ames, B. N.**, Free radicals, DNA damage and aging, in *Modern Biological Theories of Aging,* Warner, H. R., Butler, R. N., Sprott, R. L., and Schneider, E. L., Eds., Raven Press, New York, 1987, 113.

118. **Chung, M. H., Kasai, H., Nishimura, S., and Yu, B. P.**, Protection of DNA damage by dietary restriction, *Free Radical Biol. Med.,* 12, 523, 1992.

119. **Park, J. W. and Floyd, R. A.**, Lipid peroxidation products mediate the formation of 8-hydroxydeoxyguanosine in DNA, *Free Radical Biol. Med.,* 122, 245, 199.

120. **Cathcart, R., Schwiers, E., Saul, R. L., and Ames, B. N.**, Thymine glycol and thymidine glycol in human and urine: a possible assay for oxidative DNA damage, *Proc. Natl. Acad. Sci. U.S.A.,* 81, 5633, 1984.

121. **Szilard, L.**, On the nature of the aging process, *Proc. Natl. Acad. Sci. U.S.A.,* 45, 30, 1959.

122. **Gensler, H. L. and Bernstein, H.**, DNA damage as the primary cause of aging, *Q. Rev. Biol.,* 56, 279, 1981.

123. **Pacifici, R. E. and Davies, K. J. A.**, Protein, lipid and DNA repair systems in oxidative stress: the free radical theory of aging revisited, *Gerontology,* 37, 166, 1991.

124. **Davies, K. J. A., Lin, S. W., and Pacifici, R. E.**, Protein damage and degradation by oxygen radicals. IV. Degradation of denatured protein, *J. Biol. Chem.,* 262, 9914, 1987.

125. **Davies, K. J. A. and Goldberg, A. L.**, Proteins damaged by oxygen radicals and rapidly degraded in extracts of red blood cells, *J. Biol. Chem.,* 262, 8227, 1987.

126. **Davies, K. J. A. and Delsignore, M. E.**, Protein damage and degradation by oxygen radicals, *J. Biol. Chem.,* 262, 9908, 1987.

127. **Oliver, C. N., Levin, R. L., and Stadtman, E. R.**, A role of mixed-function oxidation reactions in the accumulation of altered enzyme forms during aging, *J. Am. Geriatr. Soc.,* 35, 947, 1987.

128. **Levine, R. L.**, Oxidative modification of glutamine synthetase. II. Characterization of the ascorbate model system, *J. Biol. Chem.*, 258, 11828, 1983.
129. **Davies, K. J.**, Protein damage and degradation by oxygen radicals, *J. Biol. Chem.*, 262, 9895, 1987.
130. **Pacifici, R. E., Salo, D. C., and Davies, K. J. A.**, Macroxyproteinase (MOP): a 670-kda proteinase complex that degrades oxidatively denatured proteins in red blood cells, *Free Radical Biol. Med.*, 7, 521, 1989.
131. **Starke-Reed, P. E. and Oliver, C. N.**, Oxidative modification of enzymes during aging and acute oxidative stress, in *Oxygen Radicals in Biology and Medicine*, Simic, M. G., Taylor, K. A., Ward, J. F., and von Sonntag, C., Eds., Plenum Press, New York, 1987, 537.
132. **Stadtman, E. R.**, Oxidation of proteins by mixed-function oxidation system: implication in protein turnover, ageing and neutrophil function, *Trends Biochem. Sci.*, 11, 11, 1986.
133. **Stadtman, E. R.**, Covalent modification reactions are making steps in protein turnover, *Biochemistry*, 29, 6323, 1990.
134. **Garner, M. H. and Spector, A.**, Selective oxidation of cysteine and methionine in normal and senile cataractous lenses, *Proc. Natl. Acad. Sci. U.S.A.*, 77, 1274, 1980.
135. **Stadtman, E. R.**, Protein modification in aging, *J. Gerontol.*, 43, B112, 1988.
136. **Rifkind, J. M., Wang, J. T., Mohanty, J. G., and Roth, G. S.**, The possible role of protein degradation in altered membrane structure and function, *Neurobiol. Aging*, 5, 343, 1984.
137. **Davies, K. J. A. and Goldberg, A. L.**, Oxygen radicals stimulate intracellular proteolysis and lipid peroxidation by independent mechanisms in erythrocytes, *J. Biol. Chem.*, 262, 8220, 1987.
138. **Davies, K. J. A.**, Proteolytic systems as secondary antioxidant defenses, in *Cellular Antioxidant Defense Mechanisms*, Vol. 2, Chow, C. K., Ed., CRC Press, Boca Raton, FL, 1988, 25.
139. **Salo, D. C., Pacifici, R. E., Lin, S. W., Giulivi, C., and Davies, K. J.**, Superoxide dismutase undergoes proteolysis and fragmentation following oxidative modification and inactivation, *J. Biol. Chem.*, 265, 11919, 1990.
140. **Hruszkewycz, A. M., Glende, E. A., and Recknagel, R. O.**, Destruction of microsomal cytochrome P-450 and glucose-6-phosphatase by lipids extracted from peroxidized microsomes, *Toxicol. Appl. Pharmacol.*, 46, 695, 1978.
141. **Pacifici, R. E. and Davies, K. J. A.**, Protein degradation as an index of oxidative stress, *Meth. Enzym.*, 186, 485, 1990.
142. **Tappel, A. L.**, Measurement of and protection from *in vivo* lipid peroxidation, in *Free Radicals in Biology*, Vol. IV, Pryor, W. A., Ed., Academic Press, New York, 1980, 1.
143. **Siu, G. M. and Draper, H. H.**, Metabolism of malondialdehyde *in vivo* and *in vitro*, *Lipids*, 17, 349, 1982.
144. **Sagai, M. and Tappel, A. L.**, Lipid peroxidation induced by some halomethanes as measured by *in vivo* pentane production in the rat, *Toxicol. Appl. Pharmacol.*, 49, 283, 1979.
145. **Sagai, M. and Ichinose, T.**, Age-related changes in lipid peroxidation as measured by ethane, ethylene, butane and pentane in respirated gases in rats, *Life Sci.*, 27, 731, 1980.
146. **Riely, C. A., Cohen, G., and Lieberman, M.**, Ethane evolution: a new index of lipid peroxidation, *Science*, 183, 208, 1974.
147. **Habib, M. P., Dickerson, F., and Mooradian, A. D.**, Ethane production rate *in vivo* is reduced with dietary restriction, *J. Appl. Physiol.*, 68, 2588, 1990.
148. **Haberland, M. E., Fogelman, A. M., and Edwards, P. A.**, Specificity of receptor-mediated recognition of malondialdehyde-modified low density lipoproteins, *Proc. Natl. Acad. Sci. U.S.A.*, 79, 1712, 1982.
149. **Houglum, K., Filip, M., Witztum, J. L., and Chojkier, M.**, Malondialdehyde and 4-hydroxynonenal protein adducts in plasma and liver of rats with iron overload, *J. Clin. Invest.*, 86, 1991, 1991.

150. **Valenzuela, A.,** The biological significance of malondialdehyde determination in the assessment of tissue oxidative stress, *Life Sci.,* 48, 301, 1991.

151. **Vaca, C. E., Wilhelm, J., and Harms-Ringdahl, M.,** Interaction of lipid peroxidation products with DNA. A review, *Mutat. Res.,* 195, 137, 1988.

152. **Balcavage, W. X. and Alvager, T. E.,** Reaction of malondialdehyde with mitochondrial membranes, *Mech. Ageing Dev.,* 19, 159, 1982.

153. **Mitchell, D. Y. and Petersen, D. R.,** Oxidation of aldehydic products of lipid peroxidation by rat liver microsomal aldehyde dehydrogenase, *Arch. Biochem. Biophys.,* 269, 11, 1989.

154. **Kim, J. W. and Yu, B. P.,** Characterization of age-related malondialdehyde oxidation. The effect of modulation by food restriction, *Mech. Ageing Dev.,* 50, 277, 1989.

155. **Barrera, G., Brossa, O., Fazio, V. M., Farace, M. G., Paradisi, L., Gravela, E., and Dianzani, U.,** Effect of 4-hydroxynonenal, a product of lipid peroxidation on cell proliferation and ornithine decarboxylase activity, *Free Radical Res. Comm.,* 14, 81, 1991.

156. **Canuto, R. A., Muzio, G., Biocca, M. E., and Dianzani, M. U.,** Oxidative metabolism of 4-hydroxy-2,3-nonenal during diethyl-nitrosamine-induced carcinogenesis in rat liver, *Cancer Letts.,* 46, 7, 1989.

157. **Chen, J. J., Kristal, B. S., and Yu, B. P.,** Metabolism and biological effects of 4-hydroxynonenal and malondialdehyde, *FASEB J.* 6, A1816, 1992.

Chapter 5

DNA DAMAGE AND AGING

Harris Bernstein and Helen L. Gensler

TABLE OF CONTENTS

0-8493-4518-9/93/$0.00 + $.50

I. THE DNA DAMAGE THEORY OF AGING

A. INTRODUCTION TO THE THEORY

According to the DNA damage theory of aging, first proposed by Alexander,[1] mammalian aging is due to the accumulation of DNA damages in somatic cells. The idea that damage to DNA, rather than damage to other biomolecules or structures, is the underlying cause of aging is based on the following general considerations. Because DNA encodes the genetic information of the cell, deterioration of its ability to be transcribed will lead to a decline in cellular function and lethality. By contrast, other macromolecules, such as RNA or protein, can be replaced, in principle, by new synthesis if the DNA remains undamaged. In general, cells are thought to have a considerable DNA-dependent capacity for self-renewal involving replacement and repair of worn-out components. DNA is especially vulnerable to damage because it ordinarily occurs in only two copies per diploid cell (compared with the numerous copies of most other macromolecules), and each of the many deoxyribonucleotides is a potential target of damaging agents.

The DNA damage theory was preceded by the related theory that aging is due to somatic mutation.[2-4] These two theories are similar in that both attribute aging to "errors" in DNA. However, there are very important differences between DNA damages and mutations. In contrast to mutations, DNA damages cannot be replicated (in the sense that when DNA replicates, any damage present is not itself reproduced). Therefore, DNA damages cannot be inherited over successive cell generations, whereas mutations can be inherited. Furthermore, DNA damages, in contrast to mutations, can be repaired. Because of these fundamental differences at the molecular level, the DNA damage theory of aging has a logic that is substantially different from that of the somatic mutation theory, as reviewed by Bernstein and Bernstein,[5] Gensler and Bernstein,[6] and Gensler et al.[7] (Other reviews bearing on the DNA damage theory of aging have been presented by Tice and Setlow,[8] Vijg and Knook,[9] Mullaart et al.,[10] and Ames and Gold.[11])

B. THE RELATIVE IMPORTANCE OF DNA DAMAGE AND MUTATION IN AGING

A DNA damage is a DNA alteration that has an abnormal structure. Examples include a single-strand break, a double-strand break, an interstrand cross-link, a pyrimidine dimer, an apurinic/apyrimidinic site, a cytosine deamination, an abnormal alkylation, or an adduct formed by an electrophile. A mutation, on the other hand, is a change in the DNA sequence (i.e., information content), rather than a change to an abnormal DNA structure. Examples of mutations are base-pair substitutions, addition or deletion of nucleotide pairs, or rearrangements of nucleotide sequences.

A cell with a new somatic mutation may, upon repeated cell division, give rise to a clone of cells bearing the mutation. Clones of cells that arise by somatic mutation may increase in number with age in a proliferative tissue, such as colonic epithelium.[12] Focal lesions, presumed to arise from clones of mutated cells, increase in incidence with age in mammals. Some types of focal lesions such as ulcers, cancers, and atherosclerotic plaque have major health consequences. However, these lesions do not appear to be the underlying cause of aging in humans, since the incidence of each of these is strongly influenced by environmental and lifestyle factors, and each of these conditions is a problem for only a fraction of aging individuals. In general, rapidly dividing cells, which are the ones most susceptible to mutation, show the least evidence of aging. For instance, aging occurs slowly, if at all, in hematopoietic stem cells.[13,14] On the other hand, cell types such as nerve and muscle cells, which are nondividing and thus are the least susceptible to proliferation of mutated cells, undergo conspicuous aging (see below).

The DNA damage theory of aging assumes that DNA damage, rather than mutation, is the primary cause of aging. This theory is supported by the following considerations which will be reviewed further below: (1) In some mammalian cell types, particularly in nondividing or slowly dividing cells, DNA damage accumulates with time. (2) The accumulation of DNA damage is associated with a decline in gene expression, as well as declines in cellular, tissue, and organ functions. This association is consistent with a cause-and-effect relationship between DNA damage and the functional declines that define aging. (3) An increased rate of accumulation of DNA damage appears to cause an increased rate of aging.

II. THE ROLE OF DNA DAMAGE, ESPECIALLY OXIDATIVE DAMAGE, IN AGING

DNA damage can be caused either by intrinsic intracellular processes such as oxidation, hydrolysis, and alkylation, or by extrinsic chemicals and radiation that enter the organism from the outside. Among these various possible causes of DNA damage, oxidative DNA damage produced by free radicals released during normal metabolism appears to be a major cause of aging in mammals.

A. SOURCES OF OXIDATIVE DNA DAMAGE *IN VIVO*

Oxidative DNA damage is caused by free radicals produced from molecular oxygen as a consequence of normal respiratory metabolism. The univalent pathway of oxygen reduction generates the superoxide radical (O_2^-), hydrogen peroxide (H_2O_2), the hydroxyl radical ($\cdot OH$), and water.[15] Imlay and Linn[15] have concluded that about half of oxidative DNA damage is due to $\cdot OH$.

B. TYPES OF OXIDATIVE DNA DAMAGE AND THEIR INCIDENCE

Oxygen radicals can interact with DNA at either the deoxyribose-phosphate backbone or at a base.[15] The reaction of an oxygen radical with a deoxyribose leads to fragmentation of the sugar, loss of the base to which it was bonded, and strand breakage. The reaction directly with a base, such as thymine or adenine, results in a damaged base. Some of the reaction products resulting from the oxidation of thymine are thymine glycol, methyl tartronyl urea, urea, and 5-hydroxymethyluracil. A reaction product from the oxidation of adenine is 4,6-diamino-5-formamidopyrimidine. These products are removed from DNA by specific repair enzymes and excreted in the urine. Judging from their levels in human urine, Saul et al.[16] estimated the following average rates of removal from DNA: thymine glycol (270 per cell per day), thymidine glycol (70 per cell per day), and hydroxymethyluracil (620 per cell per day). The sum of these average rates is 960 per cell per day. These molecules are only three of a considerable number of possible oxidative DNA damage products. Consequently, Saul et al.[16] commented that the total number of oxidative DNA hits per cell per day in humans may be much higher than 1000. Recently, Ames and Gold[11] estimated the total number of all types of oxidative damages to DNA per cell per day to be about 10,000 in humans and about 100,000 in rats. The difference in oxidative DNA damage incidence rates between humans and rats is consistent with the proposal that oxidative DNA damage increases in proportion to species-specific basal metabolic rates.[17]

The oxidized base 8-hydroxydeoxyguanosine (oh⁸dG) is present in the DNA of rat liver at the level of about 1.4×10^5 per cell in nuclear DNA and 4.1×10^4 per cell in mitochondrial DNA.[18] Thus, even though mitochondria are the site of respiration, about 77% of these particular oxidative damages are in nuclear DNA, reflecting the much larger target size of nuclear DNA. On the basis of these data, we can infer that, in general, the majority of oxidative DNA damages are in nuclear DNA. Fraga et al.[19] estimated that for every 54 oh⁸dG residues repaired in rat kidney, one residue remains unrepaired. They further estimated the rate of accumulation of oh⁸dG residues to be 80 per cell per day in rat kidney when both the rate of formation of damage and the rate of repair are taken into account.

Treatment of DNA *in vitro* with H_2O_2 produces DNA damages of which over 90% are altered bases (that had lost UV absorbance); about 2 to 4% are single-strand breaks; about 0.9% are double-strand breaks, and about 0.8% are interstrand cross-links.[20] If the proportion of altered bases to other damages that was measured *in vitro* also applies *in vivo,* and the minimum estimated rate of occurrence of 340 per cell per day for the non-UV absorbing thymine glycol and thymidine glycol is used as the incidence of oxidatively damaged bases, then the calculated incidence of single-strand breaks is 7 to 14 per cell per day, of double-strand breaks is 3 per cell per day, and of interstrand cross-links is 3 per cell per day. These minimum rough estimates suggest that single- and double-strand breaks, as well as interstrand cross-links, may be a significant problem.

Damages which alter the two strands of DNA at or near the same position are referred to as double-strand damages, in contrast to damages which affect only one strand and are referred to as single-strand damages. As will be discussed below, double-strand damages, such as double-strand breaks and interstrand cross-links, are more difficult to repair than are single-strand damages. Ward et al.[21] concluded, from experiments on mammalian cells treated with H_2O_2, that DNA single-strand breaks caused by hydroxyl radicals are ineffective in causing cell death, and, that to produce lethal events, "locally multiple damage sites" such as double-strand damages are required. If death of somatic cells due to DNA damage is important in aging, then double-strand damages, despite their low frequency, may be a significant factor.

C. CELLULAR DEFENSE MECHANISMS AGAINST OXIDATIVE DNA DAMAGES

There appear to be three levels of defense against the DNA damage caused by active oxygen species. These levels are (1) prevention by removal of active oxygen species before they can interact with DNA; (2) repair of DNA damages; and (3) compensation for cell loss due to lethal DNA damage through the strategy of cellular redundancy and/or replication.

1. Removal of Oxidative Free Radicals

Cellular enzymes have evolved to remove active oxygen species. These include superoxide dismutase which converts O_2^- into H_2O_2 and catalase and glutathione peroxidase which convert H_2O_2 into H_2O. The removal of active oxygen species, however, is incomplete,[22] allowing those that escape to damage cellular constituents.

2. DNA Repair

Double-stranded DNA genomes have a built-in informational redundancy because the coding sequences of the two strands are complementary. Consequently, it is possible to repair damage localized to one strand by excising the damaged sequence and replacing the lost information by copying from the complementary strand. This general process is known as excision repair. Excision repair is the most well-studied type of repair in mammals and it appears to be the principal mechanism for removing single-strand damages that, if unrepaired, would contribute to aging. The most well-understood pathways of excision repair in mammals are those initiated by specific glycosylases which remove damaged bases from the deoxyribose phosphate backbone of DNA. Numerous DNA glycosylases have been described in mammals, each one specific for a particular kind of base damage. Glycosylases which act on oxidatively altered bases are thymine-glycol glycosylase,[23-25] hydroxymethyluracil glycosylase,[25] and urea-DNA glycosylase.[23] DNA damages caused by processes other than oxidation are also removed by glycosylases. Cytosine and adenine, upon hydrolytic deamination, form, respectively, uracil and hypoxanthine. These can be removed, respectively, by uracil-DNA glycosylase[26] and hypoxanthine glycosylase.[27] Another type of damage is the methylation of adenine to form 3-methyladenine and of guanine to form 7-methylguanine. These altered bases also can be removed by glycosylases.[28]

When the damaged base is removed from the DNA by a glycosylase, an apurinic/apyrimidinic (AP) site is formed. For repair to be completed, the AP site must be removed and replaced by an undamaged correct base (one complementary to the pairing partner in the undamaged strand of DNA). AP sites are removed by a process in which the DNA strand is first cleaved, either to the 3' side or the 5' side, by an AP endonuclease. Those AP endonucleases that cleave on the 3' side are defined as being in class I and those that cleave on the 5' side are in class II. In principle, an AP site can be excised by the sequential action of a class I and class II endonuclease (or vice versa). This would leave a gap of a single nucleotide in the deoxyribose-phosphate backbone. In actuality, the excision process appears to be more complex, involving the removal of a patch of nucleotides. After an initial incision by an AP endonuclease, exonucleases can degrade the DNA in the 5' to 3' or 3' to 5' direction at the free ends created by the incision. Finally, a DNA polymerase inserts correctly paired bases in a 5' to 3' direction. The particular DNA polymerase employed is probably DNA polymerase β, which is apparently the principal repair polymerase in mammalian cells.[29] The final reaction in the pathway involves the formation of the last phosphodiester bond in the repaired strand by polynucleotide ligase. The overall consequence of an excision repair pathway is the removal of a damage in one strand of DNA and its replacement by an accurate complementary copy of the undamaged strand. This restores the original DNA sequence.

Another mechanism for removing single-strand damages is referred to as direct reversal. This mechanism depends on enzymes that can recognize some specific types of damage and then essentially reverse the damage-forming reaction to restore the intact sequence. This type of repair occurs with a narrow spectrum of damages that may have limited relevance to aging. Other repair processes, whose occurrence in mammals is only speculative (e.g., error prone repair and postreplication recombinational repair), will not be discussed here.

We noted above that double-strand damages, although infrequent, are potentially important in aging because they are difficult to repair. Since double-strand damages are ones in which both complementary strands are altered at approximately the same position, neither strand can be used as an accurate template to repair the other. Excision repair is presumably ineffective in removing double-strand damages because this type of repair depends on the intactness of the DNA strand opposite the damaged one. Therefore, to repair double-strand damages, a second DNA molecule with information homologous to that lost in the first must be available, and exchange of information between the two DNA molecules must occur. Specifically, repair can occur if the undamaged DNA duplex donates a single-stranded section to the damaged DNA molecule to allow replacement of its lost information. This process of exchange is referred to as recombinational repair. We indicated above that double-strand damages may contribute to aging. Therefore, repair of double-strand damages by recombinational repair (e.g., involving sister chromatid exchange) may be significant in resisting aging.

In general, DNA repair capacity in terminally differentiated nonproliferating cells is lower than in proliferating cells from organ systems or embryos.[5,30] Low DNA repair in nonproliferating cells may enhance DNA damage accumulation in these cells.

3. Cellular Redundancy and/or Replication

One way for a multicellular organism to cope with unrepaired DNA damages is by the use of cellular redundancy.[6] For example, in humans more cells are formed in the brain than are necessary for normal function.[31] Indeed, according to Glassman,[32] the human brain may be at least twice as large as it would have to be for short-term survival. Hofman[33] reviewed evidence that, in mammals, maximum potential life-span is proportional to the product of relative brain size (encephalization) and the reciprocal of specific metabolic rate. The inverse relationship of life-span to specific metabolic rate may reflect the correlation of specific metabolic rate with rate of oxidative DNA damage formation.[16,34] The correlation of longevity with relative brain size may reflect the advantage of a reserve supply of neurons to compensate for loss of neuron function due to DNA damage.

Another way for a population of cells to cope with unrepaired DNA damage is to replace lethally damaged cells by replication of undamaged ones. Examples of rapidly replicating cell populations are hemopoietic cells of the bone marrow and intestinal epithelial cells. The turnover time for replacing hemopoietic bone-marrow cells of the mouse is only 1 to 2 d.[35] According to extensive data compiled by Buetow,[36] bone marrow and hemopoietic cells do not decline in numbers with age in the mouse and guinea pig. Evidence reviewed by Harrison[13] indicates that mouse erythropoietic stem cells have a very large capacity for self renewal. No significant differences were found in comparisons of erythrocyte production by marrow stem cell lines from old and young adults. Thus, little, if any, of erythropoietic stem cell proliferative capacity is exhausted in the mouse by a lifetime of normal functioning. In these cells, it appears that any cell loss due to DNA damage is compensated for by replication of those cells with little or no unrepaired DNA damages.

In the epithelial lining of the mammalian small intestine, cell renewal is restricted to the crypts, where production of new cells is continuous.[37] As mice age, the number of cycling cells in the crypts decreases, and the generation time increases.[38] The decrease in cycling cells may mean that, over the long term, the rate of cell replacement by duplication in these cell populations is insufficient to keep up with the rate of occurrence of unrepaired lethal DNA damage. The increase in generation time might reflect the slowing of DNA replication past unrepaired damages.

D. ACCUMULATION OF DNA DAMAGES IN NONDIVIDING TISSUES

The DNA damage theory of aging predicts that DNA damage accumulates in cells of critical tissues, leading to aging. In this section, we review evidence showing that long-lived, nondividing, differentiated cells of the brain, muscle, the liver, and lymphocytes accumulate DNA damage with age.

1. Brain

Nine studies have shown accumulation of DNA damage in mammalian brain with age, while in four additional studies no such accumulation was observed. All but one of these studies examined whether or not single-strand DNA breaks (and/or alkali labile sites, in some cases) accumulate in the brain. Single-strand breaks can be caused by oxidative damage,[20] but also can be caused by heat.[10] The studies reporting an increase of single-strand breaks with age were carried out in mouse,[39,40-43] rat,[44] rabbit,[45] and beagle dogs.[46] The four studies finding no accumulation of single strand-breaks were done in mouse,[47-49] and rat.[50] The differences in findings may be explained by differences in method and ages of the animals used. The one study that did not involve single-strand breaks found an accumulation of 7-methylguanine with age in mouse brain.[51]

One of the more informative studies was that of Bergtold and Lett[45] on rabbit retina photoreceptor cells. They used the technique of zonal ultracentrifugation of DNA through reoriented alkaline sucrose gradients, which they regarded as the most sensitive method yet devised for measuring damage to mammalian chromosomal DNA. They found an age-related decline in median sedimentation coefficient of this DNA, indicating that strand breaks (and/or alkali-labile sites) accumulate as animals age. The oldest rabbits had an increased number of breaks in the DNA of their photoreceptor cells equivalent to the effects of several hundred rads of X-photons in young rabbits.

2. Muscle

Single-strand breaks were shown to accumulate in mouse heart muscle with age in studies by Price et al.[43] and Chetsanga et al.,[52] although not in a study by Mori and Goto.[41] Another type of damage studied was methylated guanine. Gaubatz[53] found a ninefold increase in this type of damage in mouse heart muscle as the animals aged from 2 to 39 months.

Zahn et al.,[54] studying human, rather than mouse muscle, found an increase in single-stranded regions with age. DNA damage was measured as DNA alterations that give rise to complete double-strand breaks upon treatment of purified DNA solutions with single-strand-specific nucleases. The DNA was derived from samples of muscle of persons, most of whom were undergoing surgical treatment. Three specific deoxyribonucleases were used: S_1 endonuclease, nuclease Bal 31, and pea endonuclease. Each of these nucleases yielded similar results. The lengths of the double-stranded DNA segments obtained after nuclease treatment were measured from electron micrographs. The average lengths of the DNA between two single-strand breaks were obtained by measuring 20 to 200 molecules for each sample. The 470 persons contributing to the data were 1 to 91-years old. The average length of the DNA between two single-strand breaks was found to significantly decrease with age. This indicates that single-strand regions accumulate with age in human muscle.

3. Liver

Hepatocytes are the major type of cell in the liver. These cells are able to divide, but their turnover time (defined as the time required to replace the number of cells present in the entire cell population) is long: 400 to 450 d in the rat.[35] In such slowly dividing cells, DNA damages might be expected to accumulate by analogy to neurons and muscle cells which do not divide at all and which accumulate DNA damage.

Seventeen reports have been presented on whether or not DNA damage accumulates in liver cells. In 12 of these reports, the type of damage studied was that of single-strand breaks (and/or alkali labile sites in some cases).

leading to loss of functional capacity in the brain, muscle, the liver, and lymphocytes. In the next section we review evidence for such declines.

E. THE ACCUMULATION OF DNA DAMAGE CAN REASONABLY ACCOUNT FOR THE PROGRESSIVE PHYSIOLOGICAL DYSFUNCTION THAT DEFINES AGING

1. The Decline in Transcription and Protein Synthesis with Age

Observations on changes in gene expression with age have either been made with regard to overall transcription and protein synthesis or with regard to transcription and translation of specific genes. We review the data on overall transcription and protein synthesis first. Studies in the mouse showed a decline in transcription with age in muscle and the liver[77] and the liver.[78,79] Studies in rat showed a decline in transcription in the brain,[80] muscle[81] and the liver.[82-85] Human postmortem brain was examined for intact functional mRNA.[86] The mRNA from older persons was found to stimulate protein synthesis less efficiently than did younger brain mRNA.

Reduced transcription with age should result in reduced protein synthesis. A general decline in protein synthesis with age has been demonstrated in rat brain,[87-90] muscle[81,91,92] and liver.[93] In humans, protein synthesis was observed to decline with age in the brain.[94]

We now discuss changes with age in transcription and translation of specific genes, rather than changes in general transcription and protein synthesis. In rat brain, Semsei et al.[95] found a gradual decrease (21 to 27%) in the enzymes Cu/Zn superoxide dismutase and catalase and in the corresponding mRNAs (39 to 40%) as the animals aged from about 150 to 1100 d. Five different studies have been carried out on specific gene expression in rat liver with age. Roy et al.[96] observed a gradual decline and ultimate loss of α-globulin and its mRNA as rats aged from 20 to 800 d. Richardson et al.[97] observed that, as rats aged from 180 to 880 d, the liver mRNAs for α-globulin and aldolase declined by 98% and 30%, respectively; however, albumin mRNA increased by 30%. Changes in the levels of the specific proteins were similar to the respective changes in the corresponding mRNA. In agreement with the above observations on albumin, Horbach et al.[98] found a correlated increase in albumin mRNA and protein synthesis with age, but also concluded that albumin mRNAs present in the liver of old rats are biologically less active than are those found in younger animals. Wellinger and Guigoz[99] found that as rats aged from 300 to 760 d, induced synthesis of tyrosine transferase mRNA and its protein declined 50%, but induced synthesis of tryptophan oxygenase mRNA and its protein did not decline. Semsei and Richardson[100] observed that as rats aged from 182 to 1124 d, there were declines in mRNA levels for superoxide dismutase (30%), catalase (30%), and metallothionein (50%). Thus, overall, in rat liver, expression of six genes was observed to decline with age (α-globulin, aldolase, tyrosine transferase, superoxide dismutase, catalase, and metallothionein), expression of one gene increased (albumin), and one remained unchanged (tryptophan oxygenase).

b. Muscle

Although decline of brain function may be most central to aging, the generalized atrophy occurring during senescence is most evident in skeletal muscle because it is the largest single tissue of the mammal. Skeletal muscles are composed of long, thin, muscle fibers, each of which is a single, unusually large cell formed by the fusion of numerous separate cells. The muscle fibers of aged animals were found to have ultrastructural disorganization when examined with the electron microscope. This type of disorganization has been observed in several studies summarized by Goldspink and Alnaqeeb.[116] Structural disorganization in both the muscle fiber and the neuromuscular junction corresponds well with the diminished function of the locomoter system. In addition to structural alterations in the muscle fibers, a loss of muscle fibers during aging has been found for different muscles, including the rat extensor digitorum longus muscle.[117] Lexell et al.[118] studied the effects of aging on the total number of muscle fibers in two groups of humans at autopsy. The individuals in both groups had been, prior to death, physically healthy males. The older group had a mean age of 72 years, and the younger group had a mean age of 30 years. The muscles of the older individuals were, on average, 18% smaller, and the number of fibers was, on average, about 25% less than those of the young individuals. In conclusion, there is a deterioration at the cellular and tissue level in muscle with age, and this seems to account for the most apparent physiological changes of aging muscle: a decline in strength and a slowing down of the contractile process.[116,119]

c. Liver

Evidence that the number of hepatic cells declines with age has been reviewed by Tauchi and Sato.[120] In humans, the number of hepatic cells begins to diminish when individuals reach their sixties, declines significantly in their eighties, and markedly thereafter. Changes in human liver morphology and function that occur with age have been summarized by Dice and Goff.[121] These changes include decreased weight, decreased blood flow, delayed regeneration, decreased responsiveness to certain hormones, and increased fibrosis.

d. Immune System

Aging of the mammalian immune system has been reviewed by Doggett et al.,[74] with emphasis on the cellular and molecular levels. Regulatory control of the immune system declines with age. The loosening of regulatory controls results in a reduction in suppression of autoreactivity and monoclonal gammopathy, as well as a decrease in the activation of the differentiation necessary for a primary response. According to Burnet,[122] the decline in the immune system is responsible for many of the manifestations of old age, including the characteristic vulnerability of the old to disease. Old people die more frequently from infection, in part, because their immune systems have lost their former capacity to respond briskly and to generate a long-lasting immunity to most infections they encounter. Aging in humans is accompanied by atrophy of the thymus, reduction in the circulating levels of lymphocytes, and diminution of the peripheral lymphoid tissues.[123]

e. Conclusions

For the brain, we reviewed evidence that endogenous DNA damages accumulate with age, general mRNA synthesis and protein synthesis decline, and the synthesis of critical specific mRNAs and proteins is reduced. Furthermore, cell loss occurs with age, tissue function declines, and functional impairments arise, which are directly related to the central processes of aging. The hypothesis that DNA damage is the cause of the decline in brain function with age seems to be a reasonable explanation of the evidence.

We have similarly reviewed evidence that, in muscle, DNA damage accumulates with age, transcription decreases, protein synthesis declines, cellular structure deteriorates, and cells die. These declines are accompanied by a decrease in the strength of muscles and the speed of contraction. Again, a cause-and-effect relationship between DNA damage and muscle performance provides a reasonable explanation of the evidence.

The studies on the liver, reviewed above, indicate that DNA damage accumulates with age. We suggest that this damage may account for the observed declines in transcription and expression of hepatic genes, cell loss, and degenerative changes in liver morphology and function. For lymphocytes, we reviewed evidence that DNA damage accumulates with age. We also reviewed evidence for a decline in gene expression and function of the immune system which may reflect this damage accumulation. In general, the available evidence suggests that DNA damages in the brain, muscle, the liver, and lymphocytes may cause a reduction in gene expression, leading to the declines in cellular and tissue function characteristic of aging.

F. DOWN'S SYNDROME

A prediction of the hypothesis that oxidative DNA damages are an important cause of aging is that any metabolic disorder associated with an excessive production of reactive oxygen species should also have indications of premature aging. This prediction is apparently fulfilled in individuals with Down's syndrome (DS), a condition that exhibits both increased production of oxidative radicals and features of premature aging.

1. Individuals with Down's Syndrome Experience Premature Aging

Martin[124] tabulated 162 genetic syndromes with at least some features of premature aging. The syndrome that fit the most criteria, having 15 of the 21 features of premature aging, was DS. Furthermore, Wright and Whalley[125] have reviewed evidence indicating that features of the neuropathology of DS represent an acceleration of normal aging.

2. Oxidative Damage is Elevated in Down's Syndrome, Which May Account for the Premature Aging

In persons with DS, there appears to be a higher than normal level of oxidative damage due to excess CuZn superoxide dismutase (CuZn SOD).[126] The genetic basis of DS is trisomy of the distal part of the long arm of chromosome 21. This chromosomal region contains the gene for CuZn SOD. In persons with Down's syndrome, CuZn SOD is found at levels approximately 50% higher than normal in a variety of tissues, for instance, in erythrocytes,[127] fibroblasts,[128] B and T lymphocytes,[129] and fetal brain.[130] The observed increase in CuZn SOD expression in DS individuals probably results from the trisomy, since the rate at which transcripts of chromosome 21 genes appear increases in relation to the numbers of chromosome 21 that are present.[131] CuZn SOD catalyzes the formation of H_2O_2 from O_2^- (the superoxide anion radical).[126] Although this is an essential mechanism of protection against oxygen radicals, it can also cause deleterious side effects. The harm arises from the generation of $^1O_2$ (singlet oxygen) and the highly reactive ·OH (hydroxyl radical) from H_2O_2 (by the iron-catalyzed Haber Weiss reaction).[22] These compounds are very reactive and can cause oxidative damages in DNA.

The region of chromosome 21 responsible for Down's syndrome has been located to a critical segment, less than 2000 to 3000 kilobases long.[132,133] Two unrelated persons with Down's syndrome were found to have a duplication of this limited segment in one of their two copies of chromosome 21. Three genes have been identified within this segment, the CuZn SOD gene, oncogene *ets*-2, and the cystathione-β-synthase gene.[132] Individuals with this duplication were found to have elevated CuZn SOD in their erythrocytes, indicating that the extra copy of the CuZn SOD gene leads to abnormally high expression of the enzyme. Recently, Groner et al.[134] described experiments in which the human CuZn SOD gene was allowed to overexpress in transfected rat cells and in transgenic mice. The results indicated that a number of the manifestations of Down's syndrome are induced by CuZn SOD overexpression. This evidence suggests that overexpression of CuZn SOD is involved in Down's syndrome.

Groner et al.[135] detected elevated CuZn SOD in nearly all tissues of the transgenic mice which expressed the human CuZn SOD gene. However, the levels of activity varied from tissue to tissue. Expression in the liver was low, whereas in the brain, high activity was detected. The brain may be more vulnerable to oxidative DNA damage than are other tissues, even in individuals who do not suffer from DS. *A priori,* more oxidative damage might be expected to accumulate in the brain DNA than in other tissues because little or no turnover of neuronal DNA occurs during the human life-span[136] and oxygen utilization is high. The weight of the human brain is only 2% of total body weight, but its rate of oxygen consumption accounts for 20% of the total resting consumption.[137] This disproportionate expenditure of energy may be due to the maintenance of ionic gradients across the neuronal membrane on which the conduction of impulses in the approximately 10^{11} brain neurons depends. If, as suggested by the experiments of Groner et al.,[135] the level of CuZn SOD is elevated in the brain of DS persons more than in other tissues, this would make the brains of DS persons even more vulnerable than the brains of unaffected individuals to oxidative DNA damage.

To review, the extra genetic material responsible for Down's syndrome has been localized to a limited segment of chromosome 21, which includes the CuZn SOD gene. Cells of persons with DS have a high level of CuZn SOD, a likely increased production of H_2O_2, and of the very damaging hydroxyl radical and singlet oxygen. The brain of persons with DS may be a particularly vulnerable tissue because of its high level of oxidative metabolism and its lack of cell turnover. This excess production of reactive oxygen species may cause more rapid accumulation of DNA damage in the brain, and this may account, at least in part, for the accelerated aging phenotype (particularly the neuropathological aspects) in DS.

G. INCREASED DNA DAMAGE CORRELATES WITH REDUCED LONGEVITY

The DNA damage theory of aging predicts that organisms experiencing high levels of DNA damage will age at a faster rate than will comparable organisms experiencing lower levels of DNA damage. Such comparisons can be made in three circumstances. First, among different mammalian species with differing life-spans, the capacity to repair DNA damage might be expected to correlate with life-span. Second, sublethal exposure of animals to DNA-damaging agents should shorten life-span compared to untreated animals and accelerate at least some aspects of the aging process. Third, at least some human genetic syndromes with features of premature aging should have elevated accumulation of DNA damage, excess intracellular DNA damaging agents, and/or defective DNA repair.

1. Life-Span vs. DNA Repair Capacity in Different Species

Hart and Setlow[138] determined the ability of skin fibroblasts from mammals of seven different species to perform unscheduled DNA synthesis (UDS) after UV irradiation. UDS is largely a measure of the DNA synthesis carried out during excision repair of DNA damage. The mammals studied were shrew, mouse, rat, hamster, cow, elephant, and humans. Their life-spans range from 1.5 years for the shrew to 95 years for humans. They found that DNA repair capacity, as measured by UV-induced UDS, increased systematically with life-span for the seven species. This positive correlation was striking and stimulated a series of additional studies on UV-induced DNA repair in different mammalian species. These studies amplified the initial findings and, in general, supported the existence of a positive correlation between capacity to repair UV-induced DNA damages and life-span.

Ley et al.[139] found a low, *in vivo* UV-induced DNA repair capacity of mouse skin compared to human skin,[140] thus supporting the findings on DNA repair capacity in skin fibroblasts measured *in vitro* by Hart and Setlow.[138]

Four further studies were performed with mouse strains of different longevities. Paffenholz,[141] upon testing fibroblasts from three inbred mouse strains with life-spans ranging from 300 to 900 d, observed a positive correlation of UV-induced DNA repair capacity and life-span. Hall et al.[142] measured the DNA repair capacities of lymphocytes of two mouse strains with lifespans of about 300 and 900 d, respectively. UV-induced DNA repair capacity was found to correlate positively with life-span. Hart et al.[143] measured UV-induced DNA repair capacity in the skin fibroblasts of a short-lived mouse species (3.4 years) and a closely related long-lived one (8.2 years). The rate of excision repair was 2.5-fold higher for cells of the latter, about the same as the ratio of life-spans. In contrast to the above studies, Collier et al.[144] observed no correlation between UV-induced DNA repair and life-span in embryonic cells derived from a related pair of mouse strains, one long-lived and one short-lived.

Two studies were performed with primates. Hart and Daniel[145] found an excellent correlation between UV-induced DNA repair capacity and life-span in the skin fibroblasts from six primate species. Hall et al.[146] performed a double-blind study in which they measured UV-induced repair capacity in fibroblasts cultured from punch biopsies from six primate species and in lymphocytes from the blood of nine primate species of widely different life-spans. By both types of measurement, a good linear relationship was observed between life-span and UV-induced DNA repair capacity.

In each of four further studies, a variety of different mammalian species were used. Francis et al.[147] examined UV-induced DNA repair in 21 different species of mammals, usually in skin fibroblasts. They measured both the number of repaired regions per 10^8 Da of DNA and the patch size. Their measurements showed a correlation between the number of repaired regions and life-span. Treton and Courtois[148] measured UV-induced repair capacity in the epithelial cells of the lens of five species: rat, rabbit, cat, dog, and horse. They found an excellent positive correlation between repair capacity and life-span. Maslansky and Williams[149] measured UV-induced DNA repair capacity in hepatocyte primary cultures derived from five species: mouse, hamster, rat, guinea pig, and rabbit. A positive correlation was observed between the amount of DNA repair elicited by low UV fluences and species life-span.

Kato et al.[150] investigated UV-induced DNA repair capacity in fibroblasts from 34 different species. These investigators found no correlation between repair and life-span. Tice and Setlow[8] noted that two orders of species in the study of Kato et al.[150] abolish an otherwise positive correlation. These two orders are the bats (Chiroptera) and the primates. In the data of Kato et al.,[150] the bats, which have a long life-span, had low repair synthesis. Tice and Setlow[8] argued, to account for these data, that bats have a very different metabolic regime from the other animals considered. Also, in the data of Kato et al.,[150] the primates had a short life-span, but high repair synthesis.

However, Tice and Setlow[8] noted that this result contradicts the more extensive data on primates of Hart and Daniel.[145]

Overall, and despite some contradictory data, the weight of evidence from all studies indicates a good correlation between capacity to repair UV-induced DNA damage and life-span in mammals. However, UV-induced damage is unlikely to be a primary cause of mammalian aging. UV-irradiation does not penetrate the skin and, hence, cannot be a cause of aging of other organs (such as the brain and muscle) which appear to be more central to aging of the whole animal. What then is the significance of the correlation between capacity to repair UV-induced DNA damages and life-span? Perhaps the enzymes which repair UV-induced DNA damages also repair other types of DNA damages, some of which may be important in aging. Studies of the inherited human syndrome xeroderma pigmentosum (XP) provide supporting evidence for this idea.

XP is an autosomal recessive condition. Individuals homozygous for the defective gene are hypersensitive to UV-irradiation and have a high incidence of skin cancers. Cells from persons with XP are defective in the repair of damaged DNA-containing pyrimidine dimers.[151] Persons suffering from XP may be defective in any one of nine different complementation groups (A to I), implying that DNA repair in humans involves multiple gene products. XP cells are not only deficient in repair of UV-photoproducts, i.e., pyrimidine dimers, but are also defective in repair of chemical adducts introduced by DNA-damaging agents such as acetylaminofluorene, 8-methoxypsoralen plus near UV light, and benzo(a)pyrene.[152-154] These DNA damaging agents cause major distortions in the double-helix structure. Thus, measurements of excision repair in response to UV-induced damage may reflect repair capacity for a range of bulky damages, possibly including some types important in aging. Individuals with XP defects in groups A and D have severe neurological abnormalities. This observation implies that normal individuals have the ability to repair some intrinsic DNA damage, and that this ability is critical for achieving normal neuronal function. Andrews et al.[155] and Robbins et al.[156] have suggested that defective DNA repair in individuals with XP causes premature neuron death. In fact, Andrews et al.[155] speculated that the neurological abnormalities of XP are the result of abnormal aging of the human nervous system. Therefore, in humans, UV-induced damage may indeed be repaired by a pathway that is the same as, or coordinately regulated with, a DNA repair pathway important in determining neuron survival and, hence, life-span. In summary, the reasonably well-substantiated correlation of life-span in mammals with capacity to repair UV-induced DNA damages may extend, as well, to the capacity to repair DNA damages important for aging.

2. X-Rays and Radiomimetic Chemicals Reduce Life-Span

If aging is caused by an accumulation of unrepaired DNA damages, then exposure of animals to sublethal doses of X-rays or DNA-damaging chemicals might accelerate the aging process. On the other hand, when an animal is exposed to an external DNA-damaging agent, the type of damage, the distribution of damage by cell type, and the distribution of damage over time are very likely to be different than for naturally accumulating DNA damage.

Numerous studies have shown that treatment of mammals with whole body sublethal X-irradiation shortens life-span. An early review of the subject by Casarett[157] referred to 51 separate studies. This review also indicated that in 17 of the studies it was recorded that animals dying prematurely after sublethal radiation exposure exhibited changes suggestive of premature senescence. In general, Casarett[157] concluded that the manifestations of normal and X-ray-induced premature aging were similar, but there was a paucity of strictly defined and controlled information on the subject.

In addition to the review of Casarett,[157] Alexander[1] and Walburg[158] have also reviewed and interpreted studies on the effect of ionizing radiation in relation to aging. The review of Alexander[1] led him to the conclusion that, although radiation shortens life-span, the underlying processes responsible differ significantly from the cellular and subcellular changes associated with normal aging. He thought that the accumulation of DNA damage in postmitotic cells (e.g., brain and muscle cells) was central to aging. He suggested that aging in these cells is accompanied by accumulation of DNA breaks leading to reduction in the capacity for RNA synthesis. However, he noted that the amount of radiation needed to produce this level of DNA breakage would be expected to be so high that it could not be given to mammals, because they would be killed, owing to the destruction of essential stem cells in the bone marrow and the gut. Hence, the type of killing of postmitotic cells that he viewed as central to aging would not occur under the conditions of radiation-induced life-shortening of mammals.

In the review by Walburg,[158] he noted that the key test of the hypothesis that radiation-induced life-shortening is equivalent to premature aging is whether or not the time of all causes of death advances. According to Walford, very few diseases were specifically identified as advanced in time. Also, there appeared to be an absence of radiation-induced acceleration of age changes in neuromuscular performance and behavior patterns. He concluded that radiation does not result in a generalized advancement in the rate of aging.

Although most of the studies on induction of premature aging were performed with ionizing radiation, some experiments were also done with DNA-damaging (radiomimetic) chemicals.[159-163] In general the results obtained were similar to those obtained with ionizing radiation, in that life-span was shortened, but otherwise the effects were probably not equivalent to premature aging in the simplest sense.

In conclusion, the pathological conditions associated with the life shortening caused by X-rays or DNA-damaging chemicals only partially, or poorly, mimic those of natural aging. This general observation, we think, can be explained by the assumption that the distribution of DNA damages in different tissues and over time, when introduced from exogenous sources, differs drastically from the distribution of natural DNA damages.

3. Human Genetic Syndromes with Defective DNA Repair and Features of Premature Aging

The DNA damage hypothesis of aging predicts that at least some of the human genetic syndromes with features of premature aging should also have higher than normal levels of DNA damage. We have already discussed two syndromes (DS and XP) which have both features of premature aging and evidence for elevated DNA damage. We now discuss three additional genetic syndromes which, according to Martin,[124] have numerous features of premature aging. These are Cockayne's syndrome (CS), Werner's syndrome (WS), and ataxia telangiectasia (AT).

CS is thought to be an autosomal recessive condition. This syndrome has 12 of the 21 features of premature aging listed by Martin.[124] Skin fibroblasts from individuals with CS are more sensitive to killing by UV light than are cells from normal individuals.[164-167] CS cells are also abnormally sensitive to DNA-damaging chemicals that form bulky adducts.[167,168] These observations have led to the interpretation that individuals with CS have a defect in DNA repair.[106,169]

WS, an autosomal recessive condition, is considered by some gerontologists to be a model of premature aging. It has 12 of the 21 features of premature aging listed by Martin.[124] WS cells have an increase in spontaneous chromosomal aberrations compared with normal cells.[170-173] Since chromosomal aberrations arise from DNA damage, this evidence suggests an abnormally high level of DNA damage in WS.

AT is an autosomal recessive condition that affects many systems of the body, particularly the nervous system, the immune system, and the skin. It has eight of the features of premature aging listed by Martin.[124] Cells from individuals with AT have a high frequency of spontaneous chromosomal aberrations.[174,175] Furthermore, AT cells have substantially increased sensitivity to ionizing radiation.[176-178] AT cells are also sensitive to the radiomimetic chemical, bleomycin.[179,180] Coquerelle et al.[181] have shown that γ ray- or bleomycin-induced double-strand breaks were repaired less efficiently in an AT fibroblast cell line than in normal human fibroblasts. This evidence suggests that individuals with AT are defective in repair of some type(s) of DNA double-strand breaks. A DNA repair defect could lead to a higher level of some kind(s) of spontaneous DNA damage, and this could explain the high frequency of spontaneous chromosomal aberrations.

In summary, we have reviewed evidence for higher than normal levels of DNA damage in five genetic syndromes with features of premature aging, i.e., DS, XP, CS, WS, and AT. Each of these syndromes exhibits some, but not all, features of premature aging. In one syndrome, DS, features of premature aging may be generated by excess production of oxidative free radicals that damage DNA. In two syndromes, WS and AT, an increased frequency of chromosomal aberrations suggests the presence of increased DNA damage. In three syndromes, XP, CS, and AT, there is reduced ability to repair DNA damages introduced by irradiation and/or chemicals, suggesting that natural

DNA damage, similar to the damages caused by some exogenous agents, may produce features of premature aging.

As we have argued above, neurons should be especially vulnerable to an increased level of DNA damage because neurons with lethally damaged DNA cannot be replaced by replication of undamaged cells. Thus, it is noteworthy that four of the five syndromes described above (i.e., DS, XP, CS, and AT) are characterized by neuropathology. None of the genetic syndromes described above meets all of the criteria of premature aging described by Martin.[124] If life-span is determined by multiple protective and repair processes, loss of any one of them through a genetic defect might accelerate some aspects of aging, but not others. Thus, the syndromes which we reviewed should give clues about which processes are significant for resisting aging.

III. CONCLUSIONS AND OVERVIEW

A. GAPS IN THE EVIDENCE AND FUTURE DIRECTIONS

Major gaps in our understanding of aging from the perspective of the DNA damage theory of aging remain to be filled in.

1. We do not know the distribution of types and rates of occurrence of natural DNA damages in mammalian cells. We have reviewed evidence that DNA damages caused by oxidation are important. But, we do not know how important these are relative to damages caused by other endogenous processes, such as heat-induced hydrolysis and alkylation reactions.

2. The DNA damages likely to be the most important in aging are those that accumulate over the lifetime of the organism. The rate of accumulation of a specific type of damage depends on its rate of occurrence and its rate of repair. We discussed evidence that single-strand breaks in DNA accumulate in the brain, muscle, and the liver. Other types of DNA damage have also been shown to accumulate (e.g., methylated guanine in muscle and oxidized bases and methyl adducts in the liver). However, we do not know the full spectrum of damages that accumulate, nor do we know which ones accumulate most rapidly.

3. We have reviewed evidence that treatment of mammalian cell DNA with DNA-damaging agents interferes with mRNA synthesis. We have also reviewed evidence that as mammals age, their brain, muscle, and liver accumulate DNA damage, mRNA synthesis declines, cell loss occurs, and tissue and organ function decrease. However it has not been shown that the DNA damages which accumulate in the animal are the specific cause of the declines in gene function and higher order functions that define aging. Such a cause-and-effect relationship would have to exist if the DNA damage theory of aging is valid.

4. We reviewed evidence indicating that five human genetic syndromes with features of premature aging may have elevated DNA damage.

5. **Bernstein, C. and Bernstein, H.,** *Aging, Sex, and DNA Repair,* Academic Press, San Diego, 1991, 1.

6. **Gensler, H. L. and Bernstein, H.,** DNA damage as the primary cause of aging, *Q. Rev. Biol.,* 56, 279, 1981.

7. **Gensler, H. L., Hall, J. D., and Bernstein, H.,** The DNA damage hypothesis of aging: importance of oxidative damage, in *Review of Biological Research in Aging,* Vol. 3, Rothstein, M., Ed., Alan R. Liss, New York, 1987, 451.

8. **Tice, R. R. and Setlow, R. B.,** DNA repair and replication in aging organisms and cells, in *Handbook of the Biology of Aging,* Finch, C. E. and Schneider, E. L., Eds., Van Nostrand Reinhold, New York, 1985, 173.

9. **Vijg, J. and Knook, D. L.,** DNA repair in relation to the aging process, *J. Am. Geriatr. Soc.,* 35, 532, 1987.

10. **Mullaart, E., Lohman, P. H. M., Berends, F., and Vijg, J.,** DNA damage metabolism and aging, *Mutat. Res.,* 237, 189, 1990.

11. **Ames, B. N. and Gold, L. S.,** Endogenous mutagens and the causes of aging and cancer, *Mutat. Res.,* 250, 3, 1991.

12. **Winton, D. J., Blount, M. A., and Pounder, B. A. J.,** A clonal marker induced by mutation in mouse intestinal epithelium, *Nature,* 333, 463, 1988.

13. **Harrison, D. E.,** Proliferative capacity of erythropoietic stem cell lines and aging: an overview, *Mech. Ageing Dev.,* 9, 409, 1979.

14. **Mori, M., Tanaka, A., and Sato, N.,** Hematopoietic stem cells in elderly people, *Mech. Ageing Dev.,* 37, 41, 1986.

15. **Imlay, J. A. and Linn, S.,** DNA damage and oxygen radical toxicity, *Science,* 240, 1302, 1988.

16. **Saul, R. L., Gee, P. and Ames, B. N.,** Free radicals, DNA damage and aging, in *Modern Biological Theories of Aging,* Warner, H. R., Butler, R. N., Sprott, R. S., and Schneider, E. L., Eds., Raven Press, New York, 1987, 113.

17. **Shigenaga, M. K., Gimeno, C. J., and Ames, B. N.,** Urinary 8-hydroxy-2'-deoxy-guanosine as a biological marker of *in vivo* oxidative DNA damage, *Proc. Natl. Acad. Sci. U.S.A.,* 86, 9697, 1989.

18. **Richter, C., Park, J.-W., and Ames, B. N.,** Normal oxidative damage to mitochondrial and nuclear DNA is extensive, *Proc. Natl. Acad. Sci. U.S.A.,* 85, 6465, 1988.

19. **Fraga, C. G., Shigenaga, M. K., Park, J. W., Degan, P., and Ames, B. N.,** Oxidative damage to DNA during aging: 8-hydroxy-2'-deoxyguanosine in rat organ DNA and urine, *Proc. Natl. Acad. Sci. U.S.A.,* 87, 4533, 1990.

20. **Massie, H. R., Samis, H. V., and Baird, M. B.,** The kinetics of degradation of DNA and RNA by H_2O_2, *Biochim. Biophys. Acta,* 272, 539, 1972.

21. **Ward, J. E., Blakely, W. F., and Joner, E. I.,** Mammalian cells are not killed by DNA single-strand breaks caused by hydroxyl radicals from hydrogen peroxide, *Radiat. Res.,* 103, 383, 1985.

22. **Chance, B., Sies, H., and Boveris, A.,** Hydroperoxide metabolism in mammalian organs, *Physiol. Rev.,* 59, 527, 1979.

23. **Briemer, L. H.,** Urea-DNA glycosylase in mammalian cells, *Biochemistry,* 22, 4192, 1983.

24. **Higgins, S. A., Frenkel, K., Cummings, A., and Teebor, G. W.,** Definitive characterization of human thymine glycol *N*-glycosylase activity, *Biochemistry,* 26, 1683, 1987.

25. **Hollstein, M. C., Brooks, P., Linn, S., and Ames, B. N.,** Hydroxymethyluracil DNA glycosylase in mammalian cells, *Proc. Natl. Acad. Sci. U.S.A.,* 81, 4003, 1984.

26. **Kuhnlein, U., Lee, B., and Linn, S.,** Human uracil DNA *N*-glycosidase: studies in normal and repair defective cultured fibroblasts, *Nucl. Acids Res.,* 5, 112, 1978.

27. **Karran, P. and Lindahl, T.,** Hypoxanthine in DNA: generation by heat-induced hydrolysis of adenine residues and release in free form by a DNA glycosylase from calf thymus, *Biochemistry,* 19, 6005, 1980.

28. **Margison, G. P. and Pegg, A. E.**, Enzymatic release of 7-methylguanine from methylated DNA by rodent liver extracts, *Proc. Natl. Acad. Sci. U.S.A.*, 78, 861, 1981.

29. **Kornberg, A. and Baker, T. A.**, *DNA Replication*, W. H. Freeman, New York, 1991, 207.

30. **Mitchell, D. L. and Hartman, P. S.** The regulation of DNA repair during development. *BioEssays*, 12, 74, 1990.

31. **Smith, A. and Sugar, O.**, Development of above normal language and intelligence 21 years after left hemispherectomy, *Neurology*, 25, 813, 1975.

32. **Glassman, R. B.**, An hypothesis about redundancy and reliability in the brain of higher species: analogies with genes, internal organs, and engineering systems, *Neurosci. Biobehav. Rev.*, 11, 275, 1987.

33. **Hofman, M. A.**, Energy metabolism, brain size and longevity in mammals, *Q. Rev. Biol.*, 58, 495, 1983.

34. **Adelman, R., Saul, R. L., and Ames, B. N.**, Oxidative damage to DNA: relation to species metabolic rate and life span, *Proc. Natl. Acad. Sci. U.S.A.*, 85, 2706, 1988.

35. **Bowman, P. D.**, Aging and the cell cycle *in vivo* and *in vitro*, in *Handbook of Cell Biology of Aging*, Cristofalo, V. J., Adelman, R. C., and Roth, G. S., Eds., CRC Press, Boca Raton, FL, 1985, 117.

36. **Buetow, D. E.**, Cell numbers vs. age in mammalian tissues and organs, in *CRC Handbook of Cell Biology of Aging*, Cristofalo, V. J., Ed., CRC Press, Boca Raton, FL, 1985, 1.

37. **Leblond, C. P. and Stevens, C. E.**, The constant renewal of the intestinal epithelium in the albino rat, *Anat. Rec.*, 100, 357, 1948.

38. **Lesher, S. and Sacher, G. A.**, Effects of age on cell proliferation in mouse duodenal crypts, *Exp. Gerontol.*, 3, 211, 1968.

39. **Chetsanga, C. J., Tuttle, M., Jacobini, A., and Johnson, C.**, Age-associated structural alterations in senescent mouse brain DNA, *Biochim. Biophys. Acta*, 474, 180, 1977.

40. **Modak, S. P. and Price, G. B.**, Exogenous DNA polymerase-catalyzed incorporation of deoxyribonucleotide monophosphates in nuclei of fixed mouse-brain cells, *Exp. Cell Res.*, 65, 289, 1971.

41. **Mori, N. and Goto, S.**, Estimation of the single stranded region in the nuclear DNA of mouse tissues during aging with special reference to the brain, *Arch. Gerontol. Geriatr.*, 1, 143, 1982.

42. **Nakanishi, K., Shima, A., Fukuda, M., and Fujita, S.**, Age associated increase of single-stranded regions in the DNA of mouse brain and liver cells, *Mech. Ageing Dev.*, 10, 273, 1979.

43. **Price, G. B., Modak, S. P., and Makinodan, T.**, Age-associated changes in the DNA of mouse tissue, *Science*, 171, 917, 1971.

44. **Murthy, M. R. V., Bharucha, A. D., Roux-Murthy, H., Jacob, J., and Ranjekar, P. K.**, Molecular biological models in geriatric neurobiology, in *Neuropsychopharmacology*, Deniker, P., Radowco-Thomas, C., and Villeneuve, A., Eds., Pergamon Press, Oxford, 1976, 1615.

45. **Bergtold, D. S. and Lett, J. T.**, Alterations in chromosomal DNA and aging: an overview, in *Molecular Biology of Aging: Gene Stability and Gene Expression*, Sohol, R. S., Bernbaum, L. S., and Cutler, R. G., Eds., Raven Press, New York, 1985, 23.

46. **Wheeler, K. T. and Lett, J. T.**, On the possibility that DNA repair is related to age in non-dividing cells, *Proc. Natl. Acad. Sci. U.S.A.*, 71, 1862, 1974.

47. **Fu, C. S., Harris, S. B., Wilhelmi, P., and Walford, R. L.**, Lack of effect of age and dietary restriction on DNA single-strand breaks in brain, liver, and kidney of (C3H X C57BL/10) F1 mice, *J. Gerontol.*, 46, B78, 1991.

48. **Ono, T., Okada, S., and Sugahara, T.**, Comparative studies of DNA size in various tissues of mice during the aging process, *Exp. Gerontol.*, 11, 127, 1976.

49. **Su, C. M., Brash, D. E., Turturro, A., and Hart, R. W.**, Longevity-dependent organ-specific accumulation of DNA damage in two closely related murine species, *Mech. Ageing Dev.*, 27, 239, 1984.

50. **Mullaart, E., Boerrigter, M. E. T. I., Boer, G. J., and Vijg, J.**, Spontaneous DNA breaks in the rat brain during development and aging, *Mutat. Res.*, 237, 9, 1990.
51. **Tan, B. H., Bancsath, A., and Gaubatz, J. W.**, Steady-state levels of 7-methylguanine increase in nuclear DNA of postmitotic mouse tissues during aging, *Mutat. Res.*, 237, 229, 1990.
52. **Chetsanga, C. J., Tuttle, M., and Jacobini, A.**, Changes in structural integrity of heart DNA from aging mice, *Life Sci.*, 18, 1405, 1976.
53. **Gaubatz, J. W.**, DNA damage during aging of mouse myocardium, *J. Mol. Cell. Cardiol.*, 18, 1317, 1986.
54. **Zahn, R. K., Reinmuller, J., Beyer, R., and Pondeljak, V.**, Age-correlated DNA damage in human muscle tissue, *Mech. Ageing Dev.*, 41, 73, 1987.
55. **Dean, R. G. and Cutler, R. G.**, Absence of significant age-dependent increase of single stranded DNA extracted from mouse liver nuclei, *Exp. Gerontol.*, 13, 287, 1978.
56. **Finch, C. E.**, Susceptibility of mouse liver DNA to digestion by S_1 nuclease: absence of age-related change, *Age*, 2, 45, 1979.
57. **Chetsanga, C. J., Boyd, V., Peterson, L., and Rushlow, K.**, Single-stranded regions in DNA of old mice, *Nature*, 253, 130, 1975.
58. **Lawson, T. and Stohs, S.**, Changes in endogenous DNA damage in aging mice in response to butylated hydroxyanisole and oltipraz, *Mech. Ageing Dev.*, 30, 179, 1985.
59. **Massie, H. R., Baird, M. B., Nicolosi, R. J., and Samis, H. V.**, Changes in the structure of rat liver DNA in relation to age, *Arch. Biochem. Biophys.*, 153, 736, 1972.
60. **Mullaart, E., Boerrigter, M. E. T. I., Brouwer, A., Berends, F., and Vijg, J.**, Age-dependent accumulation of alkali-labile sites in DNA of postmitotic but not in that of mitotic rat liver cells, *Mech. Ageing Dev.*, 45, 41, 1988.
61. **Park, J.-W. and Ames, B. N.**, 7-methylguanine adducts in DNA are normally present at high levels and increase on aging: analysis by HPLC with electrochemical detection, *Proc. Natl. Acad. Sci. U.S.A.*, 85, 7467, 1988.
62. **Park, J.-W. and Ames, B. N.**, Correction, *Proc. Natl. Acad. Sci. U.S.A.*, 85, 9508, 1988.
63. **Sharma, R. C. and Yamamoto, O.**, Base modification in adult animal liver DNA and similarity to radiation-induced base modification, *Biochem. Biophys. Res. Commun.*, 96, 662, 1980.
64. **Summerfield, F. W. and Tappel, A. L.**, Effects of dietary polyunsaturated fats and vitamin E on aging and peroxidative damage to DNA, *Arch. Biochem. Biophys.*, 233, 408, 1984.
65. **Yamamoto, O., Fuji, I., Yoshida, T., Cox, A. B., and Lett, J. T.**, Age dependency of base modification in rabbit liver DNA, *J. Gerontol.*, 43, B132, 1988.
66. **Crowley, C. and Curtis, H. J.**, The development of somatic mutations in mice with age, *Proc. Natl. Acad. Sci. U.S.A.*, 49, 626, 1963.
67. **Stevenson, K. G. and Curtis, H. J.**, Chromosome aberrations in irradiated and nitrogen mustard treated mice, *Radiat. Res.*, 15, 774, 1961.
68. **Curtis, H. J., Leith, J., and Tilley, J.**, Chromosome aberrations in liver cells of dogs of different ages, *J. Gerontol.*, 21, 268, 1966.
69. **Curtis, H. J. and Miller, K.**, Chromosome aberrations in liver cells of guinea pigs, *J. Gerontol.*, 26, 292, 1971.
70. **Brooks, A. L., Mead, D. K., and Peters, R. F.**, Effect of aging on frequency of metaphase chromosome aberrations in the liver of the Chinese hamster, *J. Gerontol.*, 28, 452, 1973.
71. **Curtis, H. J.**, Biological mechanisms underlying the aging process, *Science*, 141, 686, 1963.
72. **Bryant, P. E.**, 9-beta D-arabinofuranosyladenine increases the frequency of X-ray induced chromosome abnormalities in mammalian cells, *Int. J. Radiat. Biol.*, 3, 459, 1983.

73. **Natarajan, A. T., Darroudi, F., Mullenders, L. H. F., and Meijers, M.**, The nature and repair of DNA lesions that lead to chromosomal aberrations induced by ionizing radiations, *Mutat. Res.*, 160, 231, 1986.
74. **Doggett, D. L., Chang, M.-P., Makinodan, T., and Strehler, B. L.**, Cellular and molecular aspects of immune system aging, *Mol. Cell. Biochem.*, 37, 137, 1981.
75. **Turner, D. R., Morley, A. A., Seshadri, R. S., and Sorrell, J. R.**, Age-related variations in human lymphocyte DNA, *Mech. Ageing Dev.*, 17, 305, 1981.
76. **Fenech, M. and Morley, A. A.**, The effect of donor age on spontaneous and induced micronuclei, *Mutat. Res.*, 148, 99, 1985.
77. **Britton, V. J., Sherman, F. G., and Florini, J. R.**, Effect of age on RNA synthesis by nuclei and soluble RNA polymerases from liver and muscle of C57BL/6J mice, *J. Gerontol.*, 27, 188, 1972.
78. **Cutler, R. G.**, Transcription of unique and reiterated DNA sequences in mouse liver and brain tissues as a function of age, *Exp. Gerontol.*, 10, 37, 1975.
79. **Fog, R. and Pakkenberg, H.**, Age-related changes in ³H uridine uptake in the mouse, *J. Gerontol.*, 36, 680, 1981.
80. **Zs-Nagy, I. and Semsei, I.**, Centrophenoxine increases the rates of total and mRNA synthesis in the brain cortex of old rats: an explanation of its action in terms of the membrane hypothesis of aging, *Exp. Gerontol.*, 19, 171, 1984.
81. **Pluskal, M. G., Moreyra, M., Burini, R. C., and Young, V. R.**, Protein synthesis studies in skeletal muscle of aging rats. I. Alterations in nitrogen composition and protein synthesis using a crude polyribosome and pH 5 enzyme system, *J. Gerontol.*, 39, 385, 1984.
82. **Bolla, R. and Denckla, W. D.**, Effect of hypophysectomy on liver nuclear ribonucleic acid synthesis in aging rats, *Biochem. J.*, 184, 669, 1979.
83. **Castle, T., Katz, A., and Richardson, A.**, Comparison of RNA synthesis by liver nuclei from rats of various ages, *Mech. Ageing Dev.*, 8, 383, 1978.
84. **Devi, A., Lindsay, P., Raina, P. L., and Sarkar, N. K.**, Effect of age on some aspects of the synthesis of ribonucleic acid, *Nature*, 212, 474, 1966.
85. **Park, G. H. and Buetow, D. E.**, RNA synthesis by hepatocytes isolated from adult and senescent Wistar rat liver, *Gerontology*, 36, 76, 1990.
86. **Sajdel-Sulkowska, E. M. and Marotta, C. A.**, Functional messenger RNA from the postmortem human brain: comparison of aged normal with Alzheimer's disease, in *Molecular Biology of Aging: Gene Stability and Gene Expression*, Sohol, R. S., Birnbaum, L. S., and Cutler, R. G., Eds., Raven Press, New York, 1985, 243.
87. **Dwyer, B. E., Fando, J. L., and Wasterlain, C. G.**, Rat brain protein synthesis declines during postdevelopmental aging, *J. Neurochem.*, 35, 746, 1980.
88. **Ekstrom, R., Liu, D. S. H., and Richardson, A.**, Changes in brain protein synthesis during the life-span of male Fischer rats, *Gerontology*, 26, 121, 1980.
89. **Fando, J. L., Salinas, M., and Wasterlain, C. G.**, Age-dependent changes in brain protein synthesis in the rat, *Neurochem. Res.*, 5, 373, 1980.
90. **Ingvar, M. C., Maeder, P., Sokoloff, L., and Smith, C. B.**, Effects of aging on local rates of cerebral protein synthesis in Sprague-Dawley Rats, *Brain*, 108, 155, 1985.
91. **Crie, J. S., Millward, D. J., Bates, P. C., Griffin, E., and Wildenthal, K.**, Age-related alterations in cardiac protein turnover, *J. Mol. Cell. Cardiol.*, 13, 589, 1981.
92. **Sonntag, W. E., Hylka, V. W., and Meites, J.**, Growth hormone restores protein synthesis in skeletal muscle of old male rats, *J. Gerontol.*, 40, 689, 1985.
93. **Birchenall-Sparks, M. C., Roberts, M. S., Staecker, J., Hardwick, J. P., and Richardson, A.**, Effect of dietary restriction on liver protein synthesis in rats, *J. Nutr.*, 115, 944, 1985.
94. **Suzuki, K., Korey, S. R., and Terry, R. D.**, Studies on protein synthesis in brain microsomal system, *J. Neurochem.*, 11, 403, 1964.
95. **Semsei, I., Rao, G., and Richardson, A.**, Expression of superoxide dismutase and catalase in rat brain as a function of age, *Mech. Ageing Dev.*, 58, 13, 1991.

96. **Roy, A. K., Nath, T. S., Motwani, N. M., and Chatterjee, B.,** Age-dependent regulation of the polymorphic forms of alpha 2_{mu}-globin, *J. Biol. Chem.,* 258, 10123, 1983.
97. **Richardson, A., Rutherford, M. S., Birchenall-Sparks, M. C., Roberts, M. S., Wu, W. T., and Cheung, H. T.,** Levels of specific messenger RNA species as a function of age, in *Molecular Biology of Aging: Gene Stability and Gene Expression,* Vol. 29, Sohal, R. S., Birnbaum, L. S., and Cutler, R. G., Eds., Raven Press, New York, 1985, 229.
98. **Horbach, G. J. M. J., Princen, H. M. G., Van Der Kroef, M., Van Bezooijen, C. F. A., and Yap, S. H.,** Changes in the sequence content of albumin mRNA and in its translational activity in the rat liver with age, *Biochim. Biophys. Acta,* 783, 60, 1984.
99. **Wellinger, R. and Guigoz, Y.,** The effect of age on the induction of tyrosine aminotransferase and tryptophan oxygenase genes by physiological stress, *Mech. Ageing Dev.,* 34, 203, 1986.
100. **Semsei, I. and Richardson, A.,** Effect of age on the expression of genes involved in free radical protection, *Fed. Proc.,* 45, 217, 1986.
101. **Wu, W., Pahlavani, M., Cheung, H. T., and Richardson, A.,** The effect of aging on the expression of interleukin 2 messenger ribonucleic acid, *Cell. Immunol.,* 100, 224, 1986.
102. **Nocentini, S.,** Inhibition and recovery of ribosomal RNA synthesis in ultraviolet-irradiated mammalian cells, *Biochim. Biophys. Acta,* 454, 114, 1976.
103. **Hackett, P. B. and Sauerbier, W.,** The transcriptional organization of the ribosomal RNA genes in mouse L cells, *J. Mol. Biol.,* 91, 235, 1975.
104. **Giorno, R. and Sauerbier, W.,** A radiological analysis of the transcription units for heterogeneous nuclear RNA in cultured murine cells, *Cell,* 9, 775, 1976.
105. **Sauerbier, W. and Hercules, K.,** Gene and transcription unit mapping by radiation effects, *Annu. Rev. Genet.,* 12, 329, 1978.
106. **Mayne, L. V. and Lehman, A. R.,** Failure of RNA synthesis to recover after UV irradiation: an early defect in cells from individuals with Cockayne's syndrome and xeroderma pigmentosum, *Cancer Res.,* 42, 1473, 1982.
107. **Leffler, S., Pulkrabak, P., Grunberger, D., and Weinstein, I. B.,** Template activity of calf thymus DNA modified by a dihydrodiol epoxide derivative of benzo(a)pyrene, *Biochemistry,* 16, 3133, 1977.
108. **Zieve, F. J.,** Effects of the carcinogen *N*-acetoxy-2-fluorenylacetamide on the template properties of deoxyribonucleic acid, *Mol. Pharmacol.,* 9, 658, 1973.
109. **Yu, F.-L.,** Preferential binding of aflatoxin B_1 to the transcriptionally active regions of rat liver nucleolar chromatin, *Carcinogenesis,* 4, 889, 1983.
110. **Byrd, S., Reines, D., and Doetsch, P. W.,** Inhibition of transcription by oxidative DNA damage products, *FASEB J.,* 5, A439, 1991.
111. **Sabel, B. A. and Stein, D. G.,** Extensive loss of subcortical neurons in the aging rat brain, *Exp. Neurol.,* 73, 507, 1981.
112. **Brizzee, K. R.,** Pathophysiology of aging, in *Risk Factors for Senility,* Rothchild, H., Ed., Oxford University Press, New York, 1984, chap. 4.
113. **Johnson, R. J.,** Anatomy of the aging cell, in *CRC Handbook of Cell Biology of Aging,* Cristofolo, V. J., Ed., CRC Press, Boca Raton, FL, 1985, 149.
114. **Scheibel, M. E., Lindsay, R. D., Tomiyasu, U., and Scheibel, A. B.,** Progressive dendritic changes in aging human cortex, *Exp. Neurol.,* 47, 392, 1975.
115. **Glick, R. and Bondareff, W.,** Loss of synapses in the cerebellar cortex of the senescent rat, *J. Gerontol.,* 34, 818, 1979.
116. **Goldspink, G. and Alnaqeeb, M. A.,** Aging of skeletal muscle, in *Handbook of Cell Biology and Aging,* Cristofolo, V. J., Adelman, R. C., and Roth, G. S., Eds., CRC Press, Boca Raton, FL, 1985, 179.
117. **Alnaqeeb, M. A. and Goldspink, G.,** Interrelation of muscle fiber types, diameter and number in aging white rats, *J. Physiol. Proc.,* 310, 56P, 1980.

118. **Lexell, J., Henriksson-Larsen, K., Winblad, B., and Sjostrom, M.**, Distribution of different fiber types in human skeletal muscles: effects of aging studied in whole muscle cross sections, *Muscle Nerve*, 6, 588, 1983.

119. **Florini, J. R.**, Effect of aging on skeletal muscle composition and function, in *Review of Biological Research in Aging*, Vol. 3, Rothstein, M., Ed., Alan R. Liss, New York, 1987, 337.

120. **Tauchi, H. and Sato, T.**, Hepatic cells of the aged, in *Liver and Aging*, Kitani, K., Ed., Elsevier/North Holland Biomedical Press, New York, 1978, 3.

121. **Dice, F. J. and Goff, S. A.**, Aging and the liver, in *The Liver, Biology and Pathobiology*, Arias, I. M., Jakoby, W. B., Pepper, H., Schachter, D., and Schafritz, D. A., Eds., Raven Press, New York, 1986, chap. 71.

122. **Burnet, F. M.**, *Endurance of Life*, Cambridge University Press, Cambridge, 1978, 84.

123. **Burnet, F. M.**, *Immunology, Aging and Cancer*, W. H. Freeman, San Francisco, 1976, 94.

124. **Martin, G. M.**, Genetic syndromes in man with potential relevance to the pathobiology of aging, *Birth Defects: Orig. Article Ser.*, 14, 5, 1978.

125. **Wright, A. F. and Whalley, L. J.**, Genetics, aging and dementia, *Br. J. Psychiatr.*, 145, 20, 1984.

126. **Sinet, P. M.**, Metabolism of oxygen derivatives in Down syndrome, *Ann. N.Y. Acad. Sci.*, 396, 83, 1982.

127. **Kedziora, J., Bartosz, G., Gromadzinska, J., Sklodwska, M., Wesowicz, W., and Scianowski, J.**, Lipid peroxides in blood plasma and enzymatic antioxidative defense of erythrocytes in Down's syndrome, *Clin. Chim. Acta*, 154, 191, 1986.

128. **Faester, W. W., Kwok, L. W., and Epstein, C. J.**, Dosage effects for superoxide dismutase-1 in nucleated cells aneuploid for chromosome 21, *Am. J. Hum. Genet.*, 29, 563, 1977.

129. **Baeteman, M. A., Baret, A., Courtiere, A., Rebuffel, P., and Mattei, J. F.**, Immunoreactive Cu-SOD and Mn-SOD in lymphocyte subpopulations from normal and trisomy 21 subjects according to age, *Life Sci.*, 32, 895, 1983.

130. **Balazs, R. and Brooksbank, B. W.**, Neurochemical approaches to the pathogenesis of Down's syndrome, *J. Ment. Defic. Res.*, 29, 1, 1985.

131. **Kurnit, D. M.**, Down syndrome: gene dosage at the transcriptional level in skin fibroblasts, *Proc. Natl. Acad. Sci. U.S.A.*, 76, 2372, 1979.

132. **Delabar, J. M., Sinet, P. M., Chadefaux, B., Nichole, A., Gegonne, A., Stehelin, D., Fridlansky, F., Creau-Goldberg, N., Turleau, C., and deGrouchy, J.**, Submicroscopic duplication of chromosome 21 and trisomy 21 phenotype (Down syndrome), *Hum. Genet.*, 76, 225, 1987.

133. **Huret, J. L., Delabar, J. M., Marlhens, F., Aurias, A., Nichole, A., Berthier, M., Tanzer, J., and Sinet, P. M.**, Down syndrome with duplication of a region of chromosome 21 containing the CuZn superoxide gene without detectable karyotypic abnormality, *Hum. Genet.*, 75, 251, 1987.

134. **Groner, Y., Elroy-Stein, O., Avraham, K. B., Yarom, R., Schickler, M., Knobler, H., and Rotman, G.**, Down syndrome clinical symptoms are manifested in transfected cells and transgenic mice overexpressing the human Cu/Zn superoxide dismutase gene, *J. Physiol. Paris*, 84, 53, 1990.

135. **Groner, Y., Elroy-Stein, O., Avraham, K. B., Rotman, G., Bernstein, Y., Dafni, N., and Schickler, M.**, Overexpression of human CuZn SOD gene in transfected cells and transgenic mice: implication for Down syndrome pathology, *J. Cell Biochem. Suppl.*, 12A, 36, 1988.

136. **Slatkin, D. N., Friedman, L., Irsa, A. P., and Micca, P. L.**, The stability of DNA in human cerebellar neurons, *Science*, 228, 1002, 1985.

137. **Iverson, L. L.**, The chemistry of the brain, *Sci. Am.*, 241(Sept.), 134, 1979.

138. **Hart, R. W. and Setlow, R. B.**, Correlation between deoxyribonucleic acid excision-repair and lifespan in a number of mammalian species, *Proc. Natl. Acad. Sci. U.S.A.*, 71, 2169, 1974.

139. **Ley, R. D., Sedita, B. A., Grube, D. D., and Frey, R. J. M.**, Induction and persistence of pyrimidine dimers in the epidermal DNA of two strains of hairless mice, *Cancer Res.*, 37, 3243, 1977.

140. **Sutherland, B. M., Harber, L. C., and Kochevar, I. E.**, Pyrimidine dimer formation and repair in human skin, *Cancer Res.*, 40, 3181, 1980.

141. **Paffenholz, V.**, Correlation between DNA repair of embryonic fibroblasts and different life-span of 3 inbred mouse strains, *Mech. Ageing Dev.*, 7, 131, 1978.

142. **Hall, K. Y., Bergman, K., and Walford, R. L.**, DNA repair, H-2, and aging in NZB and CBA mice, *Tissue Antigens*, 17, 104, 1981.

143. **Hart, R. W., Sacher, G. A., and Hoskins, T. L.**, DNA repair in a short- and a long-lived rodent species, *J. Gerontol.*, 34, 808, 1979.

144. **Collier, I. E., Popp, D. M., Lee, W. H., and Regan, J. D.**, DNA repair in a congeneic pair of mice with different longevities, *Mech. Ageing Dev.*, 19, 141, 1982.

145. **Hart, R. W. and Daniel, F. B.**, Genetic stability *in vitro* and *in vivo*, *Adv. Pathobiol.*, 7, 123, 1980.

146. **Hall, K. Y., Hart, R. W., Benirshke, A. K., and Walford, R. L.**, Correlation between ultraviolet induced DNA repair in primate lymphocytes and fibroblasts and species maximum achievable life-span, *Mech. Ageing Dev.*, 24, 163, 1984.

147. **Francis, A. A., Lee, W. H., and Regan, J. D.**, The relationship of DNA excision repair of ultraviolet-induced lesions to the maximum life-span of mammals, *Mech. Ageing Develop.*, 16, 181, 1981.

148. **Treton, J. A. and Courtois, Y.**, Correlation between DNA excision repair and mammalian life-span in lens epithelial cells, *Cell Biol. Int. Rep.*, 6, 253, 1982.

149. **Maslansky, C. J. and Williams, G. M.**, Ultraviolet light-induced DNA repair synthesis in hepatocytes from species of differing longevities, *Mech. Ageing Dev.*, 29, 191, 1985.

150. **Kato, H., Harada, M., Tsuchiya, K., and Moriwaki, K.**, Absence of correlation between DNA repair in ultraviolet irradiated mammalian cells and life-span of the donor species, *Jap. J. Genet.*, 55, 99, 1980.

151. **Zelle, B. and Lohman, P. H. M.**, Repair of UV-endonuclease-susceptible sites in the seven complementation groups of xeroderma pigmentosum A through G, *Mutat. Res.*, 62, 363, 1979.

152. **Amacher, D. E. and Lieberman, M. W.**, Removal of acetylaminofluorene from the DNA of control and repair-deficient human fibroblasts, *Biochem. Biophys. Res. Commun.*, 74, 285, 1977.

153. **Kaye, J., Smith, C. A., and Hanawalt, P. C.**, DNA repair in human cells containing photoadducts of 8-methoxy-psoralen or angelicin, *Cancer Res.*, 40, 696, 1980.

154. **Yang, L. L., Maher, V. M., and McCormick, J. J.**, Error-free excision of the cytotoxic, and mutagenic N^2deoxyguanosine DNA adduct formed in human fibroblasts by ($+/-$) 7 beta, 8 alpha-dihydroxy-9 alpha, 10 alpha-epoxy-7,8,9,10-tetrahydrobenzo(a)pyrene, *Proc. Natl. Acad. Sci. U.S.A.*, 77, 5933, 1980.

155. **Andrews, A. D., Barrett, S. F., and Robbins, J. H.**, Xeroderma pigmentosum neurological abnormalities correlate with colony-forming ability after ultraviolet radiation, *Proc. Natl. Acad. Sci. U.S.A.*, 75, 1984, 1978.

156. **Robbins, J. H., Polinsky, R. J., and Moshell, A. N.**, Evidence that lack of deoxyribonucleic acid repair causes death of neurons in xeroderma pigmentosum, *Ann. Neurol.*, 13, 682, 1983.

157. **Casarett, G. W.**, Similarities and contrasts between radiation and time pathology, *Adv. Gerontol. Res.*, 1, 109, 1964.

158. **Walburg, H. E., Jr.**, Radiation-induced lifeshortening and premature aging, *Adv. Radiat. Biol.*, 5, 145, 1975.

159. **Alexander, P. and Connell, D. I.**, Shortening of the life-span of mice by irradiation with X-rays and treatment with radiomimetic compounds, *Radiat. Res.*, 12, 38, 1960.

160. **Conklin, J. W., Upton, A. C., Christenberry, K. W., and McDonald, T. P.**, Comparative late somatic effects of some radiomimetic agents and X-rays, *Radiat. Res.*, 19, 156, 1963.

161. **Dunjic, A.**, Shortening of the span of life of rats by 'Myleran', *Nature*, 203, 887, 1964.

162. **Kodell, R. L., Farmer, J. H., and Littlefield, N. A.**, Analysis of life-shortening effects in female BALB/C mice fed 2-acetylaminofluorene, *J. Environ. Pathol. Toxicol.*, 3, 69, 1980.

163. **Ohno, S. and Nagai, Y.**, Genes in multiple copies as the primary cause of aging, in *Genetic Effects of Aging*, Bergsma, D., Harrison, D. E., and Paul, N. W., Eds., Alan R. Liss, New York, 1978, 501.

164. **Deschavanne, P. J., Diatloff-Zito, C., Macieira-Coelho, A., and Malaise, E.-P.**, Unusual sensitivity of two Cockayne's syndrome cell strains to both UV and gamma irradiation, *Mutat. Res.*, 91, 403, 1981.

165. **Marshall, R. R., Arlett, C. F., Harcourt, S. A., and Broughton, B. A.**, Increased sensitivity of cell strains from Cockayne's syndrome to sister chromatid-exchange induction and cell killing by UV light, *Mutat. Res.*, 69, 107, 1980.

166. **Schmickel, R. D., Chu, E. H. Y., Trosko, J. E., and Chang, C.-C.**, Cockayne syndrome: a cellular sensitivity to ultraviolet light, *Pediatrics*, 60, 135, 1977.

167. **Wade, M. H. and Chu, E. H. Y.**, Effects of DNA damaging agents on cultured fibroblasts derived from patients with Cockayne syndrome, *Mutat. Res.*, 59, 49, 1979.

168. **Wade, M. H. and Chu, E. H. Y.**, Effects of DNA damaging agents on cultured fibroblasts derived from patients with Cockayne syndrome, in *DNA Repair Mechanisms*, Hanawalt, P. C., Friedberg, E. C., and Fox, C. F., Eds., Academic Press, New York, 1978, 667.

169. **Mayne, L. V., Mullenders, L. H. F., and van Zeeland, A. A.**, Cockayne's syndrome: a UV sensitive disorder with a defect in the repair of transcribing DNA but normal overall excision repair, in *Mechanisms and Consequences of DNA Damage Processing*, Friedberg, E. C. and Hanawalt, P. C., Eds., Alan R. Liss, New York, 1988, 349.

170. **Gebhart, E., Schinzel, M., and Ruprecht, K. W.**, Cytogenetic studies using various clastogens in two patients with Werner syndrome and control individuals, *Hum. Genet.*, 70, 324, 1985.

171. **Hoehn, H., Bryant, E. M., Au, K., Norwood, T. H., Boman, H., and Martin, G. M.**, Variegated translocation mosaicism in human skin fibroblast cultures, *Cytogenet. Cell Genet.*, 15, 282, 1975.

172. **Salk, D.**, Werner syndrome: a review of recent research with an analysis of connective tissue metabolism, growth control of cultured cells and chromosomal aberrations, *Hum. Genet.*, 62, 1, 1982.

173. **Stefanini, M., Scappaticci, S., Lagomarsini, P., Borroni, G., Berardesca, E., and Nuzzo, F.**, Chromosome instability in lymphocytes from a patient with Werner's syndrome is not associated with DNA repair defects, *Mutat. Res.*, 219, 179, 1989.

174. **Taylor, A. M. R., Metcalfe, J. A., Oxford, J. M., and Harnden, D. G.**, Is chromatid-type damage in ataxia telangiectasia after irradiation at G_0 a consequence of defective repair?, *Nature*, 260, 441, 1976.

175. **Webb, T., Harnden, D. G., and Harding, M.**, The chromosome analysis and susceptibility to transformation by simian virus 40 of fibroblasts from ataxia telangiectasia, *Cancer Res.*, 37, 997, 1977.

176. **Arlett, C. F. and Harcourt, S. A.**, Survey of radiosensitivity in a variety of human cell strains, *Cancer Res.*, 40, 926, 1980.

177. **Paterson, M. C., Anderson, A. K., Smith, B. P., and Smith, P. J.**, Enhanced radiosensitivity of cultured fibroblasts from ataxia telangiectasia heterozygotes manifested by defective colony-forming ability and reduced DNA repair replication after hypoxic gamma-irradiation, *Cancer Res.*, 39, 3725, 1979.

178. **Taylor, A. M. R., Harnden, D. G., Arlett, C. F., Harcourt, S. A., Lehmann, A. R., Stevens, S., and Bridges, B. A.,** Ataxia telangiectasia: a human mutation with abnormal radiation sensitivity, *Nature,* 258, 427, 1975.

179. **Lehman, A. R. and Stevens, S.,** The response of ataxia telangiectasia cells to bleomycin, *Nucl. Acids Res.,* 6, 1953, 1979.

180. **Taylor, A. M. R., Rosney, C. M., and Campbell, J. B.,** Unusual sensitivity of ataxia telangiectasia cells to bleomycin, *Cancer Res.,* 39, 1046, 1979.

181. **Coquerelle, T. M., Weibezahn, K. F., and Lucke-Huhle, C.,** Rejoining of double-strand breaks in normal human and ataxia-telangiectasia fibroblasts after exposure to ^{60}Co gamma rays, ^{241}Am alpha particles or bleomycin, *Int. J. Radiat. Biol.,* 51, 209, 1987.

Chapter 6

FREE RADICALS IN GLYCATION

Simon P. Wolff

TABLE OF CONTENTS

0-8493-4518-9/93/$0.00 + $.50
© 1993 by CRC Press, Inc.

I. THE DIABETIC COMPLICATIONS

Before the introduction of insulin, the prognosis of insulin-dependent diabetes mellitus was extremely poor, with early death from coma or infection.[1,2] It had been hoped that the discovery and introduction of insulin would permit diabetic individuals to lead normal lives. In the course of the following decades, it became apparent that this was not so. The individual with diabetes often develops complications of the disease which are a major threat to both the quality and length of life.[3,4] These complications are a wide group of clinical disorders which affect the vascular system, the kidney, the retina, the peripheral nerves, the lens, and the skin. The individual with diabetes has a 25-fold increase in the risk of blindness, a 20-fold increase in the risk of renal failure, a 20-fold increase in the risk of amputation as a result of gangrene, and a 2- to 6-fold increased risk of coronary heart disease and ischemic brain damage. Almost half of those diagnosed as diabetic before age 31 die before they reach 50, largely as a result of cardiovascular or renal complications, often with many years of crippling and debilitating disease beforehand.[5] The cause of these complications has been of considerable mystery, but various theories have been proposed relating tissue damage to chronically elevated levels of plasma and tissue glucose. This chapter discusses the idea that glucose produces deleterious changes to long-lived proteins, and that analysis of these protein modifications suggests that free radical processes operate in the causation of diabetic tissue damage.

II. GLYCATION

Glucose can slowly condense nonenzymatically with protein amino groups forming, initially, a Schiff base which may rearrange to form the Amadori adduct (Figure 1). This early stage of the reaction is called nonenzymatic glycosylation, or, more properly, "glycation."[6] The Amadori adduct is subsequently believed to degrade into alpha-ketoaldehyde compounds such as 1- and 3-deoxyglucosones (Figure 1). These secondary compounds are more protein-reactive than are the parent monosaccharide[7,8] and can react with proteins to form cross-links, as well as chromo/fluorophoric adducts called Maillard adducts (or advanced glycation end products [AGE]),[9] which result in the protein becoming "browned", fluorescent and cross-linked *in vitro*[10] (Figure 1). Evidence that at least the early stage of this reaction occurs *in vivo* was obtained through the study of minor hemoglobins which were elevated in diabetes.[11] Later, borohydride reduction of hemoglobin permitted stabilization of the Amadori adduct and its identification and quantitation using amino acid analysis.[12,13] The extent of hemoglobin glycation is now used as a cumulative index of blood-sugar levels (glycemia) over the previous few (4 to 8) weeks in the clinical management of diabetes.[14]

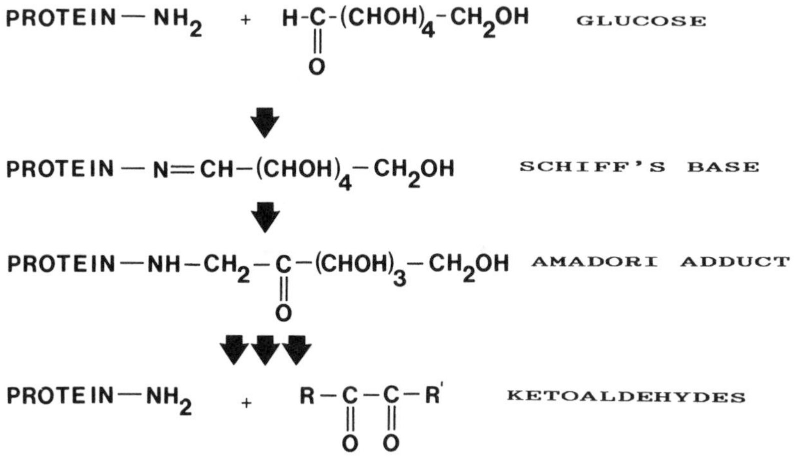

PROTEIN — NH$_2$ + H-C-(CHOH)$_4$-CH$_2$OH GLUCOSE
ǁ
O

⬇

PROTEIN — N=CH-(CHOH)$_4$-CH$_2$OH SCHIFF'S BASE

⬇

PROTEIN—NH-CH$_2$-C-(CHOH)$_3$-CH$_2$OH AMADORI ADDUCT
ǁ
O

⬇⬇⬇

PROTEIN—NH$_2$ + R-C-C-R' KETOALDEHYDES
ǁ ǁ
O O

FIGURE 1. Glycation and the Maillard reactions. The addition of glucose to protein followed by rearrangements and dehydrations. The deoxyglucosones (ketoaldehydes) react with protein to form many of the advanced glycation endproducts (AGE).

III. DIABETES AND "ACCELERATED AGING"

In diabetes, arteries and joints are prematurely stiff,[15,16] and elasticity as well as vital capacity of the lungs are prematurely decreased.[17] Collagen-associated fluorescence (370 nm excitation; 440 nm emission) increases with age and is increased in diabetic subjects,[18] more so in those with complications.[19] These changes have been postulated to result from the *in vivo* reaction of glucose with collagen, since collagen, when incubated with glucose *in vitro,* becomes browned, fluorescent, and cross-linked, as well as altered with respect to tensile properties.[20] Increases in plasma glucose concentration with age are also suggested to contribute to an increase in the glycation of long-lived proteins such as collagens and lens crystallins.[21]

Many proteins are modified adversely when incubated with glucose *in vitro.* Albumin, for example, undergoes conformational alterations and shows diminished ligand-binding capacity.[22] Similarly, superoxide dismutase (SOD) loses activity when exposed to glucose *in vitro;* higher levels of glycated erythrocyte SOD are found in aged erythrocytes and in diabetes.[23,24] Lens crystallins are glycated *in vivo* and aggregate and undergo thiol oxidation when incubated with glucose *in vitro.*[25] This has been used as an explanation for the increased cataract risk in diabetes.[26] Similarly, when low density lipoprotein (LDL) is incubated with glucose *in vitro,* it becomes poorly recognized by fibroblasts and preferentially accumulated by macrophages.[27-29] This has been suggested to contribute to plasma LDL accumulation and atherosclerosis in diabetes.

In basis, the conformational alterations and loss of cellular recognition caused by protein exposure to glucose have been postulated to result from cancellation of positive charges on the protein, to blocking of critical amino groups, loss of hydrogen bonding capacity, and the formation of complex products capable of inter- /intra-molecular cross-linking. One of the postulated cross-linking and fluorescent AGE found in hydrolysates of *in vitro* glycated protein has been identified as 2-furoyl-4[5]-[2-furanyl]-1-H-imidazole (FFI).[30] This compound has been suggested to be relevant to protein cross-linking and fluorescence *in vivo,* since a specific macrophage receptor (distinct from the well-known ''scavenger'' receptor) has been identified which recognizes proteins that have been exposed to glucose *in vitro* or to which this product is attached.[31]

IV. GLUCOSE "AUTOXIDATION"

Although this brief summary would seem to suggest that glycation and the later reactions associated with glycation are of direct pathophysiological significance, some caution needs to be observed. First, the reactions which occur when protein is exposed to glucose *in vitro* are considerably more complex than the simple addition of glucose to protein amino groups. Glucose, like other alpha-hydroxyaldehydes, can enolize and thereby reduce molecular oxygen under physiological conditions, catalyzed by transition metals, yielding ketoaldehydes and oxidizing intermediates[32,33] such as hydroxyl radicals and hydrogen peroxide (Figure 2). Evidence suggests that free radicals and hydrogen peroxide slowly produced by glucose ''autoxidation'' are a substantial cause of the structural damage which results when protein is exposed to glucose *in vitro*. For example, the conformational alterations which occur when bovine serum albumin (BSA) is exposed to glucose under physiological conditions *in vitro* are inhibited by the metal chelating agents diethylene-triaminepenta-acetic acid or ethylenediaminetetra-acetic acid. Oxidative reactions are critical for the production of glucose-induced protein alterations and seem more important than the covalent attachment of monosaccharide to protein per se.[34,35] The rate of glucose autoxidation is slow, but the amounts of ketoaldehydes and oxidizing agents formed over the typical time courses of *in vitro* glycation studies (days to weeks) are in the range consistent with protein damage and modification by this process. There is evidence to suggest that glucose is oxidized by copper ions attached to histidine residues on the protein chain leading to a localized ''site-specific'' form of protein damage.[36,37] H_2O_2 production during glucose autoxidation is low, but measurable.[38]

V. AMADORI ADDUCT AUTOXIDATION

Work by Baynes and colleagues[39] has shown that the Amadori adduct itself is able to oxidize, similarly catalyzed by transition metals, leading to the release of erythronic acid and the formation of carboxymethylated lysine

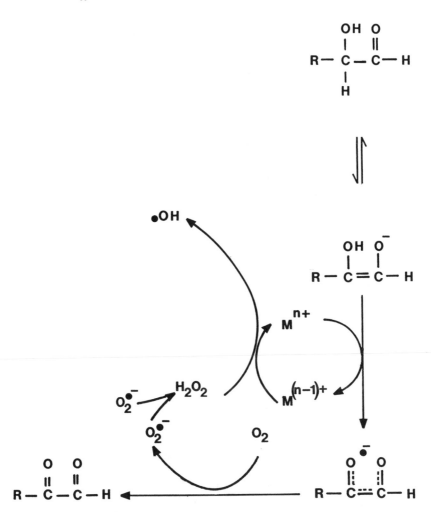

FIGURE 2. Glucose autoxidation.

(CML) residues (Figure 3). CML was originally observed in a cataractous lens hydrolysate (at levels in excess of the Amadori adduct), indicating that Amadori adduct oxidation occurs *in vivo*.[44] Further work indicated that, whereas the Amadori adduct accumulates in the lens only marginally with age, there is a strong age-dependent accumulation of CML.[40] Trace amounts of CML are present in the juvenile lens; by age 79 almost 1% of available lens protein lysine groups are present in the form of CML. This exceeds the concentration of the Amadori adduct by a factor of five. CML also accumulates in age-dependent fashion in skin collagen.[41] Here, however, the pattern is a little different. There is a modest (33%) increase in skin collagen Amadori adduct

$$LYSINE-NH-CH_2-\overset{\underset{\displaystyle \|}{O}}{C}-CHOH-(CHOH)_2-CH_2OH$$

Amadori Adduct

$$LYSINE-NH-CH_2-\underset{HO}{C}=\underset{OH}{C}-(CHOH)_2-CH_2OH$$

Postulated Enediol Intermediate

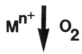 M^{n+} ↓ O_2

$$LYSINE-NH-CH_2-COOH \qquad + \qquad HOOC-(CHOH)_2-CH_2OH$$

Carboxymethyllysine *Erythronic Acid*

FIGURE 3. Oxidation of the Amadori adduct.

content from age 0 to 80. The concentration of skin collagen CML at age 80 was, however, only 0.2% of total available lysine and was less than the Amadori adduct (0.5% total lysine residues). Different mechanisms of CML formation between lens crystallin and skin collagen thus seem to be operating. Baynes and colleagues[42] have also studied skin collagen CML formation in relation to the complications of diabetes and find that CML levels are twice as high in skin collagen from diabetics compared with age-matched nondiabetics, and that the level of skin CML correlates positively with the presence of retinopathy and nephropathy, correcting for age.[43]

The identification of CML and its relationship to aging and diabetes mellitus are important findings. Although CML is present only in trace concentrations (less than 1% of total lysine groups) and cannot (by reasons of its structure) contribute to protein cross-linking or novel fluorescence,[44] its presence is strongly indicative of the idea that transition metal-catalyzed oxidations occur *in vivo*. Thus, CML accumulation may indicate either an accumulation of oxidizable substrate (i.e., the Amadori adduct in diabetes and aging) or an increased level of transition metal in a form capable of catalyzing oxidation. Although it is evident that the concentration of Amadori adduct increases in diabetes, this is not the case for the aging process, and the question of the cause of CML accumulation remains open. The possibilities are discussed further below.

above, the level of protein glycation, although increased in diabetes, is small in absolute terms. In hemoglobin, for example, only about 1% of the total amino groups are glycated at the end of the 120-d life-span of a normal red blood cell; this increases to about 2.5% in diabetes.[55] Similarly, levels of lysine glycation in plasma proteins are typically considerably less than 1%.[56] This may be substantially higher in longer-lived proteins such as collagen, but the concentration of Amadori adducts on collagen (in contrast to collagen-associated fluorescence) does not correlate with the presence of complications in individual diabetics,[57] as noted above. Levels of skin collagen Amadori adduct do not correlate with diabetic complications.

IX. RELEVANCE OF THE MAILLARD PATHWAY

Since the level of Amadori adduct does not seem to be a good predictor of diabetic tissue damage, it has been suggested that it is the Maillard (AGE) products, which contribute to protein cross-linking and fluorescence, not the Amadori adducts, which are primarily responsible for tissue damage in diabetes. Current evidence suggests that Maillard products produced by glucose *in vitro* are formed mainly from the reaction of ketoaldehyde products with protein, formed as a result of Amadori adduct oxidations and rearrangements, or transition metal-catalyzed glucose oxidation.[58,59] A great number of different products are produced when glucose is incubated with protein, but most are formed in only small yields and are subject to hydrolysis and other degradations during isolation,[60] which can lead to methodological artefacts. FFI, the recently identified AGE noted above, for example, is apparently not formed as a result of rearrangements of the Amadori adduct, but is produced as an *in vitro* artefact by the condensation of furosine (produced when glycated protein is hydrolyzed to amino acids) with the ammonia used to neutralize the hydrolysates.[61] FFI is not present *in vivo*,[62,63] and a great deal of work on this molecule (in particular, evidence relating to specific receptors for the molecule and the selectivity of antibodies raised to test its *in vivo* presence) now needs to be reappraised.

X. PENTOSIDINE: AN AUTHENTIC "AGE" MOLECULE

Although FFI may eventually materialize as a "red herring", its description and analysis has encouraged recognition of the idea that identifiable single AGE products may be extracted from tissues. Thus, recent work has led to the identification of an important authentic AGE compound with the trivial name "pentosidine". Pentosidine is a highly fluorescent cross-linking compound apparently derived from a pentose, arginine, and lysine[64,65] in an imidazo(4,5,6)pyridinium ring (Figure 5). Although initially believed actually to originate from ribose, recent work has shown that it also forms with glucose, fructose, and even ascorbate by a sequence of oxidation and decarboxylation

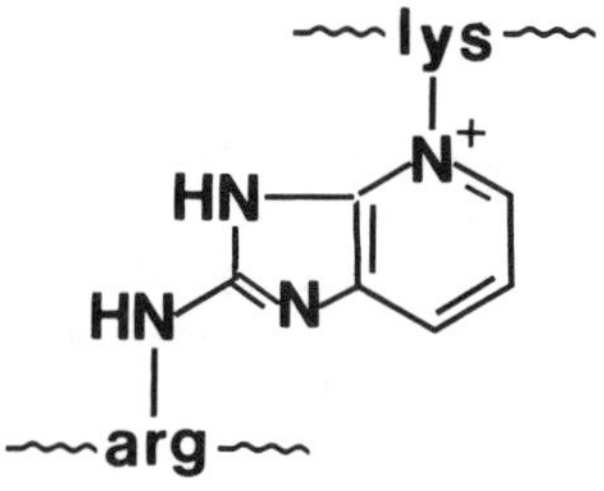

FIGURE 5.   The structure of pentosidine.

reactions.[66,67] Pentosidine increases with age and with diabetes and is not an artefact, but is present only in extremely small amounts; less than 1 in 200,000 lens crystallin lysine residues is part of a pentosidine molecule. Nevertheless, skin collagen pentosidine correlates positively with the presence of retinopathy and nephropathy in the diabetic patient and accounts for as much as 40% of total nontryptophan fluorescence in the lens.[68] Clearly, it is unlikely that fluorescence itself can be damaging, and the significance of pentosidine formation is taken to be indicative of other important (but not yet identified) protein modification reactions in diabetic tissue. Pentosidine can be referred to as a "biomarker" for related protein modifications.

XI. ARE FLUORESCENT MOLECULES PREDICTORS OF TISSUE DAMAGE?

A further complication in the analysis of tissue "browning" in diabetes is that the role of Maillard products, such as pentosidine, as causative factors in the diabetic complications is rather unclear. Although there **is** a correlation between the extent of skin collagen fluorescence and/or pentosidine with certain complications in patients, this correlation is not particularly strong ($r < 0.5$); some patients have high skin fluorescence but no diabetic complications, and vice versa.[28] Tissue fluorescence associated with products such as pentosidine are, thus, an imprecise indicator of underlying tissue damage and appears not to have a direct causative role in tissue degeneration by reason of the very low concentration of fluorescent products. Thus, although diabetes is a risk factor for cataract, there is no difference in the levels of fluorescent compounds attached to lens crystallin extracted from the cataracts of diabetic and nondiabetic patients, although the level of Amadori adducts is expectedly higher in the former group.[69] This observation suggests that it may be incorrect to assume that diabetic subjects with high fluorescence values have been exposed to a higher cumulative glycaemia than have those with lower values. It may also be wrong to assume that these fluorophores are necessarily produced by glycation. This speculation is supported by the observation that many physiologically-abundant oxidizable molecules, such as vitamin C and unsaturated fatty acids, are efficient browning and cross-linking agents *in* *vitro* when their oxidation is permitted by the presence of oxygen and trace amounts of transition metals.[70-73] For example, fluorescence and chromophore development in collagen, lens crystallin, and albumin is much more extensive with ascorbate and arachidonic acid than with glucose, and in these cases is similarly inhibited by metal-chelating agents.[74] *In vitro,* at least, browning reactions caused by a variety of aldehyde-forming molecules are dependent upon the presence of trace amounts of transition metals which catalyze the oxidative reactions required.

XII. TRANSITION METAL "DECOMPARTMENTALIZATION"

Could the presence and level of decompartmentalized transition metals *in vivo* be more important than the concentration and type of substrate available for fluorescence generation? This question was raised above with reference to Amadori adduct oxidation and the formation of CML, but becomes more pertinent when we consider the formation of pentosidine and other fluorophores. Although it is natural to believe that fluorescent molecules in diabetes would be derived from glucose reactions with protein as a result of hyperglycemia, evidence suggests that, in the case of human cataract, the major route to fluorophore and pentosidine formation is the reaction of ascorbic acid with crystallins.[75] Increased oxidation of ascorbate to dehydroascorbate and 2,3-diketogulonate followed by decarboxylation to xylosone is ostensibly the route of formation of pentosidine in human cataract (Figure 6). The formation of pentosidine under these circumstances would thus appear to be the result of a catastrophic failure of lens defense systems. The rate of ascorbate oxidation must be increased and/or the rate of reduction of dehydroascorbate to the reduced form must be decreased. There must also be a failure of the glyoxalase system to trap the ketoaldehydes 2,3-diketogulonate and xylosone. The rate of ascorbate oxidation must be relatively high, and the rate of metabolism of its oxidation products must be relatively low in order for any pentosidine to form. Of particular note is the observation that the ascorbate-dependent pathway to pentosidine formation would seem to require at least two transition metal- and oxygen-dependent steps. Baynes and colleagues[76] have similarly shown that CML is also able to form from ascorbic acid, raising the possibility that the Amadori adduct may not be the source of CML formation *in vivo*. CML, as well as pentosidine, may be the products of ascorbate oxidation.

XIII. PROTEIN MODIFICATIONS AND ASCORBATE

These observations raise serious concerns about a focus on glucose as the source of the protein modifications which are linked with long-term pathology in diabetes. Specifically, they raise the possibility that browning products, such as pentosidine, or protein-bound oxidation products, such as CML, are

ASCORBIC ACID

DEHYDROASCORBATE

2,3–DIKETOGULONATE

XYLOSONE

PENTOSIDINE

FIGURE 6.   The hypothetical route of pentosidine formation.

indirect measures of the rate of transition metal- and oxygen-dependent ox-idations *in vivo*. This conclusion may sound a little dramatic, but it is supported by several other important indirect observations.

For example, careful study of pentosidine levels in disease have shown that pentosidine levels of plasma proteins are elevated, not merely in diabetes (2.5-fold elevation), but are greatly increased also in uremia associated with end-stage renal disease (23-fold elevation).[77] Given that blood sugar levels are not elevated in uremia, it follows that factors other than hyperglycemia and glucose-derived modifications are responsible for pentosidine elevation in uremia, and not by extension, also in diabetes. Monnier[77] thus hypothesized that the increased level of dehydroascorbate in diabetes mellitus could provide an explanation for the increased levels of pentosidine in diabetes mellitus as well as in uremia.[78]

Uremia, like diabetes, is a powerful risk factor for cataract,[79] and the possibility thus arises that increased tissue pentosidine and crystallin fluo-rescence levels in cataract associated with diabetes and renal failure are the result of a systemic oxidative stress leading to high levels of dehydroascorbate in the lens. It is attractive to hypothesize that this oxidative stress could be the result of an elevated level of transition metal in a form capable of catalyzing the oxidation of ascorbic acid. Ascorbic acid is well-known to be very sus-ceptible to copper-catalyzed oxidation.[80]

XIV. TRANSITION METAL-BINDING DRUGS

Evidence consistent with increased transition metal-catalyzed oxidation as a cause of cataract is indirect. Some indications that this may be the case have, however, come from the study of inhibitors of the nicotinamide-adenine dinucleotide phosphate (reduced) (NADPH)-dependent enzyme aldose reductase. The aldose reductase inhibitors are a structurally diverse group of compounds (including flavanoids and hydantoin derivatives) which are powerful inhibitors of cataract and other complications of experimental diabetes.[81] Although believed to exert their protective effect against long-term diabetic tissue damage by blocking the accumulation of sorbitol in tissues, recent evidence has linked their effect to the inhibition of tissue browning. Suarez and colleagues,[82] for example, found that the aldose reductase inhibitor, sorbinil, inhibited collagen fluorescence in diabetic rats, an effect which they ascribed to the ability of fructose to generate fluorophores and a reduction of fructose concentration induced by the drug. This suggestion was, however, questioned by observations of the effect of sorbinil in galactosemia.

Rodents fed a diet containing high levels of galactose develop cataract which is morphologically and biochemically similar to cataract found in diabetes and which can also be blocked by aldose reductase inhibitors. There is a difference between diabetic and galactosemic cataract, however, in that there is no alteration in lens fructose levels in galactosemia. Yet sorbinil blocks crystallin fluorescence development in galactosemia[83] and prevents the accumulation of pentosidine.[84] Since there is no accumulation of fructose in galactosemia, these observations cannot be explained on any basis of fluorescence derived from fructose. A possible explanation for this effect of sorbinil was offered by the finding that some of these compounds have a secondary activity of binding free copper ions and can thereby block copper-catalyzed ascorbate oxidation.[85] The effect of these drugs in susceptible tissues in diabetes might thus be to bind free copper ions which catalyze the oxidation of ascorbic acid and other reductants. At the time of writing, there is little information about the metabolism of copper, and it is not clear how diabetes, uremia, and galactosemia could lead to an elevation of decompartmentalized redox-active copper ions. It is known, however, that total plasma copper levels are higher in diabetic individuals than in normals, and are highest in diabetics with angiopathy and alterations in lipid metabolism.[86,87] In diabetes, levels of plasma and white blood cell ascorbic acid are lower (despite similar levels of intake and excretion), and oxidation of this antioxidant to dehydroascorbate is higher than in normal individuals.[88,89] Aldose reductase inhibitors reverse the depletion of plasma ascorbic acid found in experimental diabetes, which would be consistent with a transition metal-binding effect of the drugs.[90] Oxidative stress, perhaps initiated by transition metal, may contribute to the pathogenesis of diabetes and its complications.[91,92]

XV. INFORMATION ABOUT FREE RADICALS FROM STUDIES OF GLYCATION IN DIABETES

The field of protein modification in diabetes is currently developing very rapidly. Although the focus has been on the tissue-damaging effects of chronically-elevated tissue glucose, a view is gradually emerging that free radicals and oxidative stress might have a substantial role to play in the pathogenesis of the diabetic complications. Detailed study of the chemistry of Amadori adduct formation and breakdown, as well as of the genesis of the complex browning products, indicate that transition metal-catalyzed oxidative processes appear to play a critical role and may be more than bystanders in diabetic tissue damage. Studies of glycation and the oxidation reactions associated with glycation have led to the surprising suspicion that glucose may not be a major pathogenetic factor. Yet, without these studies, there would have been no appreciation of the role of transition metals and oxidation of a wide variety of reducing agents.

A generalized theorem can now be developed which argues that diabetes is associated with a redistribution of transition metal, probably copper, into sites where the metal can catalyze the oxidation of susceptible compounds (Figure 7). The transition metal-catalyzed oxidation of low-molecular weight reductants such as ascorbate, thiols, and polyunsaturated fatty acids would contribute to oxidative stress via the production of a steady flux of hydrogen peroxide and/or lipid peroxides *in vivo*. Aldehydic products of such oxidations (such as pentosidine) appear to accumulate on long-lived proteins as an indirect measure of the rate of such oxidation. In this respect, pentosidine and similar compounds might emerge as useful markers of oxidative stress events in a wide variety of cellular insults.

XVI. CONCLUSIONS

Amadori adduct accumulation, AGE accumulation, as well as increases in tissue fluorescence, do not, in themselves, adequately explain the pathogenesis of the diabetic complications. There is, however, indirect evidence for a systemic oxidative stress in diabetic pathogenesis. Transition metal overload, with a concomitant increased oxidation rate of reducing agents and/ or lipid peroxidation, appears to be an attractive candidate for this stress.

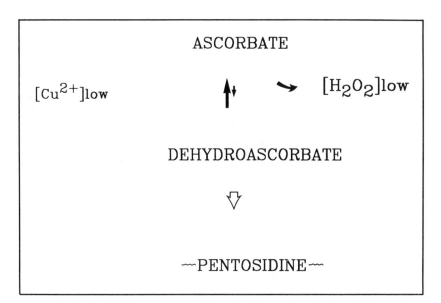

NORMAL

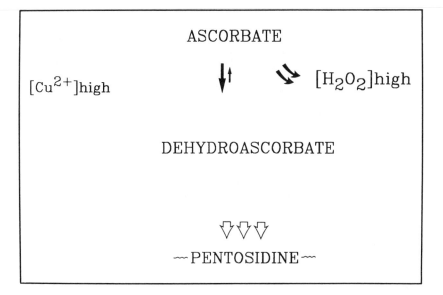

DIABETES

FIGURE 7. Decompartmentalization of transition metal in diabetes.

REFERENCES

1. **Rayfield, E. J., Ault, M. J., Keusch, G. T., Brothers, M. J., Nechemias, C., and Smith, H.,** Infection and diabetes: the case for glucose control, *Am. J. Med.,* 72, 439, 1982.
2. **Entmacher, P. S.,** Long-term prognosis in diabetes mellitus, in *Diabetes Mellitus,* Sussman, K. E. and Metz, R. J. S., Eds., American Diabetes Association, New York, 1975, 191.
3. **Entmacher, P. S., Root, H. F., and Marks, H. H.,** Longevity of diabetic patients in recent years, *Diabetes,* 13, 373, 1964.
4. **Pell, S. and D'Alonzo, C.,** Factors associated with long-term survival of diabetics, *JAMA,* 214, 1833, 1971.
5. **Deckert, T., Poulsen, J. E., and Larsen, M.,** Prognosis of diabetics with diabetes onset before the age of thirty-one, *Diabetologia,* 14, 363, 1978.
6. **Roth, M.,** "Glycated" hemoglobin, not "glycosylated" or "glucosylated", *Clin. Chem.,* 29, 1991, 1983.
7. **Njorge, F. G., Sayre, L. M., and Monnier, V. M.,** Detection of D-glucose derived pyrrole compounds during Maillard reaction under physiological conditions, *Carbohyd. Res.,* 167, 211, 1987.
8. **McLaughlin, A., Pethig, R., and Szent-Gyorgyi, A.,** Studies of the methylglyoxal-protein adduct, *Proc. Natl. Acad. Sci.,* 77, 949, 1980.
9. **Monnier, V. M.,** Toward a Maillard theory of ageing, in *The Maillard Reaction in Aging, Diabetes and Nutrition,* Baynes J. W. and Monnier, V. M., Eds., Alan R. Liss, New York, 1989, 1.
10. **Brownlee, M., Vlassara, H., and Cerami, A.,** Nonenzymatic glycosylation and the pathogenesis of the diabetic complications, *Ann. Intern. Med.,* 101, 527, 1984.
11. **Trivelli, L. A., Ranney, H. M., and Hont-Tien, L.,** Hemoglobin components in patients with diabetes mellitus, *N. Engl. J. Med.,* 284, 353, 1971.
12. **Bookchin, R. M. and Gallop, P. M.,** Structure of hemoglobin A1c: nature of the N-terminal beta chain blocking group, *Biochem. Biophys. Res. Comm.,* 32, 86, 1968.
13. **Stevens, R. J., Rouzer, C. A., and Monnier, V. M.,** Diabetic cataract formation: potential role of glycosylation of lens proteins, *Proc. Natl. Acad. Sci. U.S.A.,* 75, 2918, 1978.
14. **Kennedy, L. and Baynes, J. W.,** Nonenzymatic glycosylation and the chronic complications of diabetes: an overview, *Diabetologia,* 26, 93, 1984.
15. **Pillsbury, H. C., Hung, W., Kyle, M. C., and Freis, E. D.,** Arterial pulse waves and velocity and systolic time intervals in diabetic children, *Am. Heart J.,* 87, 783, 1974.
16. **Grgic, A., Rosenbloom, A. L., Weber, F. T., and Giordana, B.,** Joint contracture in childhood diabetes, *N. Engl. J. Med.,* 292, 372, 1975.
17. **Schuyler, M. R., Niewoehner, D. E., Inkley, S. R., and Kohn, R. R.,** Abnormal lung elasticity in juvenile diabetes mellitus, *Am. Rev. Respir. Dis.,* 113, 37, 1976.
18. **Monnier, V. M., Kohn, R. R., and Cerami, A.,** Accelerated age-related browning of human collagen in diabetes mellitus, *Proc. Natl. Acad. Sci. U.S.A.,* 81, 583, 1984.
19. **Monnier, V. M., Vishwanath, V., Frank, K. E., Elmets, C. E., Dauchot, P., and Kohn, R. R.,** Relation between complications of type I diabetes mellitus and collagen-linked fluorescence, *New Engl. J. Med.,* 314, 403, 1986.
20. **Bailey, A. J. and Kent, M. J. C.,** Non-enzymatic glycosylation of fibrous and basement membrane collagens, in *The Maillard Reaction in Aging, Diabetes and Nutrition,* Baynes, J. W. and Monnier, V. M., Eds., Alan R. Liss, New York, 1989, 109.
21. **Harding, J. J. and Furth, A.,** Why sugar is bad for you, *New Sci.,* 23rd September, 44, 1989.
22. **Shaklai, N., Garlick, R. L., and Bunn, H. F.,** Nonenzymatic glycosylation of human serum albumin alters its conformation and function, *J. Biol. Chem.,* 259, 3812, 1984.

23. **Arai, K., Maguchi, S., Fujii, S., Ishibashi, H., Oikawa, K., and Taniguchi, N.,** Glycation and inactivation of human Cu-Zn-superoxide dismutase, *J. Biol. Chem.*, 262, 16969, 1987.

24. **Arai, K., Iizuka, S., Tada, Y., Oikawa, K., and Taniguchi, N.,** Increase in the glucosylated form of erythrocyte Cu-Zn-superoxide dismutase in diabetes and close association of the non-enzymatic glucosylation with the enzyme activity, *Biochim. Biophys. Acta*, 924, 292, 1987.

25. **Monnier, V. M., Stevens, V. J., and Cerami, A.,** Non-enzymatic glycosylation, sulfhydryl oxidation, and aggregation of lens proteins in experimental sugar cataracts, *J. Exp. Med.*, 150, 1098, 1979.

26. **Harding, J. J.,** Nonenzymatic covalent post-translational modification of proteins *in vivo*, *Adv. Protein Chem.*, 129, 97, 1985.

27. **Saski, J. and Cottam, G. L.,** Glycosylation of LDL decreases its ability to interact with high-affinity receptors of human fibroblasts *in vitro* and decreases its clearance from rabbit plasma *in vivo*, *Biochim. Biophys. Acta*, 713, 199, 1982.

28. **Steinbrecher, U. P. and Witzum, J. L.,** Glucosylation of LDL to an extent comparable to that seen in diabetes slows their catabolism, *Diabetes*, 33, 130, 1984.

29. **Lopes-Virella, M. F., Klein, R. L., Lyons, T. J., and Witzum, J. L.,** Glucosylation of low density lipoprotein enhances cholesterol ester synthesis in human-monocyte derived macrophages, *Diabetes*, 37, 550, 1988.

30. **Pongor, S., Ulrich, P. C., Bencsath, F. A., and Cerami, A.,** Aging of proteins: isolation and identification of a fluorescent chromophore from the reaction of polypeptides with glucose, *Proc. Natl. Acad. Sci. U.S.A.*, 81, 2684, 1984.

31. **Vlassara, H., Brownlee, M., and Cerami, A.,** Novel macrophage receptor for glucose-modified proteins is distinct from previously described scavenger receptors, *J. Exp. Med.*, 164, 1301, 1986.

32. **Wolff, S. P., Crabbe, M. J. C., and Thornalley, P. J.,** The autoxidation of simple monosaccharides, *Experientia*, 40, 244, 1984.

33. **Wolff, S. P. and Dean, R. T.,** Glucose autoxidation and protein oxidation: the role of autoxidative glycosylation in diabetes mellitus and ageing, *Biochem. J.*, 245, 243, 1987.

34. **Wolff, S. P. and Dean, R. T.,** Aldehydes and ketoaldehydes in the non-enzymatic glycosylation of proteins, *Biochem. J.*, 249, 617, 1988.

35. **Hunt, J. V., Dean, R. T., and Wolff, S. P.,** Hydroxyl radical production and autoxidative glycosylation: glucose autoxidation as the cause of protein damage in the experimental glycation model of diabetes mellitus and ageing, *Biochem. J.*, 256, 205, 1988.

36. **Dean, R. T., Wolff, S. P., and McElligott, M. A.,** Histidine and proline are important sites of free radical damage to protein, *Free Radical Res. Commun.*, 7, 97, 1989.

37. **Hunt, J. V. and Wolff, S. P.,** The role of histidine residues in the non-enzymic covalent attachment of glucose and ascorbic acid to protein, *Free Radical Res. Commun.*, 14, 279, 1991.

38. **Jiang, Z.-Y., Woollard, A. C. S., and Wolff, S. P.,** Hydrogen peroxide production during experimental protein glycation, *FEBS Lett.*, 268, 69, 1990.

39. **Ahmed, M. U., Thorpe, S. R., and Baynes, J. W.,** Identification of N-carboxymethyllysine as a degradation product of fructoselysine in glycated protein, *J. Biol. Chem.*, 261, 4889, 1986.

40. **Dunn, J. A., Patrick, J. S., Thorpe, S. R., and Baynes, J. W.,** Oxidation of glycated proteins: age-dependent accumulation of N-epsilon(carboxymethyl)lysine in lens protein, *Biochemistry*, 28, 9464, 1989.

41. **Dunn, J. A., McCance, D. R., Thorpe, S. R., Lyons, T. J., and Baynes, J. W.,** Age-dependent accumulation of N-(carboxymethyl)lysine and N-(carboxymethyl)hydroxylysine in human skin collagen, *Biochemistry*, 30, 1205, 1991.

42. **Dyer, D. G., Dunn, J. A., Thorpe, S. R., Bailie, K. E., Lyons, T. J., McCance, D. R., and Baynes, J. W.,** Accumulation of Maillard reaction products in skin collagen in diabetes and aging, *J. Clin. Invest.*, in press.

43. **McCance, D. R., Dyer, D. G., Dunn, J. A., Bailie, K. E., Thorpe, S. R., Baynes, J. W., and Lyons, T. J.**, Maillard reaction products and their relation to complications in insulin dependent diabetes mellitus, *J. Clin. Invest.*, in press.

44. **Baynes, J. W.**, Role of oxidative stress in development of complications in diabetes, *Diabetes*, 40, 405, 1991.

45. **Cheng, R.-Z., Tsunehiro, J., Uchida, K., and Kawakishi, S.**, Oxidative damage of glycated protein in the presence of transition metal ion, *Agric. Biol. Chem.*, 55, 1993, 1991.

46. **Kawakishi, S., Tsunehiro, J., and Uchida, K.**, Autoxidative degradation of Amadori compounds in the presence of copper ion, *Carb. Res.*, 211, 167, 1991.

47. **Wolff, S. P. and Dean, R. T.**, Monosaccharide autoxidation: a potential source of oxidative stress in diabetes? Model reactions with nucleotides and protein *Bioelectrochem. Bioenerg.*, 18, 283, 1988.

48. **Gascoyne, P. R. C.**, Electron spin resonance and spectral studies of bovine serum albumin-methylglyoxal complexes., *Int. J. Quant. Chem.: Quant. Biol. Symp.*, 7, 93, 1980.

49. **Hunt, J. V. and Wolff, S. P.**, Oxidative glycation and free radical production: a causal mechanism of diabetic complications? *Free Radical Res. Commun.*, 12–13, 115, 1991.

50. **Hunt, J. V., Smith, C. C. T., and Wolff, S. P.**, Autoxidative glycosylation and possible involvement of peroxides and free radicals in LDL modification by glucose, *Diabetes*, 39, 1420, 1990.

51. **Sakurai, T., Kimura, S., Nakano, M., and Kimura, H.**, Oxidative modification of glycated low density lipoprotein in the presence of iron, *Biochem. Biophys. Res. Comm.*, 177, 433, 1991.

52. **Jessup, W., Jurgens, G., Lang, J., Esterbauer, H., and Dean, R. T.**, Interaction of 4-hydroxynonenal-modified low-density lipoproteins with the fibroblast apolipoprotein B/E receptor, *Biochem. J.*, 234, 245, 1986.

53. **Yagi, K.**, A biochemical approach to atherogenesis, *Trends Bio. Sci.*, 11, 18, 1986.

54. **Babiy, A. V., Gebicki, J. M., Sullivan, D. R., and Willey, K.**, Increased oxidizability of plasma lipoproteins in diabetic patients can be decreased by probucol therapy and is not due to glycation, *Biochem. Pharmacol.*, 43, 995, 1992.

55. **Shapiro, R., McManus, M. J., Zalut, C., and Bunn, H. F.**, Sites of non-enzymatic glycosylation of human hemoglobin A, *J. Biol. Chem.*, 255, 3120, 1980.

56. **Baynes, J. W., Watkins, N. G., Fisher, C. I., Hull, C. J., Patrick, J. S., Ahmed, M. U., Dunn, J. A., and Thorpe, S. R.**, The Amadori product on protein: structure and reactions, in *The Maillard Reaction in Aging, Diabetes and Nutrition*, Monnier, V. M. and Baynes, J. W., Eds., Alan R. Liss, New York, 1989, 43.

57. **Vishwanath, V., Frank, K. E., Elmets, C. A., Dauchot, P. J., and Monnier, V. M.**, Glycation of skin collagen in Type I diabetes mellitus: correlation with long-term complications, *Diabetes*, 35, 916, 1986.

58. **Ledl, F., Fritsch, G., Hiebl, J., Parchmayer, O., and Severin, T.**, Degradation of Maillard products, in *Amino-Carbonyl Reactions in Food and Biological Systems*, Fujimaki, M., Namiki, M., and Kato, H., Eds., Dev. Fd. Sci., Elsevier, Amsterdam, 1985, 173.

59. **Kato, H., Hayase, F., Shin, D. B., Oimimi, M., and Baba, S.**, 3-deoxyglucosone, an intermediate product of the Maillard reaction, in *The Maillard Reaction in Aging, Diabetes and Nutrition*, Baynes, J. W. and Monnier, V. M., Eds., Alan R. Liss, New York, 1989, 69.

60. **Njoroge, F. G. and Monnier, V. M.**, The chemistry of the Maillard reaction under physiological conditions: a review, in *The Maillard Reaction in Aging, Diabetes and Nutrition*, Baynes, J. W. and Monnier, V. M., Eds., Alan R. Liss, New York, 1989, 85.

61. **Njoroge, F. G., Fernandes, A. A., and Monnier, V. M.**, Mechanism of formation of the putative advanced glycosylation end product and protein crosslink 2-(2-Furoyl)-4(5)-(2-furanyl)-H-imidazole, *J. Biol. Chem.*, 263, 10646, 1988.

62. **Horiuchi, S., Shiga, M., Araki, N., Takata, K., Saitoh, M., and Morino, Y.,** Evidence against *in vivo* presence of 2-(2-furoyl)-4(5)-(2-furanyl)-1H-imidazole, a major fluorescent advanced end product generated by non-enzymatic glycosylation, *J. Biol. Chem.,* 263, 18821, 1990.

63. **Lapolla, A., Gerhardinger, C., Pelli, B., Sturaro, A., Del Favero, E., Traldi, P., Crepaldi, G., and Fedele, D.,** Absence of brown product FFI in nondiabetic and diabetic rat collagen, *Diabetes,* 39, 57, 1990.

64. **Sell, D. R. and Monnier, V. M.,** Structure elucidation of a senescence crosslink from human extracellular matrix: implication of pentoses in the aging process, *J. Biol. Chem.,* 264, 21597, 1989.

65. **Sell, D. R. and Monnier, V. M.,** End-stage renal disease and diabetes catalyze the formation of a pentose-derived cross link from aging human collagen, *J. Biol. Chem.,* 85, 380, 1990.

66. **Grandhee, S. K. and Monnier, V. M.,** Mechanism of formation of the Maillard protein crosslink pentosidine: glucose, fructose and ascorbate as pentosidine precursors, *J. Biol. Chem.,* 266, 11649, 1991.

67. **Dyer, D. G., Blackledge, J. A., Thorpe, S. R., and Baynes, J. W.,** Formation of pentosidine during non-enzymatic browning of proteins by glucose: identification of glucose and other carbohydrates as possible precursors of pentosidine *in vivo, J. Biol. Chem.,* 266, 11654, 1991.

68. **Sell, D. R., Lapolla, A., Odetti, P., Fogarty, J., and Monnier, V. M.,** Pentosidine formation in skin correlates with severity of complications in individuals with long-standing insulin-dependent diabetes mellitus, *Diabetes,* in press.

69. **Oimimi, M., Maeda, Y., Hata, F., Kitamura, Y., Matsumoto, S., Baba, S., Iga, T., and Yamamoto, M.,** Glycation of cataractous lens in non-diabetic senile subjects and in diabetic patients, *Exp. Eye Res.,* 46, 415, 1988.

70. **Gutteridge, J. M. C.,** Age pigments and free radicals: fluorescent lipid complexes formed by iron- and copper-containing proteins, *Biochim. Biophys. Acta,* 834, 144, 1985.

71. **Ortwerth, B. J., Feather, M. S., and Olesen, P. R.,** The precipitation and cross-linking of lens crystallins by ascorbic acid, *Exp. Eye Res.,* 47, 155, 1988.

72. **Koller, E., Quehenberger, O., Jurgens, G., Wolfbeis, O. S., and Esterbauer, H.,** Investigation of human plasma low density lipoprotein by three-dimensional fluorescence spectroscopy, *FEBS Lett.,* 198, 229, 1986.

73. **Ortwerth, B. J. and Olesen, P. R.,** Ascorbic acid-induced crosslinking of lens proteins: evidence supporting a Maillard reaction, *Biochim. Biophys. Acta,* 956, 10, 1988.

74. **Wolff, S. P. and Hunt, J. V.,** Is glucose the sole source of tissue browning in diabetes mellitus?, *FEBS Lett.,* 269, 258, 1990.

75. **Nagaraj, R. H., Dell, D. R., Prabhakaram, M., Ortwerth, B. J., and Monnier, V. M.,** High correlation between pentosidine crosslinks and pigmentation implicates ascorbate oxidation in human lens senescence and cataractogenesis, *Proc. Natl. Acad. Sci. U.S.A.,* 88, 10257, 1991.

76. **Dunn, J. A., Ahmed, M. U., Murtiashaw, M. H., Richardson, J. M., Walla, M. D., Thorpe, S. R., and Baynes, J. W.,** Reaction of ascorbate with lysine and protein under autoxidising conditions: formation of N-(carboxymethyl)lysine by reaction between lysine and products of autoxidation of ascorbate, *Biochemistry,* 29, 10964, 1990.

77. **Odetti, P., Fogarty, J., Sell, D. R., and Monnier, V. M.,** Chromatographic quantitation of plasma and erythrocyte pentosidine in diabetic and uremic subjects, *Diabetes,* 41, 153, 1992.

78. **Chatterjee, I. B. and Banerjee, A.,** Estimation of dehydroascorbic acid in blood of diabetic patients, *Anal. Biochem.,* 98, 368, 1979.

79. **Harding, J. J. and van Heyningen, R.,** Epidemiology and risk factors for cataract, *Eye,* 1, 537, 1987.

80. **Buettner, G. R.,** In the absence of catalytic metals ascorbate does not autoxidize at pH 7: ascorbate as a test for catalytic metals, *J. Biochem. Biophys. Res. Meth.,* 16, 27, 1988.

81. **Dvornik, D. and Porte, D.**, *Aldose Reductase Inhibition: An Approach to the Prevention of Diabetic Complications,* McGraw-Hill, New York, 1987.
82. **Suarez, G., Rajaram, R., Bhuyan, K. C., Oronsky, A. L., and Giodji, J. A.**, Administration of an aldose reductase inhibitor induces a decrease of collagen fluorescence in diabetic rats, *J. Clin. Invest.,* 82, 624, 1988.
83. **Nagaraj, R. and Monnier, V. M.**, Non-tryptophan fluorescence and high molecular weight protein formation in lens crystallins of rats with chronic galactosaemia: prevention by the aldose reductase inhibitor sorbinil, *Exp. Eye Res.,* 51, 411, 1990.
84. **Nagaraj, R. H., Prabhakaram, M., Ortwerth, B. J., and Monnie, V. M.**, Aldose reductase inhibition suppresses the advanced Maillard reaction in galactosaemic rat lens, in press.
85. **Jiang, Z.-Y., Qiong, L.-Z., Eaton, J. W., Hunt, J. V., Koppenol, W. H., and Wolff, S. P.**, Spirohydantoin inhibitors of aldose reductase inhibit iron- and copper-catalysed ascorbate oxidation *in vitro, Biochem. Pharmacol.,* 42, 1273, 1991.
86. **Mateo, M. C. M., Bustamante, J. B., and Cantalapiedra, M. A. G.**, Serum zinc, copper and insulin in diabetes mellitus, *Biomedical,* 29, 56, 1978.
87. **Noto, R., Alicata, R., and Sfogliano, L.**, A study of cupremia in a group of elderly diabetics, *Acta Diabetol. Latina* 20, 81, 1983.
88. **Jennings, P. E., Chirico, S., Jones, A. F., Lunec, J., and Barnett, A. H.**, Vitamin C metabolites and microangiopathy in diabetes mellitus, *Diabetes Res.,* 6, 151, 1987.
89. **Som, S., Basu, D., Mukherjee, S., Deb, S., Choudary, P. R., Mukherjee, S. N., Chatterjee, S. N., and Chatterjee, I. B.**, Ascorbic acid metabolism in diabetes mellitus, *Metabolism,* 30, 572, 1981.
90. **Yue, K., McLennan, S., Fisher, E., Heffernan, S., Capogreco, C., Ross, G. R., and Turtle, J. R.**, Ascorbic acid metabolism and polyol pathway in diabetes, *Diabetes,* 38, 257, 1989.
91. **Oberley, L. W.**, Free radicals and diabetes, *Free Radical Biol. Med.,* 5, 113, 1988.
92. **Wolff, S. P.**, The potential role of oxidative stress in diabetes and its complications: novel implications for theory and therapy, in *Diabetic Complications: Scientific and Clinical Aspects,* Crabbe, M. J. C., Ed., Churchill Livingstone, Edinburgh, 1987, 167.

Chapter 7

AGE-RELATED ALTERATIONS IN ANTIOXIDANT DEFENSE

Mitsuyoshi Matsuo

TABLE OF CONTENTS

0-8493-4518-9/93/$0.00 + $.50

I. OXIDATIVE STRESS AND ANTIOXIDANT DEFENSE

The Earth is surrounded by an atmosphere containing about 21% molecular oxygen. Molecular oxygen is a causative factor for oxidation, in particular an essential factor for oxygenation. Oxygenation is usually exothermic and, hence, can thermodynamically occur in every place on this planet. This means that organisms live under an oxidative environment.

Aerobic organisms obtain energy efficiently through respiration. Respiration can release much of the 686 kcal of energy produced by the complete oxidation of 1 mol glucose to carbon dioxide and water, while fermentation releases only a small fraction of 47 kcal from the conversion of 1 mol glucose to lactate. Aerobic organisms, including human beings, maintain their high activity by respiration and cannot exist without molecular oxygen. On the other hand, it has long been known that molecular oxygen is toxic. For example, anaerobes such as several *Clostridium* species are killed in the presence of molecular oxygen. Furthermore, when maintained under 100% oxygen, rats die within about 3 d. Thus, in exchange for having high activity, aerobic organisms are always exposed to oxidative stress due to molecular oxygen and related substances.

From a chemical viewpoint, respiration is a series of one-electron reductions by which molecular oxygen is converted into water. It has been suggested that in the electron transport chain of mitochondria, molecular oxygen is reduced in turn to the superoxide radical (O_2^-), hydrogen peroxide (H_2O_2), the hydroxyl radical ($HO\cdot$), and lastly to water (H_2O). The superoxide radical, hydrogen peroxide, and the hydroxyl radical are so-called active oxygen species, and the superoxide radical and the hydroxyl radical also are free radicals. If these reactive species are generated *in vivo* in the absence of any control, they must cause oxidative stress.

When oxidative stress causes lethal damage to organisms, they cannot survive. To avert damage, aerobic organisms are thought to have acquired both antioxidant defense mechanisms and oxidative damage-repairing mechanisms during evolution. Antioxidant defense is composed of both antioxidant enzymes and biological antioxidants. Antioxidant enzymes include superoxide dismutase (SOD: e.g., copper/zinc and manganese SODs) which dismutates the superoxide radical to molecular oxygen and hydrogen peroxide, catalase which decomposes hydrogen peroxide to molecular oxygen and water, glutathione peroxidase which reduces hydroperoxides to alcohols and also reduces hydrogen peroxide to water, glutathione S-transferase which reduces hydroperoxides to alcohols, and so forth.

Biological antioxidants include water-soluble antioxidants, such as glutathione (the reduced form: GSH, the oxidized form: GSSG); ascorbic acid and uric acid, and fat-soluble antioxidants, such as vitamin E (mainly α-tocopherol), ubiquinones, and carotenoids. Glutathione is one of the most abundant biological reductants and acts as a thiol reagent converting disulfides to thiols and as a substrate for antioxidant enzymes, including glutathione peroxidase and glutathione S-transferase. Ascorbic acid is another abundant biological reductant. Uric acid and carotenoids are presumed to behave as singlet-oxygen quenchers and radical scavengers. Vitamin E and ubiquinones exist mainly in biomembranes and function as radical scavengers.

Oxidative damage-repairing mechanisms are also thought to be necessary for the maintenance of homeostasis in organisms. Oxidized DNA may be repaired by the action of enzymes such as endonuclease and glycosylase. Oxidized proteins may be removed by proteases. Oxidized lipids may be reduced by glutathione peroxidase directly or after hydrolysis with phospholipase.

When antioxidant defense mechanisms and oxidative damage-repairing mechanisms work, aerobic organisms can avoid damage due to active oxygen species and free radicals. It is hardly presumed, however, that such mechanisms can absolutely prevent biological systems from damage. Based on superoxide radical generation *in vitro* in the mitochondria and microsomes of rat lungs and livers, the formation rate of oxygen radicals is estimated to be about 50 nmol/g of tissue per min or about 10^{11} radicals per cell per day.[1] Fraga et al.[2] calculated that 8.6×10^4 oxidized DNA residues are formed in one cell in a day, and estimated from a comparison of the amount of oxidized DNA residues and the number of oxygen radicals produced that one oxidized DNA residue is formed for every 7.6×10^5 oxygen radicals generated through aerobic cellular metabolism.

Active oxygen species and free radicals that escape the antioxidant mechanisms may cause oxidative damage, and oxidative damage that escapes the repair mechanisms may cause deteriorative alteration. If this is the case, unfavorable balances between oxidative stress and antioxidant defense and inabilities in repair functions may accelerate the aging rate. Active oxygen species and free radicals derived from normal metabolism may be involved in the aging process.

II. RELEVANCE TO EVOLUTION

Animals have species-specific life-spans and also species-specific metabolic rates (oxygen consumption rates). Interestingly, the maximum life-span of animal species is inversely correlated with the oxygen consumption rate, as shown in Figure 1. The longer the maximum life-span of an animal species is, the lower its oxygen consumption rate is. It is assumed that in animals having a high oxygen consumption rate, the leakage of active oxygen species from antioxidant defense mechanisms may be greater. This leads to the view that the magnitude of oxidative stress is species-specific, which produces species-specific life-spans. According to Sohal et al.,[3,4] the formation rates of the superoxide radical and hydrogen peroxide are higher in the liver mitochondria of mammalian species having shorter life-spans. For example, the production rate of the superoxide radical in rat mitochondria is about six times that in cow mitochondria.

If the amount of oxidative stress to animals depends on their oxygen consumption rate, oxidative damage may accumulate more in animals having a shorter maximum lifespan. It has been observed that in animals, trace amounts of oxidized DNA bases, such as thymine glycol and 8-hydroxy-guanine, are always excreted in urine. Ames and his associates[5,6] presumed that oxidized DNA bases result from the hazardous oxidation of DNA due to oxidative stress, and, thus, their production rates can be used as indices of oxidative damage. They reported that the excretion rates of thymine glycol and thymidine glycol into urine are 0.39 and 0.15 nmol/kg body weight per day for a white male; 1.1 and 1.0 nmol/kg body weight per day for male monkeys *Macaca fascicularis;* 5.5 and 1.7 nmol/kg body weight per day for male Sprague-Dawley rats; and 6.0 and 2.6 nmol/kg body weight per day for male C3H mice, respectively. The excretion rates of the oxidative DNA fragments into urine are higher in short-lived animals than in long-lived animals and are proportional to the oxygen consumption rate of these animals. This is consistent with the view that short-lived animals have higher oxygen consumption rates, which may cause increases in the leakage of active oxygen species from antioxidant defense and in oxidative damage.

There are interesting observations on the relationships between the maximum life-spans of animal species and the SOD activity levels in their tissues. According to Tolmasoff et al.,[7] the ratio of the specific SOD activity (units per milligram of protein) of the liver, brain, or heart homogenates in a given animal species to the specific metabolic rate (calorie per gram weight per day) of the animal species increases with its increasing maximum life-span.

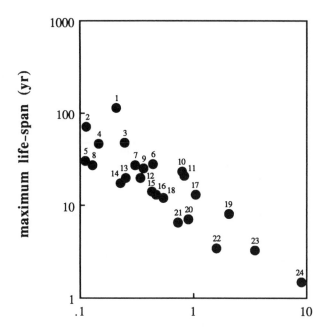

oxygen consumption rate (ml/g body wt/hr)

FIGURE 1. Maximum life-span vs. oxygen consumption rate. Numbers indicate the following species: 1, human (*Homo sapiens:* Caucasian); 2, Asian elephant (*Elephas maximus*); 3, chimpanzee (*Pan troglodytes*); 4, horse (*Equus caballus*); 5, bovine (*Bos taurus*); 6, cat (*Felis catus*); 7, chacma baboon (*Papio ursinus*); 8, European wild hog (*Sus scrofa*); 9, Atlantic bottle-nose dolphin (*Tursiops truncatus*); 10, grey squirrel (*Sciurus carolinensis*); 11, squirrel monkey (*Saimiri sciureus*); 12, dog (*Canis familaris*); 13, sheep (*Ovis aries*); 14, white-tailed deer (*Odocoileus virginianus*); 15, fox (*Vulpes vulpes*); 16, rabbit (*Oryctolagus cuniculus*); 17, red-crested barefaced tamarin (*Saguinus geoffroyi*); 18, common marmot (*Marmota marmota*); 19, deer rat (*Peromyscus maniculatus*); 20, plains pocket gopher (*Geomys bursarius*); 21, European hedgehog (*Erinaceus europaeus*); 22, mouse (*Mus musculus*); 23, short-tailed shrew (*Blarina brevicauda*); 24, sorex (life-span: *Sorex palustris,* oxygen consumption: *Sorex cinereus*). (Data for maximum life-spans and oxygen consumption rates of mammals are plotted based on: Altman, P. L. and Ditter, D. S., *Biology Data Book,* 2nd ed., Vol. I and Vol. III, *Fed. Am. Societies for Experimental Biology,* Bethesda, MD, 1972, 229; 1974, 1613; Jones, M. L., *The List of Maximum Life-Spans of Caught Mammals,* Zoological Society of San Diego, CA, 1979.)

In animals whose normal metabolism provides efficient antioxidant defense against active oxygen species, aging seems to be retarded. Ono and Okada[8] compared the brain activity levels of six enzymes, including SOD, lactate dehydrogenase, glucose-6-phosphate dehydrogenase, glutamic oxalacetic transaminase, creatine phosphokinase, and choline esterase, in each of 11 mammalian species having different maximum life-spans. Among these enzymes, only SOD shows a positive correlation between their enzyme activity levels and their maximum life-span. These findings suggest that SOD is a unique enzyme, the activity of which correlates with maximum life-span.

In order to examine the relationships between the maximum life-span and the antioxidant capacities of six different mammalian species with maximum life-spans ranging from 3.5 to 30 years, Sohal et al.[9] measured the activities of SOD, catalase, and glutathione peroxidase, and the concentrations of glutathione in the liver, heart, and brain. With relatively high correlation coefficients, the maximum life-span is positively correlated with the SOD activity level of the livers, the catalase activity level of the hearts, and the glutathione peroxidase activity levels of the brains, and negatively correlated with the glutathione concentration level of the livers and brains. Except for the above cases, however, correlations between maximum life-span and the levels of antioxidant enzyme activity and biological antioxidant concentration are insignificant.

Furthermore, Cutler[10] examined the relationships between the maximum life-span of mammalian species and the activity levels of antioxidant enzymes other than SOD. The maximum life-span is not correlated with the ratios of the catalase activity levels of the brains and kidneys or the glutathione peroxidase activity levels of the brains and livers to the specific metabolic rate, negatively correlated with the ratio of the catalase activity level of livers, and positively correlated with the ratio of the ceruloplasmin activity level of plasma. Ceruloplasmin is a copper-containing antioxidant enzyme. Cutler[10] also examined the relationships between the maximum life-span of mammalian species and the concentrations of biological antioxidants. The maximum life-span is correlated with the ratios of the α-tocopherol, urate, and carotenoid concentration levels of plasma or the ascorbate concentration level of brains to the specific metabolic rate, while it is not correlated with ratios of the ascorbate concentration levels of the livers and lenses or the glutathione concentration levels of blood, brains, and livers to the specific metabolic rate. He reported that in the brain and kidney homogentes from long-lived animals, the reaction rates and substrate concentration levels of autoxidation are lower.[11]

These observations suggest that decreases in the metabolic rate and oxidative DNA damage and an increase in antioxidant capacity are advantageous for longevity, although there are inconsistencies in the results of studies on the relationships between maximum life-span and antioxidant capacities in mammalian species. Oxidative stress may act as a life-span-shortening factor.

III. ANTIOXIDANT DEFENSE

A. RODENTS

For most laboratories, mice and rats are the only mammals which can be used for aging research because old mammals, other than these rodents, are difficult to supply and are very expensive. Thus, the observations of age-related alterations in antioxidant defense have so far been made using mice and rats.

TABLE 1
Age-Related Changes in the Superoxide Dismutase Activity Levels of Mouse Tissues

Strains	Gender	Brain	Liver	Heart	Ref.
C57BL/6J	male	↓			13
C57BL/6J	n.d.[a]	→[b]	↓[c]	→	12
LP/J	male	→	→		15
A/J	male	→	→		
CBF$_1$	male		→[e]		14
Swiss	female	↑[df] →[g]	↑[df] →[g]		19
C3B10RF$_1$	female		→		17
BALB/c	female		→		18

[a] No description.
[b] →, No change.
[c] ↓, Decrease.
[d] ↑, Increase.
[e] Purified enzyme.
[f] Based on 3-month-old mice.
[g] Based on 6-month-old mice.

1. Antioxidant Enzymes in Rodents
a. Superoxide Dismutase
1. Mice

As shown in Table 1, several reports have been published on age-related alterations in the SOD activity levels of mouse brains, livers, and hearts. Reiss and Gershon[12] reported that as C57 BL/6J mice age, the SOD activity level in liver homogenates decreases considerably, and the level of heart homogenates decreases slightly, while the level in brain homogenates remains unchanged. In comparing equal amounts of SOD activity in tissue homogenates from 8- and 28-month-old mice, a larger quantity of rabbit antiserum prepared against rat liver SOD is required to precipitate a given amount of enzyme activity from tissue homogenates of old mice than from those of young mice. There may be a considerable decline in catalytic activity per antigenic unit in the brains, livers, and hearts of old mice. Massie et al.[13] described, however, that the SOD activity level of brain homogenates from 30-month-old male C57 BL/6J mice decreases by more than 30% from that in brain homogenates from 1.7-month-old mice.

SOD was purified by gel filtration and ion exchange chromatographies from the liver cytoplasm of male CBF$_1$ mice.[14] The specific activities of purified SOD from the livers of 3- and 24-month-old mice are identical. In addition, no cross-reacting material is accumulated in the SOD from 24-month-old mice.

Kellogg and Fridovich[15] assayed the SOD activity levels of tissue homogenates from short-lived male A/J and long-lived male LP/J mice. The mean life-spans of male A/J and LP/J mice are 16 and 25 months, respectively. The SOD activity levels in the brains and livers of both strains increase for one month after birth and then remained unchanged until the end of the life-span. At nine months of age, the SOD activity levels in the brain and lung are higher in LP/J mice than in A/J mice, although no significant differences were found between the levels in the heart, kidney, liver, or spleen.

Furthermore, it has been reported that there are no differences between the liver SOD activity levels of 6- and 12-month-old female Swiss mice,[19] 12- and 24-month-old female C3B10 RF$_1$ mice,[17] or 14- and 27-month-old female BALB/c mice,[16,18] or between the brain levels in 6- and 12-month-old female Swiss mice.[19]

2. Rats

As shown in Table 2, there are many reports on age-related alterations in the SOD activity levels of rat tissues. The rat strains examined include Fischer 344, Wistar, Sprague-Dawley, and Donryu strains. It has been observed that during aging, the SOD activity levels of the brains, livers, lungs, hearts, kidneys, intestinal mucosae, and muscles remain unchanged or decrease with three exceptions: increases were found in the mitochondrial SOD activity levels of the brains and muscles and in the cytoplasmic SOD activity level of the lungs.

Richardson and his associates[20-22] reported that in male Fischer 344 rats, the cytoplasmic SOD activity levels of the brains, hearts, hepatocytes, intestinal mucosae, and kidneys decrease by 28, 52, 55, 33, and 22%, respectively, between 6- and 24 to 26 months of age, and a large decrease of about 45% in the SOD activity of hepatocytes occurs between 6 and 16 months of age. They also reported that the SOD mRNA levels of the brains, livers, hepatocytes, and kidneys decrease by 33, 37, 48, and 28%, respectively, between 5 to 6 and 23 to 26 months of age. Ansari et al.[23] observed that in male Fischer 344 rats, the total SOD activity levels of the cerebrums, basal ganglia, cerebellums, medullae, or cervical cords are not different at 3, 12, and 22 months of age. Ischiropoulos et al.[24] found that in male Fischer 344 rats, the cytoplasmic SOD activity level of the lungs increases slightly, and the mitochondrial SOD activity level of the lungs decreases between 4 to 5 and 24 months of age. Matsuo et al.[25] showed that in female Fischer 344 rats, the total SOD activity levels of the brains, livers, or lungs are not different at 8, 14, 26, and 32 months of age (Figure 2).

It has been observed that in Wistar rats, the total, cytoplasmic, and mitochondrial SOD levels of the brains, livers, lungs, hearts, and kidneys remain unchanged or decrease during aging.[12,26-34] Reiss and Gershon[26] purified cytoplasmic SOD from the livers of 6- and 27-month-old Wistar rats.

TABLE 2
Age-Related Changes in the Superoxide Dismutase Activity Levels of Rat Tissues

Strain	Gender	Enzyme source	Brain	Liver	Lung	Heart	Kidney	Intestine[a]	Muscle	Ref.
Fischer 344	male	cytoplasm	↓[b]	↓		↓	↓	↓		20,21,22
Fischer 344	male	total	→[c]							23
Fischer 344 or Sprague Dawley	male	cytoplasm			↑[d]					24
		mitochondria			↓					
Fischer 344	female	total	→	→	→					25
Wistar	male	cytoplasm	↓							27
		mitochondria	↑							
Wistar	male	cytoplasm		↓						28
		mitochondria		→						
Wistar	male	mitochondria				→				29
Wistar	male	total	↓							30
Wistar	male	total	→	→						31
Wistar	male	total			↓					32
Wistar	female	cytoplasm		↓						33
Wistar	female	total	→	↓		→	↓			34
Wistar	n.d.[e]	total	→	↓		→				12,26
Sprague Dawley	male	cytoplasm	→	→						15
		mitochondria	→	↓						
Sprague Dawley	male	cytoplasm							→	35
		mitochondria							↑	
Donryu	male	total	→	→						36

[a] Intestinal mucosa.
[b] ↓ , Decrease.
[c] → , No change.
[d] ↑ , Increase.
[e] No description.

From Matsuo, M., et al., *Mech. Ageing Dev.*, 64, 286, 1992. With permission.

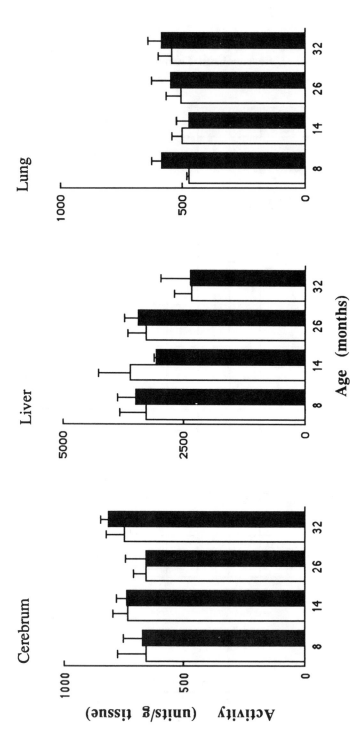

FIGURE 2. Variations in superoxide dismutase activity as a function of age. Superoxide dismutase activities in the cerebrum, liver, and lung homogenates from normal (open columns) and vitamin E-deficient (closed columns) rats are shown. Each column represents a mean value of three samples from three rats. Each small bar represents the standard error of the estimate of a mean value. (From Matsuo, M., et al., *Mech. Ageing Dev.*, 64, 277, 1992. With permission.)

The specific activity of the purified SOD from old rats is about 40% of that from young rats, in contrast with no age-dependent decrease in the specific activity of purified liver SOD from male CBF_1 mice.[14] In the SOD from old rats, antigenically cross-reacting material is accumulated, and thermostability is reduced. No differences were found, however, in the molecular weight, electrophoretic mobility, antigenicity, or inhibition constant for cyanide between the SODs from young and old rats. Interestingly, Vanella et al.[27] reported that the cytoplasmic SOD activity level of cerebral cortices in male Wistar rats decreases with advancing age, and the level at 30 months of age is about one tenth of that at 1 month of age; on the contrary, they found that the mitochondrial SOD activity level increases with advancing age, and that the level at 30 months of age is about 2.5 times that at 1 month of age.

For Sprague-Dawley rats, the cytoplasmic and mitochondrial SOD activity levels of the brains, livers,[15] and muscles[35] were measured. The cytoplasmic SOD activity of those tissues remains unchanged during aging, while the mitochondrial SOD activity level of livers decreases and that of muscles increases.

The total SOD activity levels of the brains and livers in Donryu rats remain unchanged.[36]

These results contain many conflicting findings. This may arise from differences in the strains and maintenance conditions of the mice and rats and in the experimental conditions used, because SOD is thought to be readily induced by oxidative stress.[37]

b. Catalase
1. Mice

Only a few reports have been published on age-related alterations in the catalase activity levels of mouse tissues. In female $C3B10F_1$ mice of a long-lived F_1 hybrid strain, the catalase activity level of the livers remains unchanged between 12 and 24 months of age.[17] In female BALB/c mice, however, the catalase activity level of the livers decreases between 14 and 27 months of age.[18]

2. Rats

Table 3 shows the previously reported age-related alterations in the catalase activity levels of the brains, livers, lungs, hearts, kidneys, and intestines in Fischer 344 and Wistar rats.[20-23,25,28,29,32-34,38] Rao et al.[21] reported that in male Fischer 344 rats, the catalase activity levels of the brains, livers, and kidneys decrease by 38, 55, and 50%, respectively, between 6 and 24 to 26 months of age; that of hearts increases by 38%; and that of intestinal mucosae remains unchanged. They also reported that the catalase mRNA levels of the brains, livers, hepatocytes, and kidneys decrease by 28, 39, 48, and 55%, respectively, between 5 to 6 and 23 to 26 months of age. Matsuo et al.[25] observed that in female Fischer 344 rats, the catalase activity level of the

TABLE 3
Age-Related Changes in the Catalase Activity Levels of Rat Tissues

Strain	Gender	Brain	Liver	Lung	Heart	Kidney	Intestine[a]	Ref.
Fischer 344	male	↓[b]	↓		↑[d]	↓	→[c]	20,21,22
Fischer 344	male	→						23
Fischer 344	male		↓					38
Fischer 344	female	→	↓	→				25
Wistar	male		↑[e] →[f]					28
Wistar	male			→				32
Wistar	male				↑[g]			29
Wistar	female	↓	↓		↑	↓		34
Wistar	female		↓					33

a   Intestinal mucosa.
b   ↓ , Decrease.
c   →, No change.
d   ↑ , Increase.
e   Mitochondria with peroxisomes.
f   Cytoplasm.
g   Mitochondria.

From Matsuo, M., et al., *Mech. Ageing Dev.,* 64, 287, 1992. With permission.

livers decreases by 38% between 8 to 14 and 32 months of age, although the catalase activity levels of the brains and lungs remain unchanged (Figure 3).

It has been described that in male Wistar rats, the catalase activity levels of liver cytoplasm[28] and the lungs[32] remain unchanged, and those of the liver[28] and heart[29] mitochondria increase during aging. Nohl et al.[29] reported that in male Wistar rats, the catalase activity level of heart mitochondria increases by 60% between 3 and 24 months of age. On the other hand, Cand and Verdetti[34] found that in female Wistar rats, the catalase activity level of the hearts increases by 41% between 4 and 24 months of age, although those of the brains, livers, and kidneys remain unchanged. Pieri et al.[33] found, however, that in female Wistar rats, the catalase activity level of the livers decreases by 31% between 6 and 24 months of age. It should be noted that age-related decreases in the catalase activity levels of the livers and kidneys and an age-related increase in the level of the hearts have been observed in different laboratories.

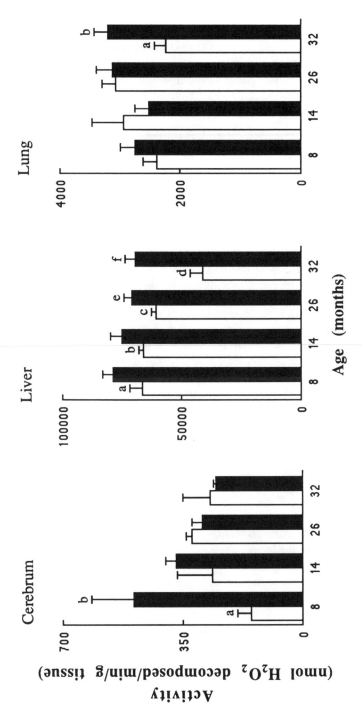

FIGURE 3. Variations in catalase activity as a function of age. Catalase activities in the cerebrum, liver, and lung homogenates from normal (open columns) and vitamin E-deficient (closed columns) rats are shown. Each column represents a mean value of three samples from three rats. Each small bar represents the standard error of the estimate of a mean value. Differences between pairs of means indicated by the following paired letters are statistically significant ($p \le 0.05$): for cerebrum, ab; for liver, ad, bd, cd, ce and df; for lung, ab. (From Matsuo, M., et al., *Mech. Ageing Dev.*, 64, 278, 1992. With permission.)

c. Glutathione Peroxidase
1. Mice
There are only a few reports on age-related alterations in the glutathione peroxidase activity levels of mouse tissues. Hazelton and Lang[39] reported that in male C57BL/6J mice, the glutathione peroxidase activity levels of the livers, hearts, and kidneys decrease by 53, 28, and 35%, respectively, between 10 and 36 months of age when hydrogen peroxide is used as the substrate, and by 48%, 34%, and 40%, respectively, when cumene hydroperoxide is used as the substrate.

2. Rats
Table 4 shows the previously reported age-related alterations in the glutathione peroxidase activity levels of tissues in Fischer 344 and Wistar rats.[21,23,25,29-34,38,40-42] Rao et al.[21] reported that in male Fischer 344 rats, the glutathione peroxidase activity levels of kidneys and intestinal mucosae decrease by 20 and 30%, respectively, between 6 and 24 to 26 months of age, and those of the brains, livers, and lungs remain unchanged. They also reported that the glutathione peroxidase mRNA level of the kidneys decreases by 15% between 16 and 26 months of age, and that the mRNA level of hepatocytes decreases by 51% between 6 and 24 months of age, although no decrease was observed in the enzyme activity between 6 and 26 months of age. The discrepancy between the age-related changes in the mRNA and enzyme activity levels of hepatocyte glutathione peroxidase could be due to changes in the translational activity of the mRNA and/or in protein turnover. In addition to the above data, there are reports that in male Fischer 344 rats, the glutathione peroxidase activity levels of the brains[23] and livers[38] remain unchanged during aging. On the other hand, Matsuo et al.[25] found that in female Fischer 344 rats, the glutathione peroxidase activity level of the livers decreases by 38% between 14 and 26 months of age and by 68% between 14 and 32 months of age, while the levels of the brains and lungs remain unchanged (Figure 4).

Barja de Quiroga et al.[31] described that in male Wistar rats, the glutathione peroxidase activity levels of the brains and livers remain unchanged between 9 and 28 months of age. Pinto and Bartley[40] described, however, that in male Wistar rats, the level in the livers increases between 4 and 18 months of age. Benzi et al.[30] observed the age-related alterations in the glutathione peroxidase activity levels of four brain regions in male Wistar rats. The glutathione peroxidase activity levels of the parieto-temporal cortices and caudate-putamina increase between 5 and 20 months of age and then remain constant, while the levels of thalami and substantia nigra tend to decrease until 20 to 25 months of age. Zhang et al.[41] examined the glutathione peroxidase activity levels of tissues in male Wistar rats at 0.5, 4, and 24 months of age, using three different substrates. The selenium-dependent activity for hydrogen peroxide is much higher than either the selenium-independent activity for cumene hydroperoxide or the activity for phospholipid hydroperoxide. The strength

TABLE 4
Age-Related Changes in the Glutathione Peroxidase Activity Levels of Rat Tissues

Strain	Gender		Brain	Liver	Lung	Heart	Kidney	Intestine[a]	Muscle	Ref.
Fischer 344	male		→[c]	→		→	↓[b]	↓		21
Fischer 344	male		→							23
Fischer 344	male			→						38
Fischer 344	female		→	↓	→					25
Wister	male		→	→						31
Wister	male		→							30
Wister	male			↑[d]						40
Wister	male				↓					32
Wister	male					↑[e]				29
Wister	male	PH[f]	→	↑	→	→	→		→	41
		+Se[g]	↓	↓	↓	↓	↓		↓	
		-Se[h]	→	↓	↓	↓	→		↓	
Wister	male				↓					42
	female				↓					
Wister	female		→	↓		→	↓			34
Wister	female			↓						33

[a] Intestinal mucosa.
[b] ↓, Decrease.
[c] →, No change.
[d] ↑, Increase.
[e] Mitochondria.
[f] Phospholipid hydroperoxide glutathione peroxidase.
[g] Se-dependent glutathione peroxidase.
[h] Non-Se-dependent glutathione peroxidase.

From Matsuo, M., et al., *Mech. Ageing Dev.,* 64, 287, 1992. With permission.

of the activity for hydrogen peroxide in tissues is in the following order: liver > kidney > heart > lung > brain = muscle. For each tissue, the selenium-dependent activity is highest in adult rats and higher in old rats than in young rats. The selenium-independent activity is found virtually only in tissues of young rats, in particular in the liver. The activity for phospholipid hydroperoxide remains constant during aging. Nohl et al.[29] showed that the selenium-dependent glutathione peroxidase activity level of heart mitochondria in male Wistar rats increases by about 40% between 3 and 24 months of age.

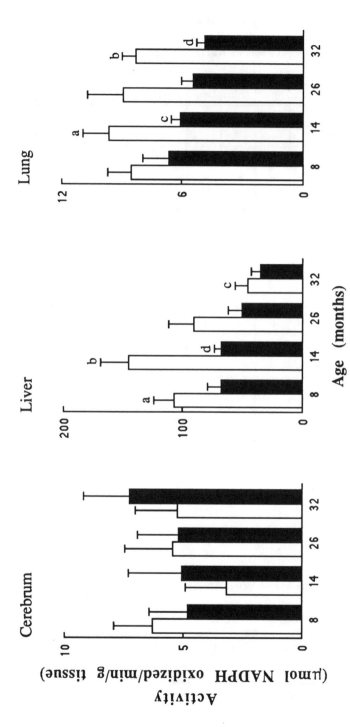

FIGURE 4. Variations in glutathione peroxidase activity as a function of age. Glutathione peroxidase activities in the cerebrum, liver, and lung homogenates from normal (open columns) and vitamin E-deficient (closed columns) rats are shown. Each column represents a mean value of three samples from three rats. Each small bar represents the standard error of the estimate of a mean value. Differences between pairs of means indicated by the following paired letters are statistically significant ($p \leq 0.05$): for liver, ac, bc, and bd; for lung, ac, bd. (From Matsuo, M., et al., *Mech. Ageing Dev.*, 64, 279, 1992. With permission.)

Cand and Verdetti[34] reported that in female Wistar rats, the glutathione peroxidase activity levels of the livers and kidneys decreases by 34 and 12%, respectively, between 4 and 24 months of age, and the levels of the brains and hearts remain unchanged. Pieri et al.[33] reported that in female Wistar rats, the glutathione peroxidase activity level of the livers decreases by 32% between 6 and 24 months of age.

Santa Maria and Machado[42] found a large difference between the glutathione peroxidase activity levels of lungs in male and female adult Wistar rats; at 24 months of age, the level in male rats is about three times that in female rats. In addition, it was found that the activity level decreases by 39% between 6 and 24 months of age in male rats, while the level remains unchanged during aging in female rats.

It appears that during aging, the glutathione peroxidase activity level of brains remains unchanged, and the level of kidneys decreases. The data for the level of other tissues are somewhat contradictory.

2. Biological Antioxidants in Rodents
a. Thiol Compounds and Other Water-Soluble Antioxidants

Thiol concentration levels of tissues are considered to be lower in old animals than in young animals.[43] It appears that in blood, cysteine and reduced glutathione concentration levels decrease with advancing age, while cystine and oxidized glutathione concentration levels increase. Abraham et al.[44] reported that the reduced glutathione concentration level of erythrocytes in male C57BL/6J mice decreases by 49% between 19 and 37 months of age. Hazelton and Lang[45] reported that the reduced glutathione concentration levels of the livers, kidneys, and hearts in male C57BL/6J mice decrease gradually with advancing age by 36, 46, and 30%, respectively, between 6 and 31 months of age. Hughes et al.[46] examined age-related alterations in thiol groups on the surface of adipocytes from the epididymal fat pads of male Wistar and Sprague-Dawley rats, using an impermeable reagent, mercury [^{3}H]dextran. The ratio of the number of thiol groups to the total number of thiol and disulfide groups decreases by two thirds with advancing age between 2 and 24 months of age, while the total number of thiol and disulfide groups remains unchanged. In adipocytes, the repair ability to reduce disulfide groups to thiol groups may be impaired in old rats. Since adipocytes are known not to proliferate throughout the life-span, they are a model system suitable for the observation of age-related alterations in cells.

Rikans and Moore[47] measured the concentrations of reduced glutathione, ascorbate, and uric acid in the livers, lungs, hearts, kidneys, brains, testes, lenses, and plasma of male Fischer 344 rats at 6, 15, and 26 months of age. The levels of reduced glutathione in the lens and kidney decrease by 50% and 20%, respectively, between 15 and 26 months of age, and those in other tissues remain unchanged. The levels of ascorbate in the liver, lung, and lens decrease by 40 to 60%, while that in the testis increases by 39% between 6 and 26 months of age. The concentration level of uric acid in the liver decreases by 25% and that in the heart, kidney, and testis increases by 88, 15, and 110%, respectively, between 6 and 26 months of age. De and Darad[28] reported that the reduced glutathione and ascorbate levels of the livers in male Wistar rats are higher in young adults than in adults.

Age-related alterations in the concentrations of these water-soluble antioxidants seem to be very complicated.

b. Vitamin E

Figure 5 shows variations in the vitamin E (α-tocopherol) concentrations of the cerebrums, livers, and lungs in normal and vitamin E-deficient female Fischer 344 rats as a function of age.[25] In order to induce vitamin E deficiency, we maintained rats under vitamin E-deficient conditions for nine weeks.

Interestingly, the vitamin E concentrations of the livers and lungs increase with advancing age, although that of cerebrums does not change. Vitamin E has been reported to increase in concentration in the livers, adrenals, and hearts of 29-month-old male and female Wistar rats,[48] in the livers of 24-month-old male Sprague-Dawley rats,[49] and in the livers and adipose tissues of 30-month-old male Fischer 344 rats.[50] Vitamin E accumulates in some rat tissues during aging.

The vitamin E concentration of tissues seems to be affected by dietary fat type.[51] When corn or coconut oil is fed to male C57BL/6Nia mice, the vitamin E levels of plasma and livers are lower in 24-month-old mice than in 3-month-old mice. However, when fish oil is fed to these mice, the vitamin E level of plasma is higher in old mice than in young mice.

Figure 6 shows that when lipid extracts from tissue homogenates are incubated under air, the length of the induction period for conjugated-diene formation in lipid extracts is proportional to the concentration of vitamin E in the tissue homogenates.[25] The induction period for conjugated-diene formation in a lipid extract (i.e., the time lag from the start of incubation to the onset of conjugated-diene formation) reflects the antioxidant capacity of the tissue homogenate from which the lipid extract has been prepared. The induction period of lipid extracts from the livers or lungs of old rats is longer than that of lipid extracts from young rats. These observations can be explained reasonably by the facts that vitamin E is an efficient, fat-soluble chain-breaking antioxidant, and that the vitamin E levels of the livers and lungs increase with advancing age.

In general, vitamin E deficiency seems to be readily induced in the liver, not so readily in the lung, and only slowly in the cerebrum (Figure 5). Muller and Goss-Sampson[52] also reported that under vitamin E-deficient conditions, the vitamin E concentration level of the livers decreases rapidly, while that of the brains decreases slowly. According to Ingold et al.,[53] the turnover rate of vitamin E is high in the lung and liver, while it is very low in the brain. The rate of vitamin E depletion in tissues under vitamin E-deficient conditions may be related to the turnover rate in tissues. During aging, the vitamin E concentration level of the brains remains unchanged, while those of the livers

treatment to mice (male LAF$_1$,[59] C57H,[60] female C3,[61] and male and female LAF$_1$ and C3H/He[62]) and rats (male and female Sprague-Dawley[63] and male Wistar[64]). There have been no reports, however, that vitamin E has a life-span-extending effect.

3. Aging Perturbation of Rodents: Food Restriction

Food restriction is well known to extend the life-span of mice and rats, and is thought to retard the aging process.[65] However, the mechanisms by which food restriction extends life-span remain unknown. Although several hypotheses have been proposed for how food restriction retards the aging process, such as by slowing growth and development,[66] by reducing body fat content,[67] or by reducing the metabolic rate,[68] they are not supported by recent studies.[69] At present, it is suggested that endocrine and neural regulation, protein turnover, gene expression, and oxidative damage may be involved in the underlying mechanisms for the retardation of the aging process by food restriction.[69]

a. Mice

Chipalkatti et al.[19] maintained female Swiss albino mice *ad libitum* and under food restriction from 3 weeks to 12 months of age. The food-restricted mice were given 50% of the diet consumed by the *ad libitum*-fed mice. The thiobarbituric acid (TBA) value, an index of *in vivo* lipid peroxidation, of liver homogenates from food-restricted mice is lower than that from *ad libitum*-fed rats. The SOD activity levels of the brains and livers of the mice at 12 months of age are lower under food restriction than under *ad libitum*.

Koizumi et al.[17] raised male long-lived C3B10RF$_1$ mice under control and restricted feedings from three weeks of age. The control mice were given about 95 kcal per week, a level less by about 20% than that of the diet consumed by *ad libitum*-fed mice. The food-restricted mice were given about 55 kcal per week. The control mice have mean and maximum lifespans of 33 and 42 months, respectively. Their mean body weight is 29 g at 24 months of age. The food-restricted mice have mean and maximum life-spans of 41 and 48 months, respectively. Their mean body weight is 22 g at 24 months of age. The TBA values of preincubated liver homogenates from the control mice are greater by 30% and 17% at 12 and 24 months of age, respectively, than are those from the food-restricted mice. Although having no effect on the SOD activity level of the livers, food restriction increases the catalase activity level of livers by 42% and 64% at 12 and 24 months of age, respectively. The mechanism for the increase in catalase activity is unknown.

b. Rats

Laganiere and Yu[70,71] maintained male Fischer 344 rats *ad libitum* and under food restriction from 6 weeks of age. The food-restricted rats were given 60% of the diet consumed by the *ad libitum*-fed rats. The mean body weight of the food-restricted rats is 64% of that of *ad libitum*-fed rats at 24 months of age. Food restriction inhibits age-related increases in the TBA values of liver mitochondria and microsomes. The glutathione reductase and glutathione S-transferase activity levels of the livers in food-restricted rats at 24 months of age are higher by 27% and 36%, respectively, than are those in *ad libitum*-fed rats, although food restriction has no effect on the SOD and glutathione peroxidase activity levels of livers. At each age, the catalase activity level of the livers in food-restricted rats is more enhanced than that in *ad libitum*-fed rats. At 24 months of age, the catalase activity and glutathione concentration levels of the livers are higher by 134 and 35%, respectively, in the food-restricted rats than in the *ad libitum*-fed rats. Although having no effect on the ascorbate concentration level of the livers, food restriction decreases the vitamin E concentration levels of liver mitochondria and microsomes.

Semsei et al.[20] used food-restricted male Fischer 344 rats fed daily 60% of the diet consumed by *ad libitum*-fed rats. The mean and 10% survivals of the food-restricted rats are about 30% greater than those of *ad libitum*-fed rats. In the livers of the food-restricted rats at 18 months of age, SOD activity and mRNA levels are higher by 59% and 51%, respectively, and catalase activity and mRNA levels are higher by 51% and 42%, respectively, as compared with those in the livers of *ad libitum*-fed rats. In addition, the transcription of SOD and catalase genes is higher in nuclei from the liver cells of the food-restricted rats than in those of *ad libitum*-fed rats. At 18 months of age, thus, food restriction results in an increased expression of SOD and catalase genes.

Pieri et al.[33] fed female Wistar rats on an every-other-day feeding schedule from 3.5 months of age. Food restriction suppresses perfectly the age-dependent increase in liver catalase activity and tends to suppress those in liver SOD and glutathione peroxidase activities.

Sagai and Ichinose[72] reported that the production of respired hydrocarbons in rats increases with advancing age. Respired hydrocarbons have been used as the indices of *in vivo* lipid peroxidation because volatile hydrocarbons are produced by the degradation of peroxidized unsaturated lipids.[73,74] It is of great interest to see whether food restriction prevents an age-dependent increase in *in vivo* lipid peroxidation. Matsuo et al.[75] measured the rates of the production of respired hydrocarbons in young and old male Fischer 344 rats fed *ad libitum* and restrictedly (for discontinuous for 3 d per week).

Figure 7 depicts the respiration rates of ethane and pentane from *ad libitum*-fed and food-restricted rats 6 to 9, 22, and 28 to 30 months old. The respiration rates of ethane and pentane from old rats are about two and five times, respectively, higher than those of the corresponding hydrocarbons from young rats. There is no difference between the respiration rates of each hydrocarbon from *ad libitum*-fed and food-restricted rats at 6 to 9 or 22 months of age. It was found, however, that the respiration rate of ethane from 28 to 30 month-old, food-restricted rats tends to be lower than that from 28 to 30 month-old, *ad libitum*-fed rats, and that the respiration rate of pentane from

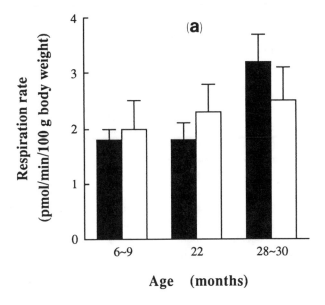

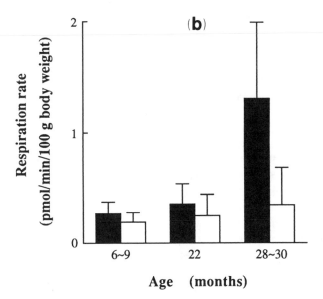

FIGURE 7. Respiration rates of ethane and pentane from *ad libitum*-fed and food-restricted rats. The respiration rates of ethane (a) and pentane (b) from 6 to 9- 22- and 28 to 30-month-old, *ad libitum*-fed (closed columns) and food-restricted (open columns) rats were measured. Each column represents a mean value for seven rats. Each small bar represents the standard deviation of a mean value. (From Matsuo, M., et al., *J. Gerontol.*, in press.)

28 to 30 month-old, food-restricted rats is significantly lower than that from 28 to 30 month-old, *ad libitum*-fed rats. The respiration rate of pentane from the old, food-restricted rats is about one fourth of that from the old, *ad libitum*-fed rats. In particular, it should be noted that the respiration rate of pentane from old, food-restricted rats was the same as that from young rats.

Long-term food restriction in rats prevents an age-dependent increase in the respiration of pentane and tends to prevent that in the respiration of ethane. Food restriction seems to suppress, at least partially, age-dependent increases in *in vivo* lipid peroxidation and, thus, might retard the aging process by keeping part of the antioxidant defense from deteriorating.

B. INSECTS

Insects provide good models for aging research on metazoans. In general, insects have short life-spans and are reared relatively easily. A large number can be maintained because of their small bodies. In adults, all somatic cells are postmitotic. They are poikilothermic animals and, hence, their life-spans can be modulated by means of the manipulation of some environmental factors, such as environmental temperature and physical activity. In addition, since gene manipulation is possible, many mutant strains are available. Age-related alterations have, so far, been investigated, using mainly the fruit fly *Drosophila melanogaster* and the housefly *Musca domestica*.

1. Antioxidant Enzymes in Insects
a. Fruit Fly

Sohal et al.[76] described that when male fruit flies Oregon R *D. melanogaster* are reared in 170-ml jars at 25°C, their 50% survival and maximum life-span are 28 and 46 d, respectively, and their total and mitochondrial SOD activity levels increase with advancing age. Massie et al.,[77,78] however, reported that the total SOD activity levels of male flies of two *D. melanogaster* strains, Oregon R and Swedish C, do not change with advancing age, and that the mitochondrial SOD activity levels of the two strains increase for the first 7 to 8 d and then tend to decrease.

Sohal et al.[76] also described that the catalase activity level of male Oregon R *D. melanogaster* increases with advancing age, but decreases after completion of the mean life-span. On the other hand, Nicolosi et al.[79] observed that the catalase activity level decreases after 35 d of age, with advancing age, and at 70 d of age to about 50% of the initial level. After catalase activity was suppressed by a 12-h treatment with 3.6 mM 3-amino-1H-1,2,4-triazole, a catalase inhibitor, in the drinking water, the ability of old flies to renew catalase activity is poorer than that of young flies.

It has been reported that in fruit flies, selenium-dependent glutathione peroxidase activity is undetectable[76,80] or low.[81-83]

The above results of two different research groups on age-related alterations in the SOD and catalase activities of fruit flies are very conflicting. These results need to be reinvestigated.

b. Housefly

Sohal and his associates have long studied age-related alterations in antioxidant defense in the housefly *M. domestica*. When male houseflies are fed on sucrose and maintained at 25°C with 40% humidity at a population density of 200 flies per 28-1 cage, their mean and maximum life-spans are 19 and 42 d, respectively.[84] Their oxygen consumption rates remain within 17 to 19 µl/h/mg wet weight until 17 d of age and then decline sharply between 17 and 19 d of age. In whole body homogenates, the levels of antioxidant capacity and oxidative stress were measured. The total SOD activity level, about 85% of which is attributed to the mitochondrial SOD activity level, decreases by about 33% between 15 and 19 d of age. The catalase activity level decreases by 33% between 5 and 12 d of age. The total glutathione and reduced glutathione concentrations decrease linearly with age and by 62% and 78%, respectively, between 9 and 18 d of age. In contrast, the peroxide concentration, shown as hydrogen peroxide equivalents, increases by 200% between 8 and 19 d of age.

Sohal and his associates examined the life-spans of houseflies whose antioxidant enzyme activity was inhibited. Houseflies were administered diethyldithiocarbamate for copper/zinc SOD inhibition[85] and 3-amino-1H-1,2,4-triazole for catalase inhibition.[86]

When a 10 mM diethyldithiocarbamate solution is administered to houseflies after emergence from pupae, the total SOD activity levels of whole body homogenates from the 10-d-old flies is lower by 34%, and, unexpectedly, the mitochondrial SOD levels are also lower by 29%. In the diethyldithiocarbamate-treated houseflies, furthermore, the catalase activity level decreases by 12% by 10 d of age, and the reduced glutathione concentration increases by 64% by 9 d of age. On the other hand, the peroxide concentration level decreases by 20% at 8 d of age. Paradoxically, the mean life-span of 10 mM diethyldithiocarbamate-treated houseflies is longer by 45% as compared to that of untreated houseflies. The increase in mean life-span is mainly due to a reduction in mortality at relatively younger ages rather than to an extension in the maximum lifespan of the population.

When a 2 mM 3-amino-1H-1,2,4-triazole solution is continuously administered to houseflies after emergence from pupae, the catalase activity levels of whole body homogenates from 3- 7- and 9-d-old flies are undetectable. In 3-amino-1H-1,2,4-triazole-treated houseflies, the total and mitochondrial SOD activity levels increase by 5 to 7% and 7 to 13% respectively; the total and oxidized glutathione concentrations increase by 8 to 25% and 8 to 23%, respectively; and the peroxide concentration increases by 12 to 46%. Treatment with 3-amino-1H-1,2,4-triazole has no effect on mean life-span.

These results indicate that either SOD inhibition or catalase inhibition perturbs the antioxidant defense system of houseflies, but neither has any effect on life-span. Houseflies seem to have the ability to counterbalance the loss of an antioxidant component by adaptive changes in antioxidant defense.

2. Biological Antioxidants in Insects

a. Fruit Fly

Reduced glutathione concentrations of whole body homogenates of male fruit flies, Oregon R *D. melanogaster,* remain stable during aging, except at the end of the life-span, when a sharp decline occurs.[76] In contrast, oxidized glutathione concentration increases throughout the life-span. Thus, the ratio of reduced glutathione concentration to oxidized glutathione concentration, an index of oxidative stress, in whole body homogenates declines with advancing age, indicating that the homeostatic balance shifts to become more prooxidizing in old flies. In addition, the ratio of the concentration of the reduced form of nicotinamide-adenine dinucleotide phosphate (NADPH) to the concentration of the oxidized form of nicotinamide-adenine dinucleotide (NADP$^+$) of whole body homogenates decreases with advancing age.[76] A decrease in the NADPH to NADP$^+$ ratio may contribute to the decrease in the reduced to oxidized glutathione ratio, since NADPH is the electron donor for the reduction of reduced glutathione to oxidized glutathione. Dietary supplementation with reduced glutathione, its precursors, and other sulfur-containing compounds have little life-span-extending effect on Oregon R *D. melanogaster.*[87] The mean and maximum life-spans of fruit flies increased by 8 to 15% and about 12%, respectively, on supplementation with 5.8 mM vitamin E in a dietary medium[88] and decreased on supplementation with 10 to 100 mM ascorbate in a dietary medium.[89]

b. Housefly

The intracellular redox potential of houseflies becomes progressively more prooxidizing or less reducing during aging.[90] With advancing age, the ratios of reduced to oxidized glutathione, NADPH to NADP$^+$ and NADH to NAD$^+$, in whole body homogenates of old houseflies decrease. In addition, the rate of hydrogen peroxide generation in mitochondria from houseflies increases linearly with age, and the rate of superoxide generation increases between 8 and 14 d of age.[91] These observations indicate that oxidative stress may be enhanced in houseflies during aging.

In order to examine the effect of a decrease in glutathione concentration level on life-span, Sohal et al.[92] administered diamide (azodicarboxylic acid bisdimethylamide), a thiol-oxidizing agent, to houseflies. When a 2 mM diamide solution is given to houseflies after emergence from pupae, the oxidized glutathione concentration of whole body homogenates from 8-d-old flies increases by 24% as compared with control levels; the level in 10- and 13-d-old flies decreases to the control level. Contrary to expectations, the reduced glutathione concentrations of whole body homogenates from the 6-8- and 13-d-old flies increased by 84%, 10%, and 34%, respectively. Since reduced glutathione is converted to oxidized glutathione *in vitro* by diamide, the administration of diamide to houseflies is expected to decrease the reduced glutathione concentration. It seems, however, that diamide enhances gluta-thione synthesis and increases the reduced glutathione concentration. Diamide administration has no effect on the mean life-span of houseflies.

As compared with the corresponding control levels, the total and mito-chondrial SOD activity levels of the diamide-treated houseflies decrease by 43 and 44%, respectively, at 7 d of age and by 24 and 12%, respectively, at 12 d of age. On the other hand, catalase activity levels are higher by 9 and 19% at 3 and 9 d of age, respectively, and peroxide concentrations increase by 38 and 19% at 3 and 9 d of age, respectively. The thiol-oxidizing agent, as well as antioxidant enzyme inhibitors, perturb the antioxidant defense of houseflies and have no effect of mean life-span.

The effects of administering 0.5% and 2% ascorbate, β-carotene, or α-tocopherol in sucrose on the life-span, SOD, and catalase activity levels, and on glutathione and peroxide concentrations of male, adult houseflies were examined.[93] Administration of antioxidants at a level of 0.5% does not affect their life-span, whereas 2% ascorbate or α-tocopherol decreases their mean life-span. Upon administration of these antioxidants, the SOD activity level decreases, and the catalase activity level remains unchanged. Total glutathione concentrations of ascorbate- or β-carotene-fed flies decrease. The peroxide concentrations of β-carotene- and α-tocopherol-fed flies increase, while those of ascorbate-fed flies decrease. These results suggest that administration of exogenous antioxidants causes a compensatory depression in endogenous an-tioxidants, which results in life-span shortening. In houseflies, there seems to exist a counterbalancing mechanism of antioxidant defense, by which, among antioxidant enzymes and biological antioxidants, the level of every antioxidant component influences the level of every other antioxidant com-ponent.

3. Aging Perturbation of Insects
a. Gene Manipulation

For studies of the function of antioxidant enzymes in the aging process, organisms that either underexpress or overexpress an antioxidant enzyme activity are expected to offer great advantages. Mutant strains of fruit flies that underexpress and overexpress SOD activity and underexpress catalase activity have been isolated.

Phillips et al.[94] reported the isolation of a *D. melanogaster* strain with a copper/zinc SOD-null mutation. This SOD-null allele was originally recovered as an ethyl methanesulfonate-induced recessive lethal mutation on a chro-mosome carrying the recessive makers *sr*, *e^s*, and *ca*. Homozygotes are viable as larvae, suggesting that SOD is not essential for cell viability per se. This SOD-null mutation causes hypersensitivity to paraquat, a superoxide radical-generating agent, indicating that the SOD-null condition leads to impaired superoxide metabolism. The primary biological consequences of the reduced superoxide-dismutation capacity of the SOD-null mutants were realized in adults as infertility and a reduction in life-span. The two SOD-null mutant parent strains and their hybrid have mean life-spans of 55, 58, and 61 d, respectively, while the SOD-null mutants have a mean life-span of 12 d. The infertility and reduced life-span of SOD-null mutants arose as a consequence of a decrease in the ability of embryos, larvae, and pupae to adequately protect developing preimaginal cells from superoxide-initiated cytotoxic damages. Another strain of SOD-null mutants has been reported to have a short mean life-span corresponding to 67% that of the wild type.[95]

Seto et al.[95] introduced the copper/zinc SOD gene, cloned from *D. melanogaster,* into the germ line of flies via P element-mediated transformation. Homozygous lines carrying additional copies of the SOD gene were recovered and characterized. The ranges of the SOD activity and transcript levels of these transformed lines are 130 to 170% and 99 to 153%, respectively, as compared with the wild type, indicating that all of the sequence information required for gene expression is contained on the inserted gene fragment. The transformed lines overexpress SOD activity, but show no increase in longevity or resistance to paraquat.

Reveillaud et al.[96] produced transgenic strains of *D. melanogaster* that overexpress copper/zinc SOD activity by microinjecting embryos with P-elements containing bovine copper/zinc SOD cDNA under the control of the *Drosophila* actin 5c gene promoter. The highest level of active enzyme activity expression in adults is 1.6 times the normal level. The expression of enzymatically active bovine SOD in the flies confers resistance to paraquat. There is a slight but significant increase in the mean life-span of several transgenic lines.

These results imply that extremely deficient SOD activity shortens the life-span of flies to a great extent, while excess SOD activity does not necessarily extend life-span.

Mackay and Bewley[97] described acatalasemic *Drosophila* mutants with reduced viability. Interestingly, only when the mutants have very low catalase activity levels of 2% or less of the control level, does their viability decrease in relation to catalase activity. Mutants with higher levels exhibit full viability, suggesting that a threshold level of catalase activity exists, above which viability is not affected. It appears that low levels of catalase activity are sufficient to scavenge endogenous hydrogen peroxide.

Data concerning aging of antioxidant enzyme-transgenic flies are not yet sufficient. Further work is needed for the elucidation of the relevance of antioxidant enzymes to the aging process.

b. Mutant Strains with Different Life-Spans

Massie et al.[78] reared two different wild-type *D. melanogaster* strains, long-lived Oregon R and short-lived Swedish C, whose life-spans differ by 40%; at 25°C, the mean and maximum life-spans of the Oregon R strain are 44 and 56 d, respectively, while those of the Swedish C strain are 26 and 40, respectively. No significant differences between total or mitochondrial SOD activity levels of fruit flies of either strain at different ages or between total or mitochondrial SOD activity levels of both strains were observed.

Sohal et al.[98] also examined the effects of genetic factors on age-related changes in antioxidant defense and oxidative stress, using the long-lived Cambridge and short-lived Thuron strains of the housefly *M. domestica.*

Under the rearing conditions used, the Cambridge strain has mean and max-imum life-spans of 20 and 37 d, respectively, and the Thuron strain has mean and maximum life-spans of 14 and 30 d, respectively. There is no difference between the SOD activity levels of the two strains. The catalase and gluta-thione reductase activities, reduced glutathione concentration, oxygen con-sumption rate, peroxide concentration, and TBA value in the Cambridge strain are higher than are the corresponding parameters in the Thuron strain.

c. Changes in Environmental Factors

Sohal et al. investigated antioxidant capacity and oxidative stress in house-flies whose life-span was modulated by changes in ambient temperature[99] or physical activity.[100] In houseflies having mean life-spans of 45 d at 20°C and 22 d at 28°C, the SOD and catalase activity levels and the reduced glutathione and peroxide concentrations were measured.[99] For 3- 8- or 25-d-old flies, there are no significant differences in either the total or mitochondrial SOD activity level between the groups reared at the two different temperatures. The catalase activity and reduced glutathione concentrations are lower by 40 to 50% and 23 to 42%, respectively, at 28°C than at 20°C. The peroxide concentration of 8-d-old flies is lower by 32% at 28°C than at 20°C.

A group of male houseflies was housed at a population density of 200 flies per 28-1 cage, the cage in which flying is possible, thus creating con-ditions of high physical activity.[100] In a second group, flying activity was prevented by confining each fly, individually, in a 250-ml bottle partitioned with a cardboard maze in such a manner that the flies were able to walk, but not to fly, due to space limitation.[100] The mean and maximum life-spans of the houseflies are 20 d and 28 d, respectively, under high-activity conditions and 33 d and 65 d, respectively, under low-activity conditions. No significant differences were found in the SOD activity levels of 7- 9- or 14-d-old flies between the high and low physical activity groups. The catalase activity level of active flies is slightly higher than that of inactive flies. The total glutathione and oxidized glutathione concentrations of active flies are higher, while the reduced glutathione concentration is similar at 7 d of age and higher at 10 and 14 d of age. The peroxide concentrations of both active and inactive flies increase with age, although the level of the former is higher at each age than that of the latter.

High ambient temperature and high physical activity are thought to be metabolic rate-increasing factors. These findings show, however, that the effects of the environmental factors on antioxidant defense and oxidative stress can not be consistently interpreted. Presumably, this reflects intricate rela-tionships between metabolic rate and environmental factors.

C. NEMATODES

The free living nematode also is an attractive model system for aging research on metazoans. The nematode offers the great advantages of short life-span, cellular simplicity, and easy cultivation.[101] In addition,

Caenorhabditis elegans offers another unique advantage of genetic manipulability,[102] and its mutant strains provide unique models.

1. Antioxidant Enzymes in Nematodes

It has been found that two nematode species, *C. elegans* and *Turbatrix aceti,* possess SOD, catalase, and glutathione peroxidase,[103-105] although the glutathione peroxidase activity level is very low.

Recently, Johnson[106,107] isolated the *age-1* mutant of *C. elegans,* whose mean and maximum life-spans are twice those of the wild type. Interestingly, the *age-1* strains exhibits about 2.5 times the copper/zinc SOD activity of a control strain, despite no increase in manganese SOD activity, and about 1.5 times the catalase activity.[108] The mutants are hyperresistant to paraquat and hydrogen peroxide. Suzuki and his associates[105] isolated a paraquat-sensitive mutant, *mev-1(kn1),* of *C.elegans,* whose SOD activity level is about half that of the wild type.

2. Biological Antioxidants in Nematodes

Vitamin E (α-tocopherol) has been reported to extend the life-span of nematodes. The mean and maximum life-spans of 465 μM 2-*ambo*-α-tocopherol-treated *C. elegans* at 20°C increase by 22 and 24%,[109] respectively, or by 15 and 12%, respectively.[110] Furthermore, the mean and maximum life-spans of 232 μM 2-*ambo*-α-tocopherol-treated *T. aceti* at 29°C increase by 34 and 7%, respectively.[111] Epstein and Gershon[112] reported that 929 μM α-tocopherolquinone, as well as α-tocopherol, increase the 50% survival and maximum life-span of *C. briggsae*. These results are somewhat strange, because α-tocopherolquinone has no antioxidant activity. Either the animals might have a reductase activity for the reduction of α-tocopherolquinone,[113] or the life-span-extending effects of these compounds might result from some function other than antioxidant action. In addition, 929 μM 2-*ambo*-α-tocopherol inhibits the growth of *C. elegans*.[110] The life-span extension of *C. briggsae* by α-tocopherol might be due to growth inhibition.

3. Aging Perturbation of Nematodes: Oxygen Effect

We examined the effects of changes in the concentration of atmospheric oxygen on the life-spans of wild type and *mev-1(kn1)* mutant *C. elegans*.[114,115] As mentioned above, the SOD activity level of the mutant is about half that of the wild type. Typical survival curves for the wild type and mutant under various concentrations of oxygen are depicted in Figure 8.

The mean and maximum life-spans of the wild type under air (21% oxygen) are 26 and 33 d, respectively. The life-spans under 1% oxygen are extended significantly (mean, 30 d; maximum, 41 d), while those under 60% oxygen are shortened considerably (mean, 23 d; maximum, 28 d). Mean and maximum life-spans under oxygen concentrations within a range of 2 and 40% oxygen remain unchanged.

On the other hand, the mean and maximum life-spans of the mutant strain under 21% oxygen are 21 and 26 d, respectively. The life-spans under 1%

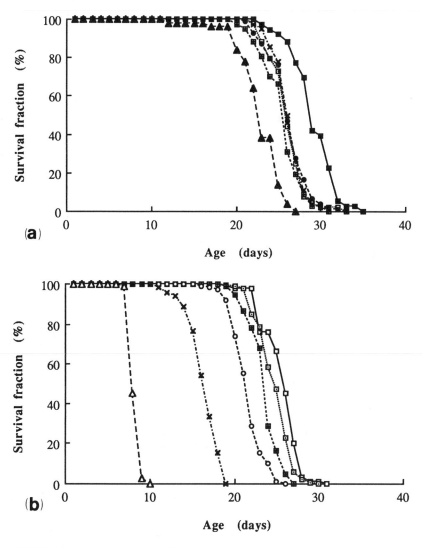

FIGURE 8. Survival curves for wild type and *mev-1(kn1)* mutant *C. elegans* under various concentrations of oxygen. From four days after hatching, the wild type (a) and mutant (b) were exposed to 1% (■, □), 2% (⊡), 8% (⊞), 21% (●, ○), 40% (×), or 60% oxygen (▲, △). (From Honda, S., et al., *J. Gerontol.,* in press.)

oxygen are also extended (mean, 26 d; maximum, 35 d), while those under 60% oxygen are greatly shortened (mean, 8 d; maximum, 10 d). The life-spans vary over a wide range of oxygen concentration.

The life-span increases under low concentrations of oxygen and decreases under high concentrations, compared with that under 21% oxygen (Figure 8). It is of great interest that the life-span not only decreases under high

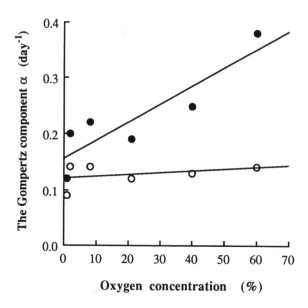

FIGURE 9. Effect of oxygen concentration on the Gompertz components of wild type and *mev-1(kn1)* mutant *C. elegans*. Gompertz analysis was carried out by means of pooling the data of the wild type (O) and mutant (●) under various oxygen concentrations. (From Honda, S., et al., *J. Gerontol.*, in press.)

concentrations of oxygen, but also increases under low concentrations. This suggests that oxygen affects the aging rate.

It is well known that one of the best criteria for the aging process is an exponential acceleration in the mortality rate M_t with chronological age t.[68] This is formulated by the Gompertz equation as follows:

$$M_t = \frac{D_{\Delta t}}{\Delta t \, L_t} = M_0 e^{\alpha t}$$

where $D_{\Delta t}$ represents the number of animals dying between age t and age t plus Δt; L_t, the number of animals alive at age t; M_0, the initial mortality rate (mortality rate at birth); and α, the Gompertz component (the acceleration rate of age-specific mortality).

In order to determine whether oxygen-induced changes in life-span result from an altered aging rate, we performed the Gompertz analysis on survival data for the wild type and *mev-1(kn1)* mutant under various concentrations of oxygen. Figure 9 depicts Gompertz components of the wild type and mutant under various oxygen concentrations. The Gompertz components for the wild type under 1, 21, and 60% oxygen are 0.09, 0.12, and 0.14 d^{-1}. The Gompertz component for the *mev-1(kn1)* mutant under 1% oxygen is 0.12 d^{-1}, smaller than that under 21% oxygen (0.19 d^{-1}), and the Gompertz component under 60% oxygen is 0.38 d^{-1}, much larger than that under 21% oxygen. These results show that, as compared with aging under 21% oxygen, the aging of the wild type and mutant strains under 60% oxygen is accelerated, and the aging of the mutant under 1% oxygen was retarded. Changes in oxygen concentration perturb the aging rate.

The mean life-span of the mutant increases by 21% under 1% oxygen and is shorter by 62% under 60% oxygen, as compared with that under 21% oxygen, while the life-span of the wild type increases by 15% under 1% oxygen and is shorter by 14% under 60% oxygen, as compared with that under 21% oxygen. The Gompertz component for the mutant decreases by 36% under 1% oxygen and increases by 100% under 60% oxygen, as compared with that under 21% oxygen, while the Gompertz component for the wild type decreases by 25% under 1% oxygen and increases by 17% under 60% oxygen, as compared with that under 21% oxygen. The effects of oxygen on the perturbation of life-span and the aging rate are more enhanced in the SOD-deficient *mev-1(kn1)* mutant than in the wild type. The genetic defect in the antioxidant defense of the mutant seems to enhance the oxygen-dependent perturbation of the aging rate.

As shown in Figure 8, the life-span of the *mev-1(kn1)* mutant increases with decreasing oxygen concentration, while the lifespan of the wild type remains unchanged within a range between 2% and 40% oxygen. Under each oxygen concentration, except 2% oxygen, the life-span of the *mev-1(kn1)* mutant is shorter than that of the wild type. The oxygen hypersensitivity of the mutant may be due to oxidative damage that results from an unfavorable balance between antioxidant defense and oxidative stress. Interestingly, under 2% oxygen, the mean and maximum life-spans of the mutant (25 and 31 d) are approximately equal to those of the wild type (26 and 33 d). Under 2% oxygen, the wild type and mutant might have a similar balance between oxidative stress and antioxidant defense.

Changes in oxygen concentration perturb the aging rate as well as the life-span of *C. elegans;* hence, oxygen acts as a life-span determinant in the nematode.

IV. CONCLUDING REMARKS

The following questions are raised through this survey of research on age-related alterations in antioxidant defense: (1) It appears that a catastrophic deterioration in overall antioxidant capacity does not occur during aging. Do age-related alterations in antioxidant defense result in a decrease in redundancy of antioxidant capacity? (2) Is there a counterbalancing mechanism of antioxidant defense, by which the level of every antioxidant component influences the level of every other antioxidant component? (3) Are there any unknown antioxidant mechanisms? (4) Does the antioxidant defense mechanism of short-lived animal species differ from the antioxidant defense mechanism of long-lived animal species? (5) Is the antioxidant defense mechanism of poikilothermic animals the same as that of homoiothermic animals? There is the possibility that the key to answering these questions might be a breakthrough for elucidating the role of antioxidant defense in the aging process. These questions are expected to be answered in the near future.

The mechanism of aging is still unknown. There must be little doubt, however, that aging is a biological phenomenon arising during evolution from interactions between genetic factors and environmental factors. Incidentally, life-span is well known to be species-specific, and a gene decreasing the aging rate has been found. On the other hand, some environmental factors evidently affect life-span, e.g., food restriction extends the life-span of mice and rats, and higher environmental temperature shortens the life-span of poikilothermic animals. Such environmental factors may affect the genetic process controlling aging. Age-related alterations in antioxidant defense are relevant to both genetic and environmental factors. A full understanding of age-related alterations in antioxidant defense may clarify the mechanism for the interaction between genetic and environmental factors of aging and, hence, may afford a clue for elucidating the aging process.

ACKNOWLEDGMENT

The author thanks Dr. Margaret Dooley Ohto for her help in preparing this manuscript.

REFERENCES

1. **Fridovich, I. and Freeman, B.,** Antioxidant defenses in the lung, *Ann. Rev. Physiol.,* 48, 693, 1986.
2. **Fraga, C. G., Shigenaga, M. K., Park, J. -W., Degan, P., and Ames, B. N.,** Oxidative damage to DNA during aging: 8-hydroxy-2'-deoxyguanosine in rat organ DNA and urine, *Proc. Natl. Acad. Sci. U.S.A.,* 87, 4533, 1990.
3. **Sohal, R. S., Svensson, I., Sohal, B. H., and Brunk, U. T.,** Superoxide anion radical production in different animal species, *Mech. Ageing Dev.,* 49, 129, 1989.
4. **Sohal, R. S., Svensson, I., and Brunk, U. T.,** Hydrogen peroxide production by liver mitochondria in different species, *Mech. Ageing Dev.,* 53, 209, 1990.
5. **Cathcart, R., Schwiers, E., Saul, R. L., and Ames, B. N.,** Thymine glycol and thymidine glycol in human and rat urine: a possible assay for oxidative DNA damage, *Proc. Natl. Acad. Sci. U.S.A.,* 81, 5633, 1984.
6. **Adelman, R., Saul, R. L., and Ames, B. N.,** Oxidative damage to DNA: relation to species metabolic rate and life span, *Proc. Natl. Acad. Sci. U.S.A.,* 85, 2706, 1988.
7. **Tolmasoff, J. M., Ono, T., and Cutler, R. G.,** Superoxide dismutase: correlation with life-span and specific metabolic rate in primate species, *Proc. Natl. Acad. Sci. U.S.A.,* 77, 2777, 1980.
8. **Ono, T. and Okada, S.,** Unique increase of superoxide dismutase level in brains of long living mammals, *Exp. Gerontol.,* 19, 349, 1984.
9. **Sohal, R. S., Sohal, B. H., and Brunk, U. T.,** Relationship between antioxidant defenses and longevity in different mammalian species, *Mech. Ageing Dev.,* 53, 217, 1990.

10. **Cutler, R. G.**, Aging and oxygen radicals, in *Physiology of Oxygen Radicals*, Taylor, A. E., Matalon, S., and Ward, P., Eds., American Physiological Society, Bethesda, 1986, 251.

11. **Cutler, R. G.**, Peroxide-producing potential of tissues: inverse correlation with longevity of mammalian species, *Proc. Natl. Acad. Sci. U.S.A.*, 82, 4798, 1985.

12. **Reiss, U. and Gershon, D.**, Comparison of cytoplasmic superoxide dismutase in liver, heart and brain of aging rats and mice, *Biochem. Biophys. Res. Commun.*, 73, 255, 1976.

13. **Massie, H. R., Aiello, V. R., and Iodice, A. A.**, Changes with age in copper and superoxide dismutase levels in brains of C57BL/6J mice, *Mech. Ageing Dev.*, 10, 93, 1979.

14. **Burrows, R. B. and Davison, P. F.**, Comparison of specific activities of enzymes from young and old dogs and mice, *Mech. Ageing Dev.*, 13, 307, 1980.

15. **Kellogg, E. W., III and Fridovich, I.**, Superoxide dismutase in the rat and mouse as a function of age and longevity, *J. Gerontol.*, 31, 405, 1976.

16. **Imre, S., Tóth, F., and Fachet, J.**, Superoxide dismutase, catalase and lipid peroxidation in liver of young mice of different ages, *Mech. Ageing Dev.*, 28, 297, 1984.

17. **Koizumi, A., Weindruch, R., and Walford, R. L.**, Influences of dietary restriction and age on liver enzyme activities and lipid peroxidation in mice, *J. Nutr.*, 117, 361, 1987.

18. **Imre, S. and Juhász, E.**, The effect of oxidative stress on inbred mice of different ages, *Mech. Ageing Dev.*, 38, 259, 1987.

19. **Chipalkatti, S., De, A. K., and Aiyar, A. S.**, Effect of diet restriction on some biochemical parameters related to aging in mice, *J. Nutr.*, 113, 944, 1983.

20. **Semsei, I., Rao, G., and Richardson, A.**, Changes in the expression of superoxide dismutase and catalase as a function of age and dietary restriction, *Biochem. Biophys. Res. Commun.*, 164, 620, 1989.

21. **Rao, G., Xia, E., and Richardson, A.**, Effect of age on the expression of antioxidant enzymes in male Fischer F344 rats, *Mech. Ageing Dev.*, 53, 49, 1990.

22. **Semsei, I., Rao, G., and Richardson, A.**, Expression of superoxide dismutase and catalase in rat brain as a function of age, *Mech. Ageing Dev.*, 58, 13, 1991.

23. **Ansari, K. A., Kaplan, E., and Shoeman, D.**, Age-related changes in lipid peroxidation and protective enzymes in the central nervous system, *Growth Dev. Aging*, 53, 117, 1989.

24. **Ischiropoulos, H., Nadziejko, C. E., and Kikkawa, Y.**, Effect of aging on pulmonary superoxide dismutase, *Mech. Ageing Dev.*, 52, 11, 1990.

25. **Matsuo, M., Gomi, F., and Dooley, M. M.**, Age-related alterations in antioxidant capacity and lipid peroxidation in brain, liver, and lung homogenates of normal and vitamin E-deficient rats, *Mech. Ageing Dev.*, 64, 273, 1992.

26. **Reiss, U. and Gershon, D.**, Rat-liver superoxide dismutase purification and age-related modifications, *Eur. J. Biochem.*, 63, 617, 1976.

27. **Vanella, A., Geremia, E., D'Urso, G., Tiriolo, P., Di Silvestro, I., Grimaldi, R., and Pinturo, R.**, Superoxide dismutase activities in aging rat brain, *Gerontology*, 28, 108, 1982.

28. **De, A. K. and Darad, R.**, Age-associated changes in antioxidants and antioxidative enzymes in rats, *Mech. Ageing Dev.*, 59, 123, 1991.

29. **Nohl, H., Hegner, D., and Summer, K.-H.**, Responses of mitochondrial superoxide dismutase, catalase and glutathione peroxidase activities to ageing, *Mech. Ageing Dev.*, 11, 145, 1979.

30. **Benzi, G., Marzatico, F., Pstoris, O., and Villa, R. F.**, Relationship between aging, drug treatment and the cerebral enzymatic antioxidant system, *Exp. Gerontol.*, 24, 137, 1989.

31. **Barja de Quiroga, G., Pérez-Cammpo, R., and López Torres, M.**, Anti-oxidant defences and peroxidation in liver and brain of aged rats, *Biochem. J.*, 272, 247, 1990.

32. **Perez, R., Lopez, M., and Barja de Quiroga, G.,** Aging and lung antioxidant enzymes, glutathione, and lipid peroxidation in the rat, *Free Radical Biol. Med.,* 10, 35, 1991.
33. **Pieri, C., Falasca, M., Marcheselli, F., Moroni, F., Recchioni, R., Marmocchi, F., and Lupidi, G.,** Food restriction in female Wistar rats. V. Lipid peroxidation and antioxidant enzymes in the liver, *Arch. Gerontol. Geriatr.,* 14, 93, 1992.
34. **Cand, F. and Verdetti, J.,** Superoxide dismutase, glutathione peroxidase, catalase, and lipid peroxidation in the major organs of the aging rats, *Free Radical Biol. Med.,* 7, 59, 1989.
35. **Lammi-Keefe, C. J., Swan, P. B., and Hegarty, P. V. J.,** Copper-zinc and manganese superoxide dismutase activities in cardiac and skeletal muscles during aging in male rats, *Gerontology,* 30, 153, 1984.
36. **Kurobe, N., Suzuki, F., Kato, K., and Sato, T.,** Sensitive immunoassay of rat Cu/Zn superoxide dismutase: concentrations in the brain, liver, and kidney are not affected by aging, *Biomed. Res.,* 11, 187, 1990.
37. **Fridovich, I.,** Superoxide dismutase, *Adv. Enzymol.,* 58, 61, 1986.
38. **Laganiere, S. and Yu, B. P.,** Effect of chronic food restriction in aging rats. II. Liver cytosolic antioxidants and related enzymes, *Mech. Ageing Dev.,* 48, 221, 1989.
39. **Hazelton, G. A. and Lang, C. A.,** Glutathione peroxidase and reductase activities in the aging mouse, *Mech. Ageing Dev.,* 29, 71, 1985.
40. **Pinto, R. E. and Bartley, W.,** The effect of age and sex on glutathione reductase and glutathione peroxidase activities and on aerobic glutathione oxidation in rat liver homogenates, *Biochem. J.,* 112, 109, 1969.
41. **Zhang, L., Maiorino, M., Roveri, A., and Ursini, F.,** Phospholipid hydroperoxide glutathione peroxidase: specific activity in tissues of rats of different age and comparison with other glutathione peroxidases, *Biochim. Biophys. Acta,* 1006, 140, 1989.
42. **Santa Maria, C. and Machado, A.,** Effects of development and ageing on pulmonary NADPH-cytochrome c reductase, glutathione peroxidase, glutathione reductase and thioredoxin reductase activities in male and female rats, *Mech. Ageing Dev.,* 37, 183, 1987.
43. **Oeriu, S.,** Proteins in development and senescence, *Adv. Gerontol. Res.,* 1, 23, 1964.
44. **Abraham, E. C., Taylor, J. F., and Lang, C. A.,** Influence of mouse age and erythrocyte age on glutathione metabolism, *Biochem. J.,* 174, 819, 1978.
45. **Hazelton, G. A. and Lang, C. A.,** Glutathione contents of tissue in the aging mouse, *Biochem. J.,* 188, 25, 1980.
46. **Hughes, B. A., Roth, G. S., and Pitha, J.,** Age-related decrease in repair of oxidative damage to surface sulfhydryl groups on rat adipocytes, *J. Cell Physiol.,* 103, 349, 1980.
47. **Rikans, L. E. and Moore, D. R.,** Effect of aging on aqueous-phase antioxidants in tissues of male Fischer rats, *Biochim. Biophys. Acta,* 966, 269, 1988.
48. **Weglicki, W. B., Luna, Z., and Nair, P. P.,** Sex and tissue specific differences in concentrations of α-tocopherol in mature and senescent rats, *Nature,* 221, 185, 1969.
49. **Braughler, J. M., Travis, M. A., and Chase, R. L.,** Letter to the editor, *Free Radical Biol. Med.,* 3, 362, 1987.
50. **Vatassery, G. T., Angerhofer, C. K., and Knox, C. A.,** Effect of age on vitamin E concentrations in various regions of the brain and a few selected peripheral tissues of the rat, and on the uptake of radioactive vitamin E by various regions of rat brain, *J. Neurochem.,* 43, 409, 1984.
51. **Meydani, S. N., Shapiro, A. C., Meydani, M., Macauley, J. B., and Blumberg, J. B.,** Effect of age and dietary fat (fish, corn and coconut oils) on tocopherol status of C57BL/6Nia mice, *Lipids,* 22, 345, 1987.
52. **Muller, D. P. R. and Goss-Sampson, M. A.,** The neurobiology of vitamin E deficiency, in *Clinical and Nutritional Aspects of Vitamin E,* Hayaishi, O. and Mino, M., Eds., Elsevier, Amsterdam, 1987, 183.
53. **Ingold, K. U., Burton, G. W., Foster, D. O., Hughes, L., Lindsay, D. A. and Webb, A.,** Biokinetics of and discrimination between dietary *RRR-* and *SRR-*α-tocopherols in the male rat, *Lipids,* 22, 162, 1987.

54. **Masugi, F. and Nakamura, T.**, Effect of vitamin E deficiency on the level of superoxide dismutase, glutathione peroxidase, catalase and lipid peroxide in rat liver, *J. Vitamin Nutr. Res.*, 46, 187, 1976.

55. **Chen, L. H., Thacker, R. R., and Chow, C. K.**, Tissue antioxidant status and related enzymes in rats with long-term vitamin E deficiency, *Nutr. Rep. Int.*, 22, 873, 1980.

56. **Murty, H. S., Caasi, P. I., Brooks, S. K., and Nair, P. P.**, Biosynthesis of heme in the vitamin E-deficient rat, *J. Biol. Chem.*, 245, 5498, 1970.

57. **Chow, C. K., Reddy, K., and Tappel, A. L.**, Effect of dietary vitamin E on the activities of the glutathione peroxidase system in rat tissues, *J. Nutr.*, 103, 618, 1973.

58. **McCay, C. M., Sperling, G., and Barnes, L. L.**, Growth, ageing, chronic diseases, and life span in rats, *Arch. Biochem.*, 2, 469, 1943.

59. **Harman, D.**, Free radical theory of aging: effect of free radical inhibitors on the life span of male LAF_1 mice — second experiment, *Gerontologist*, 8 (III), 13, 1968.

60. **Ledvina, M. and Hodáňvá, M.**, The effect of simultaneous administration of tocopherol and sunflower oil on the life-span of female mice, *Exp. Gerontol.*, 15, 67, 1980.

61. **Kohn, R. R.**, Effect of antihistamines on life-span of C57BL mice, *J. Gerontol.*, 26, 378, 1971.

62. **Blacket, A. D. and Hall, D. A.**, The effects of vitamin E on mouse fitness and survival, *Gerontology*, 27, 133, 1981.

63. **Berg, B. N.**, Study of vitamin E supplements in relation to muscular dystrophy and other diseases in aging rats, *J. Gerontol.*, 14, 174, 1959.

64. **Porta, E. A., Joun, N. S., and Nitta, R. T.**, Effects of the type of dietary fat at two levels of vitamin E in Wistar male rats during development and aging. I. Life span, serum biochemical parameters and pathological changes, *Mech. Ageing Dev.*, 13, 1, 1980.

65. **Weindruch, R. and Walford, R. L.**, *The Retardation of Aging and Disease by Dietary Restriction*, Charles C. Thomas, Springfield, IL, 1988.

66. **McCay, C. M., Crowell, M. F., and Maynard, L. A.**, The effect of retarded growth upon the length of life span and upon the ultimate body size, *J. Nutr.*, 10, 63, 1935.

67. **Berg, B. N. and Simms, H. S.**, Nutrition and longevity in the rat. II. Longevity and onset of disease with different levels of intake, *J. Nutr.*, 71, 255, 1960.

68. **Sacher, G. A.**, Life table modifications and life prolongation, in *Handbook of the Biology of Aging*, Finch, C. E. and Hayflick, L., Eds., Van Nostrand Reinhold, New York, 1977, 582.

69. **Masoro, E. J.**, Food restriction in rodents: an evaluation of its role in the study of aging, *J. Gerontol.*, 43, B59, 1988.

70. **Laganiere, S. and Yu, B. P.**, Anti-lipoperoxidation action of food restriction, *Biochem. Biophys. Res. Commun.*, 145, 1185, 1987.

71. **Laganiere, S. and Yu, B. P.**, Effect of chronic food restriction in aging rats. II. Liver cytosolic antioxidants and related enzymes, *Mech. Ageing Dev.*, 48, 221, 1989.

72. **Sagai, M. and Ichinose, T.**, Age-related changes in lipid peroxidation as measured by ethane, ethylene, butane and pentane in respired gases of rats, *Life Sci.*, 27, 731, 1980.

73. **Riely, C. A., Choen, G., and Lieberman, M.**, Ethane evolution: a new index of lipid peroxidation, *Science*, 183, 208, 1974.

74. **Frankel, E. N.**, Volatile lipid oxidation products, *Prog. Lipid Res.*, 22, 1, 1982.

75. **Matsuo, M., Gomi, F., Kuramoto, K., and Sagai, M.**, Food restriction suppresses an age-dependent increase in the exhalation rates of pentane from rats: a longitudinal study, *J. Gerontol.*, in press.

76. **Sohal, R. S., Arnold, L., and Orr, W. C.**, Effect of age on superoxide dismutase, catalase, glutathione reductase, inorganic peroxides, TBA-reactive material, GSH/GSSG, $NADPH/NADP^+$ and $NADH/NAD^+$ in *Drosophila melanogaster*, *Mech. Ageing Dev.*, 56, 223, 1990.

77. **Massie, H. R., Aiello, V. R., and Williams, T. R.**, Changes in superoxide dismutase activity and copper during development and ageing in the fruit fly *Drosophila melanogaster*, *Mech. Ageing Dev.*, 12, 279, 1980.

78. **Massie, H. R., Williams, T. R., and Aiello, V. R.,** Superoxide dismutase activity in two different wild-type strains of *Drosophila melanogaster, Gerontology,* 27, 205, 1981.
79. **Nicolosi, R. J., Baird, M. B., Massie, H. R., and Samis, H. V.,** Senescence in *Drosophila.* II. Renewal of catalase activity in flies of different ages, *Exp. Gerontol.,* 8, 101, 1973.
80. **Smith, J. and Shrift, A.,** Phylogenetic distribution of glutathione peroxidase, *Comp. Biochem. Physiol.,* 63B, 39, 1979.
81. **Simmons, T. W., Jamall, I. S., and Lockshin, R. A.,** The effect of selenium deficiency on peroxidative injury in the housefly, *Musca domestica:* a role for glutathione peroxidase, *FEBS Lett.,* 218, 251, 1987.
82. **Simmons, T. W., Jamall, I. S., and Lockshin, R. A.,** Selenium-independent glutathione peroxidase activity associated with glutathione S-transferase from the housefly, *Musca domestica, Comp. Biochem. Physiol.,* 94B, 323, 1989.
83. **Ahmed, S., Beilstein, M. A., and Pardini, R. S.,** Glutathione peroxidase activity in insects: a reassessment, *Arch. Insect Biochem. Biophys.,* 12, 31, 1989.
84. **Sohal, R. S., Farmer, K. J., Allen, R. G., and Cohen, N. R.,** Effect of age on oxygen consumption, superoxide dismutase, catalase, glutathione, inorganic peroxides and chloroform-soluble antioxidants in the adult male housefly, *Musca domestica, Mech. Ageing Dev.,* 24, 185, 1983.
85. **Sohal, R. S., Farmer, K. J., Allen, R. G., and Ragland, S. S.,** Effects of diethyl-dithiocarbamate on life span, metabolic rate, superoxide dismutase, catalase, inorganic peroxides and glutathione in the adult male housefly, *Musca domestica, Mech. Ageing Dev.,* 24, 175, 1984.
86. **Allen, R. G., Farmer, K. J., and Sohal, R. S.,** Effect of catalase inactivation on levels of inorganic peroxides, superoxide dismutase, glutathione, oxygen consumption and life span in adult housefly *(Musca domestica), Biochem. J.,* 216, 503, 1983.
87. **Massie, H. R. and Williams, T.,** Effect of sulfur-containing compounds on the life span of *Drosophila, Age,* 8, 128, 1985.
88. **Miquel, J., Binnard, R., and Howard, W. H.,** Effects of DL-α-tocopherol on the life-span of *Drosophila melanogaster, Gerontologist,* 13, (3; II), 37, 1973.
89. **Massie, H. R., Baird, M. B., and Piekieniak, M. J.,** Ascorbic acid and longevity in *Drosophila, Exp. Gerontol.,* 11, 37, 1976.
90. **Sohal, R. S., Toy, P. L., and Farmer, K. J.,** Age-related changes in the redox status of the housefly, *Musca domestica, Arch. Gerontol. Geriat.,* 6, 95, 1987.
91. **Sohal, R. S. and Sohal, B. H.,** Hydrogen peroxide release by mitochondria increases during aging, *Mech. Ageing Dev.,* 57, 187, 1991.
92. **Allen, R. G., Farmer, K. J., and Sohal, R. S.,** Effect of diamide administration on longevity, oxygen consumption, superoxide dismutase, catalase, inorganic peroxides and glutathione in the adult housefly, *Musca domestica, Comp. Biochem. Physiol.,* 78C, 31, 1984.
93. **Sohal, R. S., Allen, R. G., Farmer, K. J., Newton, R. K., and Toy, P. L.,** Effects of exogenous antioxidants on the levels of endogenous antioxidants, lipid-soluble fluorescent material and life span in the housefly, *Musca domestica, Mech. Ageing Dev.,* 31, 329, 1985.
94. **Phillips, J. P., Campbell, S. D., Michaud, D., Charbonneau, M., and Hilliker, A. J.,** Null mutation of copper/zinc superoxide dismutase in *Drosophila* confers hypersensitivity to paraquat and reduced longevity, *Proc. Natl. Acad. Sci. U.S.A.,* 86, 2761, 1989.
95. **Seto, N. O. L., Hayashi, S., and Tener, G. M.,** Overexpression of Cu-Zn superoxide dismutase in *Drosophila* does not affect life-span, *Proc. Natl. Acad. Sci. U.S.A.,* 87, 4270, 1990.
96. **Reveillaud, I., Niedzwiecki, A., Bensch, K. G., and Fleming, J. E.,** Expression of bovine superoxide dismutase in *Drosophila melanogaster* augments resistance to oxidative stress, *Mol. Cell. Biol.,* 11, 632, 1991.

97. **Mackay, W. J. and Bewley, G. C.,** The genetics of catalase in *Drosophila melanogaster:* isolation and characterization of acatalasemic mutants, *Genetics,* 122, 643, 1989.

98. **Sohal, R. S., Farmer, K. J., and Allen, R. G.,** Correlates of longevity in two strains of the housefly, *Musca domestica, Mech. Ageing Dev.,* 40, 171, 1987.

99. **Farmer, K. J. and Sohal, R. S.,** Effects of ambient temperature on free radical generation, antioxidant defenses and life span in the adult housefly, *Musca domestica, Exp. Gerontol.,* 22, 59, 1987.

100. **Sohal, R. S., Allen, R. G., Farmer, K. J., and Procter, J.,** Effect of physical activity on superoxide dismutase, catalase, inorganic peroxides and glutathione in the adult male housefly, *Musca domestica, Mech. Ageing Dev.,* 26, 75, 1984.

101. **Russell, R. L. and Jacobson, L. A.,** Some aspects of aging can be studied easily in nematodes, in *Handbook of the Biology of Aging,* 2nd ed., Finch, C. E. and Schneider, E. L., Eds., Van Nostrand Reinhold, New York, 1985, 128.

102. **Johnson, T. E.,** *Caenorhabditis elegans* offers the potential for molecular dissection of the aging processes, in *Handbook of the Biology of Aging,* 3rd ed., Schneider, E. L. and Rowe, J. W., Eds., Academic Press, San Diego, 1990, 45.

103. **Anderson, G. L.,** Superoxide dismutase activity in dauer larvae *Caenorhabditis elegans* (Nematode: Rhabditidae), *Can. J. Zool.,* 60, 288, 1982.

104. **Blum, J. and Fridovich, I.,** Superoxide, hydrogen peroxide, and oxygen toxicity in two free-living nematode species, *Arch. Biochem. Biophys.,* 222, 35, 1983.

105. **Ishii, N., Takahashi, K., Tomita, S., Keino, T., Honda, S., Yoshino, K., and Suzuki, K.,** A methyl viologen-sensitive mutant of the nematode *Caenorhabditis elegans, Mutation Res.,* 237, 165, 1990.

106. **Friedman, D. B. and Johnson, T. E.,** A mutation in the *age-1* gene in *Caenorhabditis elegans* lengthens life and reduces hermaphrodite fertility, *Genetics,* 118, 75, 1988.

107. **Johnson, T. E.,** Increased life-span of *age-1* mutants in *Caenorhabditis elegans* and low Gompertz rate of aging, *Science,* 249, 908, 1990.

108. **Vanfleteren, J. R.,** Oxidative stress and aging in *Caenorhabditis elegans,* private communication, 1992.

109. **Harrington, L. A. and Harley, C. B.,** Effect of vitamin E on life-span and reproduction in *Caenorhabditis elegans, Mech. Ageing Dev.,* 43, 71, 1988.

110. **Zuckerman, B. M. and Geist, M. A.,** Effects of vitamin E on the nematode *Caenorhabditis elegans, Age,* 6, 1, 1983.

111. **Kahn, M. and Enesco, H. E.,** Effect of α-tocopherol on the life-span of *Turbatrix aceti, Age,* 4, 109, 1981.

112. **Epstein, J. and Gershon, D.,** Studies on ageing in nematodes. IV. The effect of antioxidants on cellular damage and life-span, *Mech. Ageing Dev.,* 1, 257, 1972.

113. **Hughes, P. E. and Tove, S. B.,** Identification of an endogenous electron donor for biohydrogenation as α-tocopherolquinone, *J. Biol. Chem.,* 255, 4447, 1980.

114. **Honda, S. and Matsuo, M.,** Life-span shortening of the nematode *Caenorhabditis elegans* under higher concentrations of oxygen, *Mech. Ageing Dev.,* 63, 235, 1992.

115. **Honda, S., Ishii, N., Suzuki, K., and Matsuo, M.,** Oxygen-dependent perturbation of life-span and aging rate in the nematode, *J. Gerontol.,* in press.

Chapter 8

FREE RADICALS, EXERCISE, AND AGING

Mohsen Meydani and William J. Evans

TABLE OF CONTENTS

I. INTRODUCTION

Skeletal muscle mass decreases with advancing age. Whether this reduced muscle mass is a result of an age-associated decrease in activity or a change in muscle function is unclear. However, the age-dependent decline of muscle mass is associated with reduced aerobic capacity and muscle strength. As the age of humans exceeds 75 years, the decline in exercise capacity is accelerated.[1] The change in functional capacity becomes more prominent when older people are under physical stress. The response of older individuals to an oxidative stress induced by physical work will depend on overall health status, which is governed by several functional systems in the body, including the neuronal, hormonal, cardiovascular, immunological, and musculoskeletal systems. It has been suggested that exercise training and lifelong physical activity may contribute to a slower decline of age-associated functional systems and may prevent or delay the onset of degenerative diseases.[2] However, the impact of lifelong physical activity on longevity is yet to be determined.

Exercise influences oxidative metabolism and produces reactive oxygen species, which appear to play a key role in changing the membrane fatty acid composition, permeability and leakage of enzymes, and chemotactic factors, all of which elicit sets of metabolic events that lead to muscle fiber degradation and the repair process. The free radical theory of aging hypothesizes that the aging process and associated degenerative conditions are the cumulative results of random free radical reactions which occur within cells and organisms.[3] The production of free radicals is a continuous biological process, involving a number of defensive enzymatic and nonenzymatic systems. At least one aspect of the aging process shares a common biochemical entity with exercise-induced oxidative stress. Therefore, the interplay of exercise in the aging process and age-associated disease is the subject of interest for scientists in the field of exercise and aging and for health-conscious people and professionals. This chapter briefly reviews the major sites of free radical generation during exercise and examines the role of enzymatic and nonenzymatic antioxidant defense systems in exercise-induced oxidative stress. The impact of exercise in old age and the role of training adaptation and metabolic events that may lead to improvement of the health and physical strength of elderly people are also briefly discussed.

II. EXERCISE-INDUCED OXIDATIVE STRESS, GENERATION OF FREE RADICALS

Free radicals are atoms and molecules having an unpaired electron, i.e., O_2^-, $HO^{\cdot}$, and include organic radicals such as $R^{\cdot}$, $RO^{\cdot}$, $RO_2^{\cdot}$. Free radicals can damage molecules that are important in cellular function, thereby leading to a total loss of cellular function. These deleterious free radical reactions can also be produced by various environmental factors.[4,5] Superoxide radicals are formed during the reduction of oxygen which occurs in the inner mitochondrial membrane. These radicals can trigger chain reactions in the fatty acids of phospholipids, thereby leading to membrane lipid peroxidation and the loss of membrane bilayer organization, which is necessary for membrane-bound enzyme and receptor function.[3] In oxidative stress conditions, higher levels of oxygen radicals are produced, exceeding the cellular antioxidant defense system, resulting in the peroxidation of polyunsaturated fatty acids (PUFA) in membrane structures. Lipid peroxidation also releases reactive free radicals and toxic aldehydes, which then can completely inactivate enzymes and other cell components.[6] There are multiple enzymatic and nonenzymatic antioxidant defense systems in cells that protect the membranes and other cell organelles from the damaging effects of free radical reactions.

Strenuous and exhaustive exercise, as well as unaccustomed exercise, induce oxidative damage and result in muscle injury.[7,8] Prolonged submaximal exercise has been demonstrated to result in elevated whole body (indicated by increased exhaled pentane, but not ethane)[9] and skeletal muscle[10] levels of lipid peroxidation by-products. These studies seem to indicate that the greatly increased oxygen consumption (up to a 100-fold increase in skeletal muscle) of exercise produces superoxide radicals which are associated with a host of deleterious effects. Several *in vivo* and *in vitro* animal and human studies have shown direct and indirect evidence of free radical generation during and following exercise. The initial and early events in muscle injury have been described as autogenous[11] and occur before phagocytic cells enter the injury sites. In addition to high specific tension, the metabolic events could be the initial stimuli in exercise-induced injury. Loss of Ca^{2+} homeostasis seems to be a key event in the damaging process. Depletion of cellular thiols and increase of intracellular Ca^{2+} may potentiate free radical generation, membrane lipid peroxidation, and leakage of intracellular enzymes. The source of free radicals in exercise-induced oxidative stress has been suggested to be of (1) mitochondrial origin, where oxygen radicals may escape scavenging enzymes of mitochondria and leak into the cytosol; (2) capillary endothelium, where the hypoxia/reoxygenation condition is created during exercise;[12] (3) inflammatory cells, where superoxide production is elicited by mediator generated during exercise.

A. MITOCHONDRIAL PRODUCTION OF SUPEROXIDES

Energy in mitochondria through the respiratory chain is converted into ion gradients and adenosine triphosphate (ATP). ATP provides energy for muscle contraction. The energy conversion in mitochondria is coupled with oxygen utilization and is known as respiratory control. The respiratory control capacity has been shown to decrease when animals were subjected to exhaustive exercise.[10,13] Local stores of glycogen and fat are the energy sources for continuous regeneration of ATP during exercise that requires molecular oxygen as an electron accepter for the oxidation process in the critic acid cycle and in the electron transport chain of mitochondria. Molecular oxygen contains two unpaired electrons which, through reduction with four electrons and hydrogen ion, forms water. This process occurs in the mitochondria, with cytochrome oxidase as the final catalyst. A small fraction of molecular oxygen (2 to 5%) is reduced by a pathway which proceeds in a stepwise one-electron reduction to produce a highly reactive superoxide radical (O_2^-), which then can undergo further reduction to form hydroxyl radical ($^\cdot OH$), hydrogen peroxide (H_2O_2), and, finally, water.[14] These are normally produced during cellular metabolism, and their continuous reactions with other cellular components have been suggested to contribute to the aging process.[3] During intensive exercise due to probable loss of cytochrome oxidase activity,[15] the level of molecular oxygen that is required to be reduced through four-electron reduction exceeds the muscle mitochondria respiratory capacity. This condition leads to the univalent reduction of molecular oxygen through semiquinones, an alternate electron acceptor in the inner mitochondrial membrane, and generates superoxide radicals.[15-17]

Several lines of evidence support the theory of mitochondrial production of free radicals during exercise. Oxygen radicals are known to originate from ubiquinone oxidation in the respiratory electron transport system located in the inner mitochondrial membrane.[16,17] Evidence demonstrating mitochondrial involvement in the production of superoxide radicals during exercise arises from the work of Davies et al.,[10] who showed that exhaustive exercise in rats resulted in a marked reduction in the respiratory control indices of mitochondrial enzymes, (pyruvate-malate, glutamate, and succinate), suggesting an increasing inner membrane leakiness to protons, and a decreasing energy-coupling efficiency due to exercise.

Since free radicals have a short half-life, direct detection of radicals has been always regarded as strong evidence, rather than the determination of end-products. The direct evidence showing that exercise induces radicals emerges from increased electron paramagnetic resonance (EPR) and electron spin resonance (ESR) signals from exercised muscle. Davies et al.[10] found a two to threefold increase in EPR signals of $R^\cdot$ in muscle homogenates prepared from rats that were exercised to exhaustion. Jackson et al.,[18] using ESR techniques, found that muscle contraction generated by electrical stimulation exhibited an increase of 70% in the ESR signal, which is composed of semiquinone type radicals. Most recently, Kumar et al.[19] have found an ESR signal of free radical from exercised heart homogenate of rat which was not present when the rats were supplemented with a free radical quencher such as vitamin E. The increase in EPR and ESR signals does not yet provide evidence that free radicals are the consequence of damage, or that the higher concentration was the cause of damage. Whether the increase in radicals is primary or secondary to the exercise-induced damage has yet to be determined.

B. GENERATION OF SUPEROXIDES IN HYPOXIA AND REOXYGENATION

Reactive oxygen species are generated during ischemia/hypoxia and subsequent reperfusion/reoxygenation. In this process, ATP is depleted and intracellular calcium is increased, leading to cellular necrosis, which is known as the oxygen paradox. The presently accepted mechanism for the generation of oxygen free radicals through hypoxia and reoxygenation is that, during hypoxia, xanthine is formed from the degradation of ATP, and, during the reoxygenation upon the mild proteolysis, xanthine dehydrogenase is converted to xanthine oxidase, which then generates oxygen radical and uric acid from xanthine.[14,20] Following exercise, due to the action of capillary xanthine oxidase, the concentration of hypoxanthine (a precursor for xanthine) and uric acid in plasma increases.[21,22] Xanthine oxidase has been reported to be present in the endothelial cells of capillaries in skeletal muscle.[23] Hellsten-Westing et al.[24] have indicated that the time delay of increase in plasma uric acid that they observed during the 800 m run might be the time required for the conversion of xanthine dehydrogenase to oxidase form. During the intensive exercise, muscles suffer a temporary ATP imbalance, causing a malfunctioning of ion pumps and, thus, an increase of intracellular calcium. Protease becomes activated with increased intracellular Ca^{2+}, which in turn converts xanthine dehydrogenase to xanthine oxidase. Therefore, temporary ATP imbalance leads to a metabolic stress and simulates an ischemia and reperfusion condition. Even though the net result is the increase of oxygen free radicals, the skeletal muscles may not be the only tissues to generate free radicals by ATP degradation during the exercise. Skeletal muscles have a low activity of xanthine dehydrogenase and oxidase.[25] Therefore, Sahlin et al.[26] suggested that the generation of hypoxanthine occurs in exercising muscle, whereas the transformation to xanthine and the production of superoxides and uric acid may occur in other tissues, such as the vascular endothelium. Blockage of the muscle microvasculature by neutrophil and decrease in blood flow and partial oxygen pressure during intensive exercise may create a hypoxic condition. A hypoxic condition may also be created in the internal organs from which the blood flow may be shifted to exercising skeletal muscle. Following the reoxygenation which occurs after exercise, these organs may experience a similar condition of hypoxia/reoxygenation which then contributes to the overall oxygen radical formation.

C. SUPEROXIDE PRODUCTION BY INFLAMMATORY CELLS

Inflammatory cells are another source of free radicals following exercise. In addition to the direct damaging effect of superoxide radicals on muscle tissue, these radicals are involved in the inflammatory process, which is a secondary phenomena to the exercise-induced oxidative stress. Following exercise, infiltration of neutrophils and phagocytic cells in exercised muscles has been observed in animals and humans.[27,28] Activation of chemotactic factors by superoxide radical, similar to early manifestation of the acute phase response in infection, has been suggested to occur following exercise.[29] Products of lipoxygenase pathway in muscle are chemotactic for immune cells. Several studies have also demonstrated that, following exercise, immune complements are activated, which is an initial event in the inflammatory response.[8] This process is then followed by the mobilization and activation of neutrophils,[30] production of acute phase proteins, and accumulation of monocytes and macrophages at the site of injury. Neutrophils contain several enzymes, such as myeloperoxidase and nicotinamide-adenine dinucleotide phosphate (reduced) (NADPH) oxidase, that generate radicals such as $NO^{\cdot}$, $HO^{\cdot}$, and H_2O_2, and hypochlorous acid.[14] Neutrophils and monocytes release these superoxide anions and degradative enzymes, such as elastase[31] and lysozyme,[32] that further break down muscle to be phagocytized by macrophage and monocytes,[8] and this will be followed by the production of growth factors for new muscle fiber regeneration. As a part of the inflammatory response, activated neutrophils and macrophages produce both superoxide anions and hydrogen peroxide at the site of damaged muscle, which, in turn, is directly responsible for the disruption of phospholipid bilayer and lipid peroxidation.

III. ENZYMATIC AND NONENZYMATIC DEFENSE SYSTEMS

With the normal metabolic activity, cells are generating plenty of oxygen radicals that, if not removed, can cause oxidative damage. This accounts for up to 2 to 5% of cellular reactions that utilize molecular oxygen as an electron acceptor. Intensive exercise which increases total oxygen uptake by more than tenfold, can potentially be harmful to the exercising muscles and other organs. The double bonds of fatty acids in phospholipid of membrane are the major targets for free radical damage. Mammalian cells are well equipped with both enzymatic and nonenzymatic protection systems that eliminate these noxious radicals. The enzymatic system includes superoxide dismutase (SOD), catalase, and glutathione peroxidase (GSH-Px). These enzymes, in a cooperative interaction with other enzymes and reducing agents, provide an added layer of cellular protection. SOD converts superoxide radical to H_2O_2, and catalase converts H_2O_2 to molecular oxygen and water. Manganese-based SOD is found exclusively in mitochondria, whereas, copper- and zinc-based SOD are present in the cytosol.[33] The selenium containing enzyme GSH-Px uses glutathione as a hydrogen donor and converts H_2O_2 and organic hydroperoxides to water and the corresponding alcohol, respectively. The majority of superoxide radicals that are produced in mitochondria are reduced by mitochondrial SOD, and only a small fraction may diffuse out to the cytosol.[34] Catalase is predominantly located in peroxisome, whereas GSH-Px, as well as glutathione tripeptide, are found in mitochondria and cytosol.[35]

Exercise has been shown to influence the activity of these scavenging enzymes in muscle and other tissues. Animal studies demonstrated that exercise training and exhaustive exercise increases SOD activity in skeletal and heart muscle.[36-38] Jenkin et al.[39] reported an increase of Cu-Zn SOD activity in human skeletal muscle after training. In contrast, Alessio and Goldfarb,[40,41] found that total SOD activity was not affected by either acute or chronic exercise. While 1-h treadmill running in rat has been shown to have little effect on skeletal muscle SOD, it did increase activity of hepatic SOD.[42,43] The partial occupancy of the enzyme by the substrate and an increase of substrate concentration have been suggested as a mechanism for the increase of SOD activity.[44]

Although the increase of SOD activity by exercise training appears to be a part of the adaptive response, Higuchi et al.[38] indicated that a small increase of mitochondrial SOD (37%) in fast-twitch red type muscle of rat after training was accompanied with a twofold increase in those constituents of the mitochondrial respiratory chain that are capable of producing a higher level of superoxides. Thus, this finding indicated that the small increase in mitochondrial SOD activity by endurance training is unlikely to provide adequate protection against free radical damage. Furthermore, Higuchi et al.[38] pointed out that by training, the adapted muscle did not show an increase in capacity of other enzymes, such as cystolic SOD or catalase, to eliminate free radicals. Thus, endurance exercise-trained muscle is prone to accelerated aging.

Most of the reviewed literature reported no change in muscle catalase with exercise and training. An increase of hepatic catalase activity with an acute bout of exercise without affecting skeletal muscle catalase activity in rat has been reported by Ji et al.[42,43] However, Alessio and Goldfarb[40] and Quintanilha et al.[37] reported increased activity of this enzyme in rat muscle following exercise training. A change in the binding characteristics to membranes or the release from proxisome has been proposed as a possible mechanism for the increased activity of this enzyme.[40]

Exercise training has been shown to decrease both mitochondrial and cystolic activity of GSH-Px in rat liver,[42,43] whereas mitochondrial activity of this enzyme was found increased twofold in skeletal muscle by training. Similar increase of GSH-Px activity in heart and skeletal muscle has been reported from rats that were exercised to exhaustion.[37] In contrast, others[45,46] reported no effect on the activity of this enzyme in the skeletal muscle by training or by an acute bout of exercise. Robertson et al.[47] reported that the activity of catalase and GSH-Px in erythrocyte was significantly correlated with the weekly training distance. They found that the total erythrocyte glutathione content was higher in training subjects, and an increase in the reduced form of glutathione was accounted for by this observation. Erythrocyte of seven trained athletes after completion of a half-marathon showed no significant change in SOD, catalase, and GSH-Px activity.[48] While the level of reduced glutathione (GSH) in erythrocytes was decreased up to 24 h, vitamin E level progressively increased up to 48 h, post-race. Gohil et al.[49] found a 60% decrease of GSH and a 100% decrease of oxidized glutathione (GSSG) in whole blood during prolonged, submaximal exercise. Furthermore, Kretzchmar et al.[50] reported a decrease of GSH without change in GSSG in plasma after acute physical exercise.

Vitamin E is the major lipophilic chain-breaking antioxidant in cells, which protects membrane PUFA from lipid peroxidation. Mitochondria contains a significant portion of tissue vitamin E in the inner membrane.[51] The high content of vitamin E in the mitochondria provides a primary line of defense against superoxide radicals generated from the respiratory chain reaction in mitochondria. Evidence for the involvement of free radicals in exercise-induced damage emerges from animal studies testing the effect of exercise in vitamin E-deficient or supplemented systems, both *in vivo* and *in vitro*.

In vitamin E-deficient animals, exercise has been reported to increase susceptibility to free radical damage, which resulted in a greater fragility of lysosomal membrane and a marked depression of muscle mitochondrial respiratory control and premature exhaustion.[10,37,52] In untrained rats, it has been shown that a single bout of exercise at 70% of VO_{2max} decreased vitamin E content of the quadricept muscle by 30%.[53] Endurance training in rats has been shown to reduce muscle vitamin E, regardless of whether the rats were fed vitamin E-deficient or vitamin E-sufficient diets.[54] Vitamin E deficiency has also been demonstrated to decrease the endurance capacity of animals, indicating a higher requirement for vitamin E with exercise training.[10,52] Furthermore, Gohil et al.[55] demonstrated that muscle mitochondria and ubiquinone content were increased without a concurrent increase in vitamin E concentration. They concluded that exercise training may decrease muscle vitamin E concentration, and may be predisposed to oxidative stress. Kumar et al.[19] recently reported that exercise decreased serum and heart muscle vitamin E levels in Wistar rats, and that dietary vitamin E supplementation protected against oxidative stress induced by exercise. Their results reiterated that this protection is not mediated through the improvement of antioxidant enzyme systems like SOD, catalase, or GSH-Px. The decrease in the number of muscle fibers, the irregular appearance of Z-band arrangements in fibers, and the increase of plasma CK have also been demonstrated in vitamin E-deficient rats following exercise.[56,57] In addition to its critical antioxidant role, vitamin E may function to stabilize membranes and to maintain cellular homeostasis. Accumulation of intracellular Ca^{2+} is a crucial step in muscle injury. Increased enzyme efflux from vitamin E-depleted muscle has been demonstrated by Jackson et al.[58] When isolated muscle fiber was supplemented with large amounts of vitamin E, the toxic effect of a higher intracellular Ca^{2+} level and the leakage of enzymes were decreased.[59] This protective effect of vitamin E against the cytotoxicity of Ca^{2+} may not be solely mediated by its antioxidant function.

A change in plasma and tissue vitamin E due to heavy and unaccustomed exercise has been reported. Pincemail et al.[60] reported an increase of plasma and erythrocyte vitamin E during intensive exercise in humans and suggested that the mobilization of vitamin E from other tissue into plasma and erythrocytes could help to prevent lipid peroxidation from occurring in exercising skeletal muscle. Earlier studies have reported no beneficial effect of vitamin E supplementation on human exercise performance.[61,62] Even though physical performance has not been measured, recent reports point to some protection by vitamin E supplementation against exercise-induced oxidative stress.

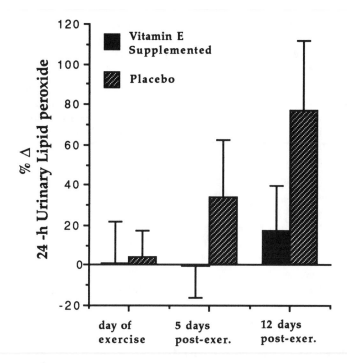

FIGURE 1.   Effect of vitamin E supplementation on 24-h urinary lipid peroxide excretion in >55-year-old subjects following eccentric exercise.

Vitamin E supplementation is shown to be effective in reducing plasma lipid peroxides,[63] pentane exhalation,[64,65] and urinary thiobarbituric (TBA)-adducts following heavy exercise[66] (Figure 1). An increase in the concentration of vitamin C in plasma and lymphocyte following a 21-km race was suggested to be associated with exercise-induced stress and an increase in plasma cortisol levels.[67]

Animal and human studies indicate that in response to training or an acute bout of exercise, the activity of antioxidant enzymes in muscle mitochondria may increase. However, unproportional production of mitochondrial super-oxide radicals generated by exercise may exceed this enzymatic antioxidant protection and predispose to free radical injury. Therefore, additional protection provided by nonenzymatic antioxidants may prevent muscle from exercise-induced free radical damage and accelerated aging.

IV. EXERCISE AND MUSCLE DAMAGE

Muscle contraction and shortening produce a concentric action; however, when skeletal muscle lengthens as it produces force, the result is an eccentric muscle action. An example of this is lifting a weight (concentric action) and lowering it (eccentric action). At the same power output, the oxygen cost of eccentric exercise is lower than that of concentric exercise.[68] Despite the lower oxygen cost, eccentric exercise has been demonstrated to be a potent cause of muscle damage,[69,70] delayed onset muscle soreness, and increased circulating creatine kinase (CK) activity.[71]

Running a marathon can cause extensive skeletal muscle damage.[72,73] Warhol and co-workers[73] showed a characteristic pattern of muscle damage, with tearing of sarcomeres at the Z-band level, followed by movement of fluid into the muscle cells in biopsies taken in the days following the race. Mitochondrial and myofibrillar damage showed progressive repair by three to four weeks after the marathon. Late biopsies (8 to 12 weeks after the race) showed central nuclei and satellite cells, characteristic of a regenerative response. The damage seen by these investigators is very similar to the ultrastructural changes in skeletal muscle resulting from eccentric exercise.

The extent of the ultrastructural evidence of damage is greater well after the initial damaging exercise. Friden et al.[74] found more damaged muscle fibers 3 d after, when compared to that seen only 1 h after high tension eccentric exercise. Newham and co-workers[69] also showed that eccentric exercise caused immediate damage, but the biopsies taken 24 to 48 h after the exercise showed more marked damage. These data are indicative of an ongoing process of skeletal muscle repair consisting of an increased degradation of damaged proteins and an increased rate of protein synthesis.

Following only one bout of high intensity eccentric exercise,[71] previously sedentary men showed a prolonged increase in the rate of muscle protein breakdown, evidenced by an increase in urinary 3-methylhistidine/creatinine, which peaked 10 d later. In addition, an increase in circulating interleukin-1 (IL-1) levels in these subjects was seen 3 h after the exercise. Endurance trained men, performing the same exercise, did not display increased circulating IL-1 levels. However, their preexercise plasma IL-1 levels were significantly higher than those seen in the untrained subjects.

V. ACUTE AND CHRONIC RESPONSE TO MUSCLE DAMAGE

Damage to tissue, as well as infection, stimulate a wide range of defense reactions, known as the acute phase response.[75] The acute phase response is critical for its antiviral and antibacterial actions, as well as for promoting the clearance of damaged tissue and subsequent repair. Within hours of injury or exercise,[76] the number of circulating neutrophils can increase many fold. Neutrophils migrate to the site of injury, where they phagocytize tissue debris and release factors known to increase protein breakdown, such as lysozyme and oxygen radicals.[77] Greater neutrophil increases have been observed after eccentric exercise than after concentric exercise.[78] While neutrophils have a relatively short half-life (1 or 2 d) within tissue,[79] the life-span of monocytes may be one to two months after migration to damaged tissue.[80] Substantial monocyte accumulation in skeletal muscle was found after completion of a marathon. Following eccentric exercise, monocyte accumulation in muscle was not seen until 4 to 7 d later.[28,81] In addition to the capability to phagocytize damaged tissue, monocytes secrete cytokines such as IL-1 and tumor necrosis factor (TNF). These and other cytokines mediate a wide range of metabolic events, having an effect on virtually every organ system in the body. Fielding et al.[82] found that, following downhill running, muscle IL-1β was increased by 135% immediately and 250% 5 d later. Intramuscular neutrophil accumulation was positively correlated with muscle IL-1β. In addition, they noted a significant relationship between the percentage of damage Z-bands (from ultrastructural analysis) and neutrophil accumulation, indicating that the tissue accumulation of neutrophils following eccentric exercise may be associated with observed exercise-induced muscle injury. Whether the injury releases a chemoattractant that leads to increased muscle neutrophils or whether invading neutrophils release oxygen radicals that lead to further damage is unclear.

Elevated cytokine levels during infection or injury have different and selective effects. IL-1 mediates an elevated core temperature during infection.[30] In laboratory animals, IL-1 and TNF increase muscle proteolysis and liberation of amino acids,[83] possibly providing substrate for increased hepatic protein synthesis. While circulating IL-1 has been shown to increase acutely as a result of eccentric exercise,[84] by 24 h after the exercise, it returned to resting levels. Biopsies of the vastus lateralis taken before, immediately after, and 5 d after downhill running, showed an immediate and prolonged increase in IL-1β.[85] This study implicates muscle IL-1β in the postexercise change in protein metabolism.

VI. EXERCISE-INDUCED OXIDATIVE STRESS AND AGING

Physical performance and functional capacity decrease with aging. These changes are in part related to the decrease of muscle mass and whole body protein which occurs with aging. There are a few studies that have examined the association of aging and exercise-induced oxidative stress and the role of the antioxidant defense system in aged skeletal muscle. Lammi-Keefe et al.[86] have found that the activity of SOD enzyme increases in several skeletal and heart muscles of rats with an increase in age of up to 23 months. Ji et al.[87] reported an increased activity of several enzymes involved in oxygen free radical metabolism in skeletal muscle with age. These include major antioxidant enzymes, i.e., SOD, catalase, and GSH-Px. In addition, the activity of GSH-S-transferases, glutathione reductase, and glucose-6-phosphate dehydrogenase enzymes, which are supporting enzymes in the cellular antioxidant function, were also higher in the middle-aged and senescent rats compared to young rats. Interestingly, the enhanced activity of enzymes was accompanied by the presence of a higher level of lipid peroxides in muscle homogenate and mitochondria from senescent rats. Ji et al.[87] suggested that in response to the increasing mitochondrial and cystolic free radical reaction, rather than the weakening of antioxidant enzyme system with aging, the enzymatic antioxidant defense system may increase in skeletal muscle. These findings indicate that muscle tissue can up-regulate the activity of these enzymes during aging.

Zerba et al.[88] have observed that old mouse muscle is more susceptible to injury and is damaged more severely by lengthening contractions, and demonstrated a lower maximum isotonic force when compared to young and adult mice. They found no differences in the degree of injury between young and adult mice, indicating that muscle susceptibility to injury increases in the late life-span. As indicated, the activity of antioxidant enzymes in muscle may increase with aging, but the efficiency of these enzymes to protect against oxidative injury might become low, or may not meet the high demand for protection at the oxidative stress condition. Although Zerba et al.[88] did not measure muscle SOD activity, they found that pretreatment of old mice with SOD provided an immediate protection against injury, indicating that during the lengthening contraction, in addition to mechanical injury, oxidative damage contributes to the initial injury, and that additional antioxidant protection may be beneficial.

The plasma level of reduced glutathione has been shown to decrease with age in both untrained and well-trained individuals.[50] Kretzchmar et al.[50] also found that well-trained individuals of age 36 to 57 years had a higher reduced glutathione level in circulating blood than did untrained individuals of the same age. Therefore, exercise training could be an effective means to restore the age-dependent decline in plasma glutathione and to enhance resistance to oxidative stress. Animal experiments have pointed out that dietary antioxidants might play a significant role in the prevention of injury resulting from oxidative stress. Supplemental vitamin E has been shown to prevent exercise-induced free radical formation in cardiac muscle of rat.[19] Cannon et al.[76] found that following an eccentric bout of exercise, young subjects (<30 years) had a higher plasma CK concentration and a greater number of neutrophils in circulating blood than did older subjects (>55 years). Supplementation with 800 IU vitamin E per day in older subjects for seven weeks tended to eliminate these differences from young subjects. Measuring plasma lipid peroxides did not show the effect of exercise or vitamin E supplementation between the two age groups. This was probably due to rapid clearance of lipid peroxides from plasma. A variety of factors may contribute to eliminate or neutralize lipid peroxides following exercise. These include the induction of enzymatic antioxidants, the mobilization of antioxidants from other tissues, and the elimination of end-products from breath and urine. From the above study, Meydani et al.[66] reported that following exercise, the excretion of lipid peroxides in urine increased in both age groups (Figure 2). They found that the excretion of these products in urine was greatest in the placebo groups at 12 d postexercise, and vitamin E supplemented subjects excreted a lower level of these compounds. This indicates that vitamin E supplementation has suppressed oxidative damage induced by eccentric exercise. Furthermore,

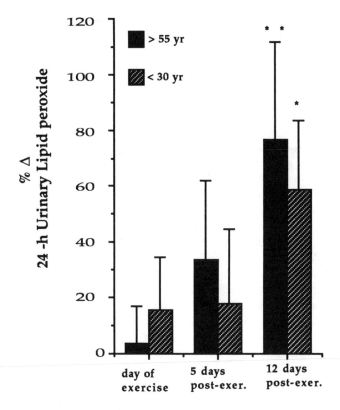

FIGURE 2. Effect of eccentric exercise on 24-h urinary lipid peroxide excretion in young (<30 years) and old (>55 years) subjects.

they found that the protective effect of vitamin E was more prominent in older subjects. The delayed increase in urinary lipid peroxides coinsided with an increased protein breakdown, as indicated by urinary excretion of 3 methylhistidine.[89] Davies et al.[10] has suggested that oxidatively modified proteins are more rapidly and selectively degraded by intracellular proteolytic systems. This process may be further accelerated by oxygen free radical species produced by mononuclear cells and neutrophils infiltrating damaged muscle tissue in order to clear debris.[10,77] The catabolic breakdown of protein and the anabolic utilization of amino acid products for remodeling and the generation of new fibers is a continuous process which may last for several weeks after initial muscle injury.[8] Therefore, the increased excretion of urinary TBA-adducts, which are in part derived from lipid peroxidation, appear to parallel the proteolytic process that was also elevated 12 d postexercise.[89]

These studies indicated that there is an increased susceptibility to muscle injury with aging. Decline in muscle mass and reduced functional capacity in older age, in combination with decreased biochemical defense system, make the elderly more susceptible to oxidative stress and injury. Mild exercise training in older age can prevent loss of lean body and muscle mass, increase functional capacity, and decrease susceptibility to muscle injury. In addition, adequate dietary intake and supplemental micronutrients, especially those of antioxidants, should be regarded as important factors against free radicals and in slowing down the age-dependent decline of functional capacity.

VII. AGING AND ADAPTATION TO EXERCISE

Eccentric exercise increases both circulating and skeletal muscle neutrophil levels.[85] Figure 3 is a micrograph of a vastus lateralis biopsy taken only 45 min after 45 min of downhill running and clearly demonstrates the presence of neutrophils. As stated earlier, muscle neutrophils and mononuclear cells can serve as a source of oxygen free radicals, which may partially cause the delayed increase in ultrastructural damage.[10] Free radical processes may also be directly related to delayed functional impairment in muscle following damage. Zerba and co-workers[88] examined the extensor digitorum longus muscles from young, adult, and old mice following *in situ* muscle damage by lengthening contractions. Muscle injury was assessed by measurement of maximum isometric tetanic force (P_o), as well as by morphological damage. Three days after the injury, muscle P_o of the old mice was approximately 15% lower than that of the young and adult mice. They also found that mice treated with a free radical scavenger, polyethylene glycol-superoxide dismutase (PEG-SOD), showed less delayed injury and significantly greater muscle P_o. Interestingly, they found that PEG-SOD afforded some protection from damage 10 min after exercise in the old animals. These data indicate that muscles of old mice are more susceptible to muscle damage from lengthening contraction than are young and adult muscles; a free-radical scavenger provides some measure of protection from delayed muscle damage; and free-radicals, as well as mechanical forces, contribute to the initial damage.

Manfredi and co-workers[90] found significantly greater amounts of ultrastructural muscle damage in older men performing 45 min of high-intensity eccentric exercise compared to the damage seen in younger men performing eccentric exercise at a similar intensity. Old skeletal muscle may be more susceptible to eccentric exercise-induced injury for the following reasons: (1) Byrnes and co-workers[91] have demonstrated that one bout of eccentric exercise significantly reduced muscle damage following subsequent bouts of exercise for up to six weeks. When compared to younger individuals, older men typically are less active and fit,[92] and thus, the lower amounts of physical activity in the elderly may increase the degree of eccentric exercise-induced muscle damage. (2) Skeletal muscle in older individuals may have more intrinsic damage than that seen in younger subjects prior to exercise. Armstrong et al.[93] noted that even among muscle fibers recruited, some showed more damage than others, and they suggested that some muscle fibers may be more susceptible to injury than other fibers. Muscle from older subjects may have more of these susceptible fibers. This intrinsic damage seen in

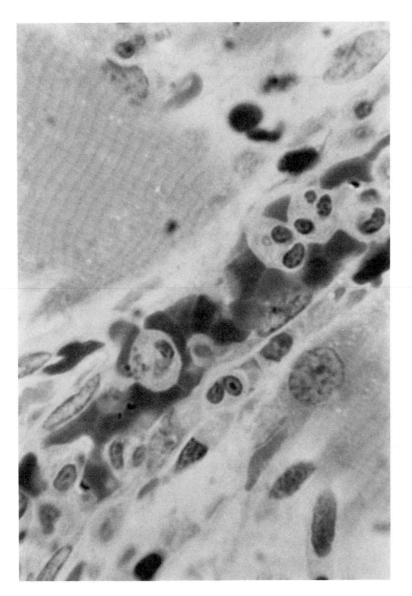

FIGURE 3. Photomicrograph of vastus lateralis biopsy 45 min after exercise, showing a substantial increase in muscle neutrophil content.

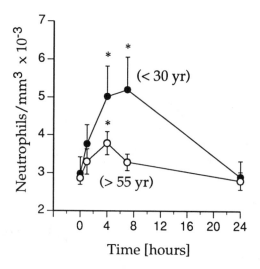

FIGURE 4. Circulating neutrophil counts before and after 45 min of downhill running in old (>55 years) and young (<30 years) men. Neutrophilia increased as a result of exercise and was significantly different between old and young.

older subjects may be due to the accumulation of oxidized forms of proteins.[94] Rates of skeletal muscle lipid peroxidation (as well as antioxidant enzyme activities) have been demonstrated to increase with advancing age.[95] The accumulation of oxidized proteins in muscle may indicate that, with age, there is a greater increase in the rate of lipid peroxidation than the increase seen in the activities of antioxidant enzymes.

Cannon et al.[76] saw a greatly attenuated neutrophil response (Figure 4) in untrained older men (>55 years) when compared to younger men (<30 years) during the 24 h period following 45 min of downhill running. In addition, the delayed increase in plasma CK activity was also significantly lower in the older men. This may be due to a reduced ability of the elderly to mount an acute-phase response to muscle damage. In this study, vitamin E supplementation (800 IU per day for two months prior to the exercise) had the effect of significantly increasing the postexercise rise in circulating neutrophils and CK activity in the older subjects only. There was no effect on the response of the younger men, in that after vitamin E supplementation, no significant age-associated differences occurred in their response to exercise. At the time of peak concentrations in the plasma, CK correlated ($r = 0.751$, $p < 0.001$) with superoxide release from neutrophils. The association of this circulating skeletal muscle enzyme with neutrophil mobilization and function supports the concept that neutrophils are involved in the delayed increase in muscle membrane permeability after damaging exercise. These data indicate that vitamin E supplementation may affect the rate of repair of skeletal muscle following muscle damage, and that these effects may be more pronounced in older subjects.

VIII. CONCLUSION

The age-associated decrease in functional capacity is due, in part, to reduced muscle mass and strength. Catabolic and anabolic processes that occur in skeletal muscle during and following exercise are under the influence of various mediators in which oxygen free radicals are major contributors. During exercise-induced oxidative stress, oxygen free radicals are released in muscles from mitochondrial oxidative phosphorylation and/or from inflammatory cells, which may trigger and stimulate a host of metabolic events that involve the antioxidant defense system. With increasing age, the balance between the antioxidant defense system and the deleterious action of oxygen radicals becomes more sensitive to physical stress. There is evidence that the age-related increase in antioxidant enzyme activity is not sufficient to compensate for increases in the rate of lipid peroxidation. This fragile balance implies that the elderly are more susceptible to oxidative muscle damage following the stress of physical activity. Exercise training, in addition to increasing muscle mass and oxidative capacity, improves immune function and mediators that are involved in muscle adaptation. Furthermore, exercise training increases enzymatic antioxidant defense against oxygen free radicals. Since the overall rate of lipid peroxidation in muscles of old age is higher than is enzymatic antioxidant protection, there is increasing evidence that the elderly may benefit from dietary antioxidants.

REFERENCES

1. **Jette, A. M. and L. G. B.,** The framingham disability study. II. Physical disability among the aging, *Am. J. Public Health,* 71, 1211, 1981.
2. **Fiatarone, M. A.,** Exercise, in *Endocrinology and Metabolism in the Elderly,* Moreley, J. E. and Koreman, S., Eds., Blackwell Scientific, Oxford, 1992.
3. **Harman, D.,** Free radicals and the origination, evolution and present status of free radical theory of aging, in *Free Radicals in Molecular Biology, Aging and Disease,* Ravenswood Press, New York, 1984, 1.
4. **Harman, D.,** Free radical theory of aging: beneficial effect of antioxidant on the lifespan of male NZB mice; role of free radical reactions in the deterioration of the immune system with aging and in the pathogenesis of systemic lupus erythematous, *Age,* 3, 64, 1980.
5. **Samarajski, T., Ordy, J. M., and Rudy-Reimer, P.,** Lipofuscin pigment accumulation in the nervous system of aging, *Anat. Rec.,* 160, 555, 1987.
6. **Halliwell, B.,** Oxidants and human disease; some new concepts, *FASEB J.,* 1, 358, 1987.
7. **Packer, L.,** Vitamin E, physical exercise and tissue damage in animals, *Med. Biol.,* 62, 105, 1984.
8. **Evans, W. and Cannon, J. G.,** The metabolic effect of exercise-induced muscle damage, in *Exercise and Sports Sciences Review,* Holloszy, J. O., Ed., Williams & Wilkins, London, 1991, 99.

9. **Gee, D. L. and Tappel, A. L.**, The effect of exhaustive exercise on expired pentane as a measure of *in vivo* lipid peroxidation in the rat, *Life Sci.*, 28, 2425, 1981.

10. **Davies, K. J. A., Quintanilha, A. T., Brooks, G. A., and Packer, L.**, Free radicals and tissue damage produced by exercise, *Biochim. Biophys. Res. Commun.*, 107, 1198, 1982.

11. **Armstrong, R. B.**, Initial events in exercise-induced muscular injury, *Med. Sci. Sports Exercise*, 22, 429, 1990.

12. **Sjodin, B., Hellsten-Westing, Y., and Apple, F. S.**, Biochemical mechanisms for oxygen free radical formation during exercise, *Sports Med.*, 10, 236, 1990.

13. **Quintanilha, A. T., Packer, L., Szyszlo-Davies, J. M., Racanel-li, T. L., and Davies, K. J. A.**, Membrane effects of vitamin E deficiency: bioenergetic and surface charge density studies of skeletal muscle and liver mitochondria, *Vitamin E: Biol. Hematol. Clin. Aspects*, 393, 32, 1982.

14. **Bast, A., Haenin, G. R. M. M., and Doelman, C. J. A.**, Oxidants and antioxidants: state of the art, *Am. J. Med.*, 91 (Supp. 3C), 2S, 1991.

15. **Soussi, B., Idstrom, J. P., Schersten, T., and Bylund-Fellenius, A. C.**, Cytochrome C oxidase and cardiolipin alterations in response to skeletal muscle ischaemia and reperfusion, *Acta Physiol. Scand.*, 138, 107, 1990.

16. **Boveris, A., Cadenas, E., and Stoppani, A. O. K.**, Role of ubiquinone in mitochondrial generation of hydrogen peroxide, *Biochem. J.*, 156, 435, 1976.

17. **Gollnick, P. D., Bertocci, L. A., Kelso, T. B., Witt, E. H., and Hodgson, D. R.**, The effect of high intensity exercise on the respiratory capacity of skeletal muscle, *Eur. J. Physiol.*, 415, 407, 1990.

18. **Jackson, M. L., Edwards, R. H. T., and Symons, M. C. R.**, Electron spin resonance studies of intact mammalian skeletal muscle, *Biochem. Biophys. Acta*, 847, 185, 1985.

19. **Kumar, C. T., Reddy, V. K., Prasd, M., Thyagaraju, K., and Reddanna, P.**, Dietary supplementation of Vitamin E protects heart tissue from exercise-induced oxidant stress, *Mol. Cell Biochem.*, 111, 109, 1992.

20. **McCord, J. M.**, Oxygen-derived free radicals in postischemic tissue injury, *N. Engl. J. Med.*, 312, 159, 1985.

21. **Brooke, M. H., Patterson, V. H., and Kaiser, K. K.**, Hypoxanthine and McArdle disease: a clue to metabolic stress in the working forearm, *Muscle Nerve*, 6, 204, 1983.

22. **Sollevi, A.**, Cardiovascular effects of adenosine in man possible clinical implication, *Prog. Neurobiol.*, 27, 319, 1986.

23. **Jarsch, E.-D., Grund, C., Bruder, G., Heid, H. W., Keenan, T. W., and Franke, W. W.**, Localization of xanthine oxidase in mammary-gland epithelium and capillary endothelium, *Cell*, 25, 67, 1981.

24. **Hellsten-Westing, Y., Ekblom, B., and Sjodin, B.**, The metabolic relation between hypoxanthine and uric acid in man following maximal short-distance running, *Acta Physiol. Scand.*, 137, 341, 1989.

25. **Wajner, W. E. and Henricksson, R. A.**, Distribution of xanthine dehydrogenase and oxidase activities in human and rabbit tissues, *Biochem. Soc. Trans.*, 16, 358, 1988.

26. **Sahlin, K., Ekberg, K., and Cizinsky, S.**, Changes in plasma hypoxanthine and free radical markers during exercise in man, *Acta Physiol. Scand.*, 142, 275, 1991.

27. **Salminen, A.**, Lysosomal changes in skeletal muscles during the repair of exercise injuries in muscle fibres, *Acta Physiol. Scand.*, 539, 1, 1985.

28. **Jones, D. A., Newsham, D. J., Round, J. M., and Tolfree, S. E. J.**, Experimental human muscle damage; morphological changes in relation to other indices of damage, *J. Physiol.*, 375, 435, 1986.

29. **Petrone, W. F., English, D. K., Wong, K., and McCord, J. M.**, Free radicals and inflammation: superoxide dependent chemotactic factor in plasma, *Proc. Natl. Acad. Sci. U.S.A.*, 77, 1159, 1980.

30. **Cannon, J. G. and Kluger, M. J.**, Endogenous pyrogen activity in human plasma after exercise, *Science*, 220, 617, 1983.

31. **Kokot, K., Schaefer, R. M., Teschiner, M., Plass, G. U. R., and Heidland, A.,** Activation of leukocytes during prolonged physical exercise, *Adv. Exp. Med. Biol.*, 240, 57, 1988.

32. **Morozov, V. I., Priiatikin, S., and Nazarov, I. B.,** Secretion of lysozome by blood neutrophils during physical exertion, *Fiziol Zh SSSR Im I M Sechenova*, 75, 334, 1989.

33. **Weisiger, R. A. and Fridorvich, I.,** Mitochondrial superoxide dismutase site of synthesis and intramitochondrial localization, *J. Biol. Chem.*, 248, 4793, 1973.

34. **Nohl, H. and Hegner, D.,** Do mitochondria produce oxygen radicals *in vivo?*, *Eur. J. Biochem.*, 82, 563, 1986.

35. **Mbemba, F., Houbion, A., Raes, M., and Remacle, J.,** Subcellular localization and modification with ageing of glutathione, glutathione peroxidase and glutathione reductase activities in human fibroblasts, *Biochem. Biophys. Acta*, 838, 211, 1985.

36. **Jenkin, R. R.,** Free radical chemistry: relationship to exercise, *Sports Med.*, 5, 156, 1988.

37. **Quintanilha, A. T.,** Effect of physical exercise and/or vitamin E on tissue oxidative metabolism, *Biochem. Soc. Trans.*, 12, 403, 1984.

38. **Higuchi, M., Cartier, L. J., Chen, M., and Holloszy, J. O.,** Superoxide dismutase and catalase in skeletal muscle: adaptive response to exercise, *J. Gerentol.*, 40, 281, 1985.

39. **Jenkin, R. R., Friendland, R., and Howald, H.,** The relationship of oxygen uptake to superoxide dismutase and catalase in human skeletal muscle, *Int. J. Sports Med.*, 5, 11, 1984.

40. **Alessio, H. M. and Goldfarb, A. H.,** Lipid peroxidation and scavenger enzymes during exercise: adaptive response to training, *J. Appl. Physiol.*, 64, 1333, 1988.

41. **Alessio, H. M., Goldfarb, A. H., and Cutler, R. G.,** MDA content increases in fast- and slow-twitch skeletal muscle with intensity of exercise in a rat, *Am. J. Physiol.*, 255, C874, 1988.

42. **Ji, L. L., Stratman, F. W., and Lardy, H. A.,** Antioxidant enzyme systems in rat liver and skeletal muscle, *Arch. Biochem. Biophys.*, 263, 150, 1988.

43. **Ji, L. L., Stratman, F. W., and Lardy, H. A.,** Enzymatic down regulation with exercise in rat skeletal muscle, *Arch. Biochem. Biophys.*, 263, 137, 1988.

44. **Vihko, V., Salminen, A., and Rantamaki, J.,** Oxidative lysosomal capacity in skeletal muscle of mice after endurance training of different intensities, *Acta Physiol. Scand.*, 104, 74, 1978.

45. **Brady, P. S., Brady, L. J., and Ullrey, D. E.,** Selenium, vitamin E and the response to swimming stress in the rat, *J. Nutr.*, 109, 1103, 1979.

46. **Salminen, A. and Vihko, V.,** Endurance training reduces the susceptibility of mouse skeletal muscle to lipid peroxidation *in vitro*, *Acta Physiol. Scand.*, 117, 109, 1983.

47. **Robertson, J. D., Maughan, R. J., Duthie, G. G., and Morrice, P. C.,** Increased blood antioxidant systems of runners in response to training load, *Clin. Sci.*, 80, 611, 1991.

48. **Duthie, G. G., Robertson, J. D., Maughan, R. J., and Morrice, P. C.,** Blood antioxidant status and erythrocyte lipid peroxidation following distance running, *Arch. Biochem. Biophys.*, 282, 78, 1990.

49. **Gohil, K., Viguie, C., Stanley, W. C., Brooks, G. A., and Packer, L.,** Blood glutathione oxidation during human exercise, *J. Appl. Physiol.*, 86, 115, 1988.

50. **Kretzchmar, M., Muller, D., Hubscher, J., Marin, E., and Klinger, W.,** Influence of aging, training and acute physical exercise on plasma glutathione and lipid peroxides in man, *Int. J. Sports Med.*, 12, 218, 1991.

51. **Buttriss, J. L. and Diplock, A. T.,** The relationship between alpha-tocopherol and phospholipid fatty acids in rat liver subcellular membrane fraction, *Biochem. Biophys. Acta*, 962, 81, 1988.

52. **Gohil, K., Packer, L., de Lumen, G., Brooks, G. A., and Terblanche, S. E.,** Vitamin E deficiency and vitamin C supplements: exercise and mitochondrial oxidation, *J. Appl. Physiol.,* 60, 1986, 1986.

53. **Bowles, D. K., Torgan, C. E., Kehrer, J. P., Ivy, J. L., and Starnes, J. W.,** Effects of acute, submaximal exercise on skeletal muscle vitamin E, *Free Radical Res. Commun.,* 14, 139, 1991.

54. **Aikawa, K. M., Quintanilha, A. T., de Lumen, B. O., Brooks, G. A., and Packer, L.,** Exercise endurance-training alters vitamin E tissue levels and red-blood-cell hemolysis in rodents, *Biosci. Rep.,* 4, 253, 1984.

55. **Gohil, K., Rothfuss, L., Lang, J., and Packer, L.,** Effect of exercise training on tissue vitamin E and ubiquinone content, *J. Appl. Physiol.,* 63, 1638, 1987.

56. **Amelink, G. J., Van der Wal, W. A. A., Wokke, J. H. J., van der Asbeck, B. S., and Bar, P. R.,** Exercise-induced muscle damage in the rat: the effect of vitamin E deficiency, *Eur. J. Physiol.,* 419, 304, 1991.

57. **Amemiya, T.,** Differences in muscular changes in rats with vitamin E and with selenium deficiency, *Int. J. Vit. Nutr. Res.,* 57, 139, 1987.

58. **Jackson, M. J., Jones, D. A., and Edwards, R. H. T.,** *Vitamin E and Skeletal Muscle. Biology of Vitamin E,* Vol. 101, Symp. edition, Pitman Press, London 1983, 224.

59. **Phoenix, J., Edwards, R. H. T., and Jackson, M. J.,** Inhibition of Ca^{2+}-induced cytosolic enzyme efflux from skeletal muscle by vitamin E and related compounds, *Biochem. J.,* 257, 207, 1989.

60. **Pincemail, J., Camus, D. C. G., Pirnay, F., Bouchez, R., Massaux, L., and Goutier, R.,** Tocopherol mobilization during intensive exercise, *Eur. Appl. Physiol.,* 57, 189, 1988.

61. **Lawrence, J. D., Bower, R. C., Riehl, W. P., and Smith, J. P.,** Effect of alpha-tocopherol acetate on the swimming endurance of trained swimmers, *Am. J. Clin. Nutr.,* 28, 205, 1975.

62. **Nagawa, T. K., Aoki, H. J., Maeshima, T., and Hiozawa, K.,** The effect of vitamin E on endurance, *Asian Med. J.,* 11, 619, 1968.

63. **Sumida, S., Tanaka, K., Kitao, H., and Nakadomo, F.,** Exercise-induced lipid peroxidation and leakage of enzymes before and after vitamin E supplementation, *Int. J. Biochem.,* 21, 835, 1989.

64. **Simon-Schnass, I. and Pabst, H.,** Influence of vitamin E on physical performance, *Int. J. Vit. Nutr. Res.,* 58, 49, 1988.

65. **Dillard, C. J., Litov, R. E., Savin, W. M., Dumelin, E. E., and Tappel, A. L.,** Effect of exercise, vitamin E, and ozone on pulmonary function and lipid peroxidation, *J. Appl. Physiol.,* 45, 927, 1978.

66. **Meydani, M., Cannon, J. G., Burrill, J., Orencole, S. F., Fielding, R. A., Fiatarone, M. A., Blumberg, J. B., and Evans, W.,** Protective effect of vitamin E on exercise-induced oxidative damage in young and elderly subjects, *Free Radical Biol. Med.,* 9, 109, 1990.

67. **Gleeson, M., Robertson, J. D., and Maughan, R. J.,** Influence of exercise on ascorbic acid status in man, *Clin. Sci.,* 73, 501, 1987.

68. **Asmussen, E.,** Observations on experimental muscular soreness, *Acta Rhum. Scand.,* 2, 109, 1956.

69. **Newham, D. J., McPhail, G., Mills, K. R., and Edwards, R. H. T.,** Ultrastructural changes after concentric and eccentric contractions of human muscle, *J. Neurol. Sci.,* 61, 109, 1983.

70. **O'Reilly, K. P., Warhol, M. J., Fielding, R. A., Frontera, W. R., Meredith, C. N., and Evans, W. J.,** Eccentric exercise-induced muscle damage impairs muscle glycogen repletion, *J. Appl. Physiol.,* 63, 252, 1987.

71. **Evans, W. J., Meredith, C. N., Cannon, J. G., Dinarello, D. A., Frontera, W. R., Hughes, V. A., Jones, B. H., and Knuttgen, H. G.,** Metabolic changes following eccentric exercise in trained and untrained men. *J. Appl. Physiol.,* 61, 1864, 1986.

72. **Hikida, R. S., Staron, R. S., Hagerman, F. C., Sherman, W. M., and Costill, D. L.,** Muscle fiber necrosis associated with human marathon runners, *J. Neurol. Sci.,* 59, 185, 1983.

73. **Warhol, M. J., Siegel, A. J., Evans, W. J., and Silverman, L. M.,** Skeletal muscle injury and repair in marathon runners after competition, *Am. J. Pathol.,* 118, 331, 1985.

74. **Friden, J., Seger, J., Sjostrom, M., and Ekblom, B.,** Adaptive response in human skeletal muscle subjected to prolonged eccentric training, *Int. J. Sports Med.,* 4, 177, 1983.

75. **Kampschmidt, R.,** Leukocytic endogenous mediator/endogenous pyrogen., in *The Physiologic and Metabolic Responses of the Host.,* Powanda, M. C. and Canonico, P. G., Eds., Elsevier, Amsterdam, 1982, 55.

76. **Cannon, J. G., Orencole, S. F., Fielding, R. A., Meydani, M., Meydani, S., Fitarone, M. A., Blumberg, J. B., and Evans, W. J.,** Acute phase response in exercise: interaction of age and vitamin E on neutrophils and muscle enzyme release, *Am. J. Physiol.,* 259, R1214, 1990.

77. **Babior, B. M., Kiphes, R. S., and Curnutte, J. T.,** Biological defense mechanisms. The production by leukocytes of superoxide, a potential bacterial agent, *J. Clin. Invest.,* 52, 741, 1973.

78. **Smith, J. K., Grisham, M. B., Granger, D. N., and Korthuis, R. J.,** Free radical defense mechanisms and neutrophil infiltration in postischemic skeletal muscle, *Am. J. Physiol.,* 256, H789, 1989.

79. **Bainton, D. F.,** Phagocytic cells: developmental biology of neutrophils and eosinophils, in *Inflammation: Basic Principles and Clinical Correlates,* Gallin, J. I., Goldstein, I. M., and Snyderman, R., Ed., Raven Press, New York, 1988, 265.

80. **Johnston, R. B.,** Monocytes and macrophages, *N. Engl. J. Med.,* 318, 747, 1988.

81. **Round, J. M., Jones, D. A., and Cambridge, G.,** Cellular infiltrates in human skeletal muscle: exercise induced damage as a model for inflammatory muscle disease?, *J. Neurol. Sci.,* 82, 1, 1987.

82. **Fielding, R. A., Manfredi, T. J., Ding, W., Fiatarone, M. A., Evans, W. J., and Cannon, J. G.,** Increased inflammatory mediators and eccentric exercise-induced muscle damage, *Med. Sci. Sports Exercise,* 24, S23, 1992.

83. **Nawabi, M. D., Block, K. P., Chakrabarti, M. C., and Buse, M. G.,** Administration of endotoxin, tumor necrosis factor, or interleukin 1 to rats activates skeletal muscle branched-chain α-keto acid dehydrogenase, *J. Clin. Invest.,* 85, 256, 1990.

84. **Evans, W. J., Fisher, E. C., Hoerr, R. A., and Young, V. R.,** Protein metabolism and endurance exercise, *Phys. Sports Med.,* 11, 63, 1983.

85. **Cannon, J. G., Fielding, R. A., Fiatarone, M. A., Orencole, S. F., Dinarello, C. A., and Evans, W. J.,** Interleukin-1β in human skeletal muscle following exercise, *Am. J. Physiol.,* 257, R451, 1989.

86. **Lammi-Keefe, C. J., Swan, P. B., and Hegarty, P. V. J.,** Copper-Zinc and maganese superoxide dismutase activities in cardiac and skeletal muscles during aging in male rats, *Gerontology,* 30, 153, 1984.

87. **Ji, L. L., Dillon, D., and Wu, E.,** Alteration of antioxidant enzymes with aging in rat skeletal muscle and liver, *Am. J. Physiol.,* 258, R918, 1990.

88. **Zerba, E., Komorowski, T. E., and Faulkner, J. A.,** Free radical injury to skeletal muscles of young, adult, and old mice, *Am. J. Physiol.,* 258, C429, 1990.

89. **Cannon, J. G., Meydani, S. N., Fielding, R. A., Fitarone, M. A., Meydani, M., Orencole, F. M. S. F., Blumberg, J. B., and Evans, W. J.,** Acute phase response in exercise. II. Associations between vitamin E, cytokines, and muscle proteolysis, *Am. J. Physiol.,* 260, R1235, 1991.

90. **Manfredi, T. G., Fielding, R. A., O'Reilly, K. P., Meredith, C. N., Lee, H. Y., and Evans, W. J.,** Serum creating kinase activity and exercise-induced muscle damage in older men, *Med. Sci. Sports Exercise,* 23, 1028, 1991.

91. **Byrnes, W. C., Clarkson, P. M., White, J. S., Hsieh, S. S., Frykman, P. N., and Maughan, R. J.,** Delayed onset muscle soreness following repeated bouts of downhill running, *J. Appl. Physiol.,* 59, 710, 1985.

92. **Meredith, C. N., Frontera, W. R., Fisher, E. C., Hughes, V. A., Herland, J. C., Edwards, J., and Evans, W. J.,** Peripheral effects of endurance training in young and old subjects, *J. Appl. Physiol.,* 66, 2844, 1989.

93. **Armstrong, R. B., Ogilvie, R. W., and Schwane, J. A.,** Eccentric exercise-induced injury to rat skeletal muscle, *J. Appl. Physiol.,* 54, 80, 1983.

94. **Oliver, C. N., Ahn, B., Moerman, E. J., Goldstein, S., and Stadtman, E.,** Age-related changes in oxidized proteins, *J. Biol. Chem.,* 262, 5488, 1987.

95. **Ji, L. L., Dillon, D., and Wu, E.,** Alteration of antioxidant enzymes with aging in rat skeletal muscle and liver, *Am. J. Physiol.,* 258, R918, 1990.

Chapter 9

FREE RADICALS AND AGE-RELATED DISEASES

Denham Harman

TABLE OF CONTENTS

0-8493-4518-9/93/$0.00 + $.50

I. INTRODUCTION

Aging is the accumulation of changes responsible for both the sequential alterations[1,2] that accompany advancing age and the associated progressive increases in the chance of disease and death. The chance of death serves as a measure of the number of such accumulated changes, i.e., of physiologic age, while the rate of change of this parameter with time measures the rate of accumulation, i.e., the rate of aging. The production of these changes can be attributed to the environment and disease and to an inborn aging process(es).

The chance of death for man — readily obtained from vital statistics data — drops precipitously after birth to a minimum figure around puberty, and then increases with age to a value beyond which it rises almost exponentially[1-5] at a rate characteristic of man, so that few individuals reach age 100, and none live beyond about 115 years.[6] That is, the chance that a combination of aging changes capable of causing death will occur in a given individual increases progressively with time beyond some age. Improvements in general living conditions — better nutrition, medical care, etc. — decrease the chance of death[2,5] in the young more than in the old, illustrated in Figure 1 by the curves of the logarithm of the chance of death vs. age for Swedish females for various periods from 1751 to 1988.[4,7]

Today in the developed countries, the chance of death rises almost exponentially after about age 28.[3,7,8] These chances are now near limiting values; only 2 to 3% of a cohort die before age 28, while average life expectancies at birth — determined by the chances for death — in the U.S.[3,9] (Figure 2), as well as in other developed countries, approach plateau values of around 75 years for males and 80 years for females. Thus, as living conditions in a population approach optimum, the curve of the chance of death vs. age shifts towards a limit, determined by the irreducible production of aging changes associated with environment and disease plus those formed by the inborn aging process. The contributions of the aging process to aging changes, small early in life, rapidly increase with age due to the exponential nature of the process.

The aging process is now the major risk factor for disease and death after around age 28 in the developed countries. The importance of this process to our health and well-being is obscured by the protean nature of its contributions to nonspecific change and to disease pathogenesis. As "risk factors" for diseases are detected and minimized, the chance of death decreases toward that determined by the aging process, while the associated average life expectancy at birth approaches a maximum of about 85 years.[10-12] Average life expectancy at birth in the developed countries is today about ten years less than the potential maximum, largely due to premature deaths from cancer and cardiovascular diseases. Conquest of these two disorders would increase average life expectancy at birth by about three and six years, respectively.[13]

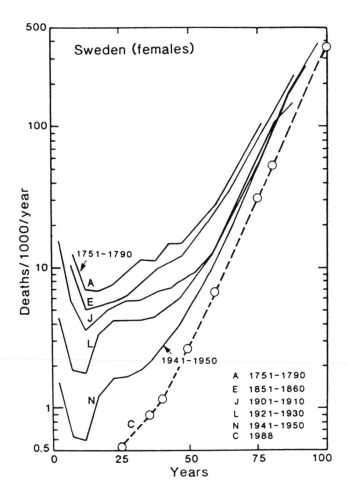

FIGURE 1. Age-specific death rates of Swedish females from 1751 to 1950 (Adapted from Jones, H. R., *Handbook of Aging and the Individual,* Birren, J. E., Ed., Chicago University Press, Chicago, 1959, 336; **Sveriges Officiella Statistik,** Statistika Centralbyran, Stockholm, 1988.)

Significant increases in average life expectancy at birth in the developed countries can now be achieved only by slowing the intrinsic aging process. Because the average period of senescence is not known, average life-span at birth serves as a measure of the span of healthy, productive life, i.e., the functional life-span.

II. FREE RADICAL THEORY OF AGING

Many theories have been advanced to account for the aging process.[14] The free radical theory[15-18] shows promise of application today. It arose from

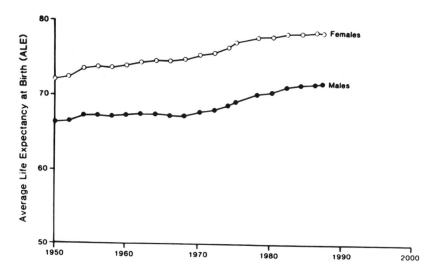

FIGURE 2.   Average life expectancy at birth since 1950 in the U.S.

a consideration of aging phenomenon from the premise[19] that a single common process, modifiable by genetic and environmental factors, was responsible for the aging and death of all living things. The theory postulates that aging is caused by free radical reactions, i.e., these reactions may be involved in production of the aging changes associated with the environment, disease, and the intrinsic aging process. It predicts that the life-span of an organism can be increased by slowing the rate of initiation of random free radical reactions and/or decreasing their chain lengths. The former should be achieved by decreasing ingestion of easily oxidized dietary components, caloric intake, and temperature; the latter should be achieved by increasing the concentrations of free radical reaction inhibitors in the organism or by increasing the resistance of its constituents to free radical attack. Studies are in accord with these predictions.

III. THE "FREE RADICAL" DISEASES

The reason for the increasing incidence of disease with advancing age has long been of interest. A disease is a combination of changes — usually forming a readily recognized pattern — that have detrimental effects on function, and in some cases may lead to death. A plausible explanation[20] for the association of age and disease is based on the observation that free radical reactions are implicated[20-22] in the pathogenesis of a growing number of disorders.

The ubiquitous free radical reactions would be expected to produce progressive adverse changes that accumulate with age throughout the body. The "normal" sequential alterations with age can be attributed to those changes more-or-less common to all persons. Superimposed on this common pattern of change are patterns that should differ from individual to individual owing to genetic and environmental differences that modulate free radical reaction damage. The superimposed patterns of change may become progressively more discernable with time, and some may eventually be recognized as diseases at ages influenced by genetic and environmental risk factors. Aging may also be viewed as a disease, differing from others in that the aging pattern is universal. The probability of developing any one of the "free radical" diseases should be decreased by lowering the free radical reaction level by any means, e.g., food restriction, antioxidants, and in the case of a specific disease, lowered further by decreases in contributing environmental factors — for example, cholesterol in atherosclerosis.

The above discussion indicates that the relationship between aging and diseases in which free radical reactions are involved is a direct one. The growing number of "free radical" diseases includes the two major causes of death, cancer and atherosclerosis.

Some of the data implicating free radical reactions in cancer, atherosclerosis, amyloidosis, the immune deficiency of age, and senile dementia of the Alzheimer type (SDAT), are presented briefly below.

A. CANCER

Cancer initiation and promotion[23,24] is associated with chromosomal defects[25] and oncogene activation.[26,27] Ionizing radiation is a "complete carcinogen", being both initiator and promoter. It is a reasonable possibility that some endogenous free radical reactions, like those initiated by ionizing radiation, will result in tumor formation.[16,28] Support for this possibility is extensive and includes the following:

1. The incidence of mammary carcinoma in C3H female mice increases as the amount and/or degree of unsaturation of the dietary fat is increased,[29] i.e., in parallel with the expected increases in endogenous free radical reactions. In women, the future risk of breast cancer is lower the higher the plasma level of vitamin E.[30]
2. In areas where the selenium intake is relatively high, the incidence of some forms of cancer tends to be low;[31,32] serum selenium levels are also inversely correlated with cancer incidence.[33] Presumably, this effect is mediated, at least in part, through a reduction in free radical reactions. Selenium is a component of glutathione peroxidase, an enzyme that decreases free radical damage by reducing H_2O_2 to water and organic hydroperoxides to alcohols.

The increasing incidence of cancer with age is of particular interest. This increase is probably due, at least in part, to the increasing level of endogenous free radical reactions with advancing age,[15,34,35] resulting in an increased rate of mutation in proto-oncogenes and tumor-suppressing genes,[36,37] coupled with the progressive diminishing capacity of the immune system[38] to eliminate the altered cells.

Thus, it is likely that the probability of developing many, if not all, types of human cancer can be decreased by lowering the free radical reaction level by eating diets selected to minimize adverse free radical reactions in the cells and tissues, e.g., diets low in calories and components such as polyunsaturates and copper, and supplemented by one or more free radical reaction inhibitors.

B. ATHEROSCLEROSIS

Atherosclerosis is the major cause of death in developed countries. Atherosclerotic lesions tend to form in areas of the vascular tree that have been subjected to injury.[39-43] The usual distribution of lesions is apparently largely the same as the localized sites of endothelial cell injury and/or increased permeability caused by a "suction effect" owing to decreased lateral wall pressure resulting from local hemodynamic factors. Injuries produced by other means are also sites of increased permeability.[42,44] It is a reasonable possibility that increased exposure of components of the arterial wall in the areas of increased permeability to serum-derived irritants might result in local tissue damage at a rate that exceeded the repair capacity of the inflammatory response, thus leading to chronic progressive change in the arterial wall.

A possible constant source of compounds capable of causing vessel injury is the reaction of molecular oxygen with the polyunsaturated substances present in serum and arterial wall lipids.[15,45] The oxidation products — including peroxides and compounds of higher molecular weight formed through oxidative polymerization, as well as substances arising from the reaction of intermediate lipid-free radicals with proteins and other substances — may be produced in amounts large enough to significantly contribute, directly or indirectly, to atherogenesis.

The first steps in atherogenesis may include interaction of localized oxidized low-density lipoproteins with endothelial cells,[46] followed by induction of mononuclear leukocyte adhesion molecules[47] that aid to localize monocytes to the endothelial surface. The adherent monocytes migrate through the endothelium, change their phenotypic expression to become tissue macrophages, and then take up oxidized lipoproteins to become foam cells. The foam cells constitute the fatty streak, the first manifestation of atherosclerosis.

Support for the possibility that free radical reactions are involved in atherogenesis includes the extensive atherosclerosis seen in patients with homocystinuria and/or hyperhomocysteinemia,[48,49] which may be related to the formation of superoxide radicals during the ready oxidation by O_2 of homocysteine to homocystine.[49] Xanthine oxidase has been implicated in atherogenesis;[50] if so, it is probably related to superoxide production during the action of the enzyme.[51] The enhanced atherogenesis observed in chronic renal dialysis patients[52] may also be due to free radical-induced endothelial cell injury; white cells tend to aggregate under these circumstances and release H_2O_2, O_2^-, and $HO^{\cdot}$.[53] In addition, the free radical reactions initiated by ionizing radiation also result in atherosclerosis,[54,55] while the plasma selenium concentration in patients with arteriographically defined coronary atherosclerosis is inversely correlated with the severity of the coronary lesions.[56] Furthermore, plasma concentrations of vitamins C, E, and of carotene have been found to be significantly inversely related to the risk of angina in man.[57,58]

Taken as a whole,[43,59-62] studies on the pathogenesis of atherosclerosis are compatible with the possibility that the disease is basically due to free radical reactions largely involving dietary-derived lipids in the arterial wall and serum that yields peroxides and other substances. These compounds induce endothelial cell injury and produce changes in other components of the arterial wall that collectively initiate and help to sustain an inflammatory reaction in the wall that interacts, in turn, with serum-derived lipids.

C. ESSENTIAL HYPERTENSION

Blood pressure normally rises with age.[63,64] Diastolic pressure usually plateaus around 45 to 50 years of age, whereas systolic pressure continues to increase.[65] At any given age, increases in blood pressure over the "normal" for that age are associated with increased morbidity and mortality risks. Based on a 50% or greater increase in mortality in adults, the following operational criteria have been proposed for hypertension:[66] men under 45 years old, 130/90; men over 45 years, 140/95; women at any age 160/95. About 5% of all causes of hypertension result from bilateral renal parenchymal disease, 5% from a number of other disorders, while 90% are due to unknown causes, i.e., essential hypertension.

The incidence of essential hypertension, based on the above or other criteria, rises steadily with age.[66] Thus, the rate of increase in blood pressure for a fraction of the population,[66] about 15 to 20%, is greater than normal and varies between individuals, those with the highest rates meeting the criteria for hypertension at earlier ages.

Two major vascular changes are associated with the increased peripheral resistance of hypertensive individuals:[67] (1) hyperplastic arteriolosclerosis, the most prevalent lesion and (2) hyaline sclerosis, a common lesion associated with age and other disorders. Hyperplastic arteriolosclerosis begins with hypertrophy of smooth muscle in the medial layer and may progress to subintimal fibrosis and hyalinization and eventual obliteration of the lumen. However, it is likely[68] that these alterations in the small vessels are more an adaptation to the increased blood pressure, and that the blood pressure level is determined by other factors within the cardiovascular system.

Blood pressure is determined by the balance between the factors that affect blood flow, vascular resistance, and sodium and water handling.[69] The vasoconstrictive/antinatrinetic factors include: (1) renin-angiotensin system, (2) sympathoadrenal system, (3) endothelium, (4) vasopressin,

(5) thromboxane/leukotrienes, and (6) serotonin. The vasodilator/natriuretic factors include: (1) atrial natriuretic peptide, (2) prostaglandins E_2 and I_2, (3) endothelium-dependent relaxant factor (NO), (4) kallikrein-kinin system, and (5) dopamine.

The endothelium-derived O_2^- has also been found to be a vasocontracting factor.[70] This radical may play a significant role in essential hypertension.[71] As expected,[71] the blood pressure of spontaneously hypertensive rats (SHR), but not that of normal rats, was decreased by superoxide dismutase. The O_2^- was apparently formed by xanthine oxidase.[71] In accord, oxypurinol, an inhibitor of xanthine oxidase, decreased the blood pressure of SHR rats, but not that of normal rats. Likewise, in accord, the serum uric acid in the SHR rats was higher than in normal rats; hyperuricemia is frequently observed in essential hypertension.[72] Furthermore, since O_2^- inactivates[71] the endothelial-dependent relaxing factor NO, it may be responsible for the observation that endothelium-mediated vasodilation is impaired in patients with essential hypertension.[73]

In view of the above, the pressor effect of catecholamines on blood pressure may be due to O_2^- formed during the ready reaction of these compounds with O_2.

D. AMYLOIDOSIS

Amyloid is an aggregation of twisted β-pleated sheet fibrils, formed from various proteins by several different mechanisms, that is associated with a small amount (about 10%) of a nonfibrillary glycoprotein called amyloid P component;[74] the fibrils are readily proteolyzed in the absence of this material.

An observation made during the course of a study of the effect of antioxidants on the life-span of male LAF_1 mice[75] has shed some light on the etiology of murine amyloidosis and its association with age. A quinoline derivative, ethoxyquin, almost completely prevented spontaneous amyloidosis in these mice; butylated hydroxytoluene (BHT) was less effective. The two antioxidants also inhibited development of amyloidosis when added to the diet of casein-injected C3HeB/FeJ male mice.[76] Plasma electrophoretic studies of the casein-injected mice showed that ethoxyquin, and to a lesser extent BHT, depressed the appearance of a protein fraction in the α_1-glycoprotein region. This suggests that the antioxidants inhibited the rate of oxidative breakdown of unknown substances, possibly of the connective tissues or of cell surface components such as the amyloid precursor protein (APP) of Alzheimer's disease, to form amyloid fibrils. The slower rate of formation of the fibrils may have allowed them to be proteolyzed before there was time for them to aggregate to form amyloid and to then be stabilized against further degradation by the amyloid P component.

Although the details of the inhibiting effect of antioxidants on amyloid formation in the two mouse strains remains to be clarified, it is apparent that a free radical(s) reaction is involved in pathogenesis, and that this can be inhibited by dietary antioxidants. Whether free radical reaction inhibitors can also inhibit formation of the amyloid observed in Alzheimer's disease and other disorders remains to be determined.

E. IMMUNE DEFICIENCY OF AGE

Cellular and humoral immune responses decline with age.[38] Studies with BC3F$_1$ mice show that old mice have only 10% of the humoral capacity and 25% of the cell-mediated capacity of young animals.

A number of antioxidants have been shown to enhance both humoral and cellular immune responses,[77] indicating that some endogenous free radical reactions have adverse effects on the immune system. With increasing age, the level of more-or-less random free radical reactions seems to increase, as indicated by the increase in exhalation of hydrocarbons[35] and of oxidized proteins[34] with age and by the concomitant decline in the serum concentration of mercaptans.[78,79] Thus, part of the decline of the immune system with age may be attributed to increasing levels of free radical reactions.

F. SENILE DEMENTIA OF THE ALZHEIMER'S TYPE

This is the major cause of dementia.[80] Most cases are sporadic;[80] a minority are familial.[81-84] The major risk factor for SDAT is age; the prevalence increases exponentially with age.[85]

The major morphologic changes in the brain in Alzheimer's disease[80,85-88] include cortical atrophy, loss of neurons, and the presence of neurofibrillary tangles and neuritic plaques. Although the extent of these changes varies, they occur in all cases of Alzheimer's disease; small numbers of neurofibrillary tangles and neuritic plaques are also seen in the majority of normal elderly individuals.

Neurofibrillary tangles are insoluble deposits found in neuronal cell bodies and neuronal "ghosts". The tangles are bundles of submicroscopic filamentous structures (each of which is about 10 nm in diameter) that are wound around each other in a helical fashion — the so-called paired helical filament (PHF). A neuritic plaque is composed of a cluster of degenerating nerve terminals, both dendritic and axonal, and a core of amyloid protein; the appearance of degenerating mitochondria in axon terminals is apparently the first indication of plaque formation.[88] Neuritic plaques and neurofibrillary tangles are distributed in the brains of persons with Alzheimer's disease in a pattern that is similar to neuronal cell loss.

The dementia of Alzheimer's disease is related to neuronal cell loss[80] and, in particular, to the associated loss of synapses[89,90] or to the presence of neurofibrillary tangles.[91] Individuals with SDAT have excessive loss of neurons in at least four neurotransmitter systems.[92-96] The neuronal loss in these four systems is associated with pigment formation; lipofuscin in the acetylcholine and serotonin systems; and neuromelanin, melanized lipofuscin,[97] in the norepinephrine and dopamine systems.

Lipofuscin (age pigment) accumulates with age in the various areas of the human central nervous system (CNS) in parallel with the activities of oxidative enzymes.[98] The rate of lipofuscin formation can be increased in the rat[99] by raising the level of free radical reactions, e.g., by vitamin E deficiency, or by increasing the degree of unsaturation of the lipid membranes.[100] The fatty acid composition of the rat brain is essentially independent of the fatty acid composition of dietary lipids, except for the content of 22:6ω3 and its precursors.[101-102] Both linolenic acid (18:3ω3) and docosahexanoic acid (22:6ω3) are avidly taken up from the diet by rats and reflected in increasing brain levels of 22:6ω3[103-106] — largely at the expense of 22:5ω6, individual differences being determined by diet and genetic influences. Brain 22:6ω3 is tenaciously retained;[102] this highly unsaturated fatty acid is concentrated in the phospholipids of neurons, both in the perikaryon[105] and in the synaptic area.[105-108]

There is a sex difference in the rate of incorporation of dietary 22:6ω3 and its precursors into brain lipids in rats, being higher in females.[101] This sex difference may be a factor in the higher incidence of senile dementia and earlier onset of brain atrophy in women.[109]

Cell loss in the human brain apparently occurs beyond some threshold of lipofuscin accumulation,[110] possibly due to adverse effects of lipofuscin on cell function and/or of the free radical reactions involved in formation of the pigment.

Lipofuscin is a product of the cellular recycling system.[99] Cellular components that are no longer needed or have been altered, for example, by oxidation change, are "marked" and then broken down and reused by the cell. Proteins "marked" by oxidative changes[34,111-114] — such marking increases, exponentially with age[34,114] — are highly susceptible to proteolysis.[113,115] The "cellular recycling system" becomes less effective with age[99] — probably due, at least in part, to the increasing level of free radical reactions with advancing age[15,34,35] — so that eventually there may be time for the "marked" components to be converted to forms that are resistant to cellular breakdown. These altered components gradually accumulate, forming lipofuscin.

SDAT pathology may be a consequence of the cellular recycling system, the age of onset of symptoms being determined by the free radical reaction level in the involved cells.

In SDAT, the cells apparently accumulate lipofuscin at a greater than normal rate, as indicated by the higher rate of neuronal loss.[80,85-88] In view of the mode of formation of lipofuscin, individuals with SDAT may have elevated levels of free radical reactions in the neurons associated with SDAT; in sporadic SDAT this may be a consequence of abnormal mitochondria[116] — because of its high polyunsaturated fatty acid content, free radical damage to the brain should be greater than elsewhere, while in familial SDAT, it may be a result of a higher rate of oxidation "marking" of the abnormal amyloid precursor protein (APP). If so, the higher than normal progressively increased rate of formation of altered cellular components with age coupled with the decreasing capacity of the cellular recycling system might, in time, overwhelm the cellular disposal system, leading to the accumulation of altered cellular constituents. These may give rise to the changes associated with SDAT, such as neurofibrillary tangles, to more lipofuscin, and eventually to earlier-than-normal cell death. The abnormal phosphorylation of tau,[117,118] a major component of the PHF, and the presence of hydroxyproline in the PHF,[119] suggest that constituents of the PHF have been altered and marked for disposal, but accumulated because the disposal system was inadequate. The presence of ubiquitin[120,121] in neurofibrillary tangles also indicates that components of the lesions were marked for disposal.

In the synaptic area, the increasing higher-than-normal rate of free radical activity might be expected to lead to an earlier accumulation of peroxidatively damaged synaptic components and eventually to synaptic destruction. The plaque amyloid could result, at least in part, from oxidative/proteolytic alteration of the amyloid precursor protein (APP) during breakup of the synaptic area. In addition, the cellular recycling system may also contribute to plaque amyloid, for it has been shown to convert APP to a number of derivatives, including potentially amyloidogenic forms;[122] whether this process is involved in murine amyloidosis, inhibited by antioxidants,[75] is not known. The fibrils, easily proteolyzed,[123] could aggregate and be stabilized against further proteolyte breakdown, possibly by serum amyloid P.[123-125] The prominent presence of amyloid in neuritic plaques has prompted many studies because of the possibility that it might be involved in the pathogenesis of SDAT.[126,127] Supporting this possibility, amyloid fibrils have been reported to have a toxic effect on neurons,[128] while in familial Alzheimer's disease, mutations have been found in the APP.[81-84] In the latter case, SDAT may result from increased free radical activity secondary to increased oxidative "marking" of the mutated APP. The toxicity of fibrils is not likely to contribute significantly to the pathogenesis of SDAT, for the diffuse deposits of amyloid fibrils — preamyloid — seen in SDAT,[129] Downs syndrome,[130] and hereditary cerebral hemorrhage with amyloidosis of the Dutch type[83] contain few or no degenerating neurites or reactive glial cells.

The above discussion suggests that decreasing endogenous free radical reaction levels by dietary modulation and/or antioxidant supplements may slow formation of changes associated with SDAT and put off, in time, clinical manifestation of this disorder.

IV. COMMENT

A beautiful coherent picture[15] is emerging from studies on the origin of life, mutation, radiation biology, aging, degenerative diseases, and free radical reactions in biological systems. It would appear that life originated as a result of free radical reactions, selected free radical reactions to play major metabolic roles, and assured evolution by also employing them to provide for mutation, aging, and death. Increases in life-span apparently evolved in parallel with the ability of organisms to cope with damaging chemical reactions, including free radical reactions. It would be remarkable that life, with its beautiful order, should owe its origin to, and be sustained by, a class of chemical reactions whose outstanding characteristic is their unruly nature.

The data supporting the free radical theory of aging indicate that aging is the sum of the deleterious free radical reactions going on continuously throughout the cells and tissues. The process may never have changed; in the beginning, the free radical reactions were initiated primarily by ultraviolet radiation from the sun, and now free radicals arise from within from enzymatic and nonenzymatic free radical reactions. In mammalian species, mitochondria are the major source of damaging free radical reactions. These reactions also damage mitochondria, resulting in progressive increases in such reactions owing to lower ATP production and enhanced O_2^- formation. Antioxidants that can slow mitochondrial aging, at concentrations that do not also significantly depress function, should increase the maximum life-span.

Chronic disorders now decrease the quality of life of numerous older persons, while the need of many of them for services and medical care from society imposes a significant and growing burden on the remainder of the population. Amelioration of these two interrelated problems should be possible by application of measures to slow the aging process. Successful efforts to increase the life-span of animals, based on the free radical theory of aging, resulted in shortened senescent periods; the average life-spans at birth were increased, while maximum life-span rose little, if at all. Successful efforts in the future to increase the maximum life-span will most likely also decrease the fraction of the life-span occupied by the senescent period.

It is reasonable to expect, on the basis of present data, that the healthy, active life-span can be increased 5 to 10 or more years by keeping body weight down, at a level compatible with a sense of well-being, while ingesting diets adequate in essential nutrients but designed to minimize random free radical reactions in the body. Such diets would contain minimal amounts of components prone to enhance free radical reactions, for example, copper and polyunsaturated lipids, and increased amounts of substances capable of decreasing free radical reaction damage, such as α-tocopherol, ascorbic acid, selenium, and the effective "natural" antioxidants present in some foods, e.g., fruits and vegetables, as well as one or more synthetic antioxidants.

REFERENCES

1. **Kohn, R. R.**, Aging and age-related diseases: normal processes, in *Relation Between Normal Aging and Disease,* Johnson, H. A., Ed., Raven Press, New York, 1985, 1.
2. **Upton, A. C.**, Pathobiology, in *The Biology of Aging,* Finch, C. E. and Hayflick, L., Eds., Von Nostrand Reinhold, New York, 1977, 513.

3. National Center for Health Statistics (1988) *Vital Statistics of the United States,* U.S. Dep. Health Human Serv., Hyattsville, MD, PHS Publ. No. 88–1104, Life Tables, Vol. 2, Sect. 6, 1985, 9.
4. **Jones, H. R.,** The relation of human health to age, place, and time, in *Handbook of Aging and the Individual,* Chicago University Press, Chicago, 1955, 333.
5. **Dubin, L. I., Lotha, A. J., and Spiegel, M.,** *Length of Life: a Study of the Life Table, Ronald Press,* New York, 1949, 141.
6. **Comfort, A.,** *The Biology of Senescence,* 3rd ed., Elsevier, New York, 81.
7. Sveriges Officiella Statistik, *Befolkningsforandringer* 1987, Statistiska Centralbyran, Stockholm, 1988, 114.
8. Office Federal de la Statistique, *Suisse — Table de Mortalite* 1986–1987, Swiss Government, Berne, Switzerland, 1988.
9. National Center for Health Statistics, *Annual Summary of Births, Marriages, Divorces, and Deaths: United States 1988,* U.S. Dep. Health Human Serv., Hyattsville, MD, PHS Publ. No. 89–1120, Monthly Vital Statistics 37, No. 13, 1989, 19.
10. **Woodhall, B. and Joblon, S.,** Prospects for future increases in average longevity, *Geriatrics,* 12, 586, 1957.
11. **Fries, J. F.,** Aging, natural death, and the compression of morbidity, *N. Engl. J. Med.,* 303, 130, 1980.
12. **Olshansky, S. J., Carnes, B. A., and Cassel, C.,** In search of Methuselah: estimating the upper limits to human longevity, *Science,* 250, 634, 1990.
13. National Center for Health Statistics, *U.S. Decennial Life Tables for 1979–1981,* Curtin, L. R. and Armstrong, R. J., Eds., U.S. Dep. Health Human Serv., PHS Publ. No. 88–1150-2, Vol. 1, No. 2, 1988, 56.
14. **Harman, D.,** The aging process: major risk factor for disease and death, *Proc. Natl. Acad. Sci. U.S.A.,* 88, 5360, 1991.
15. **Harman, D.,** Free radical theory of aging: role of free radicals in the origination and evolution of life, aging, and disease processes, in *Free Radicals, Aging, and Degenerative Diseases,* Johnson, J. E., Jr., Walford, R., Harman, D., and Miquel, J., Eds., Alan R. Liss, New York, 1986, 3.
16. **Harman, D.,** Aging: a theory based on free radical and radiation chemistry, *J. Gerontol.* 11, 298, 1956.
17. **Harman, D.,** Role of free radicals in mutation, cancer, aging, and the maintenance of life, *Radical Res.,* 16, 753, 1962.
18. **Harman, D.,** The aging process, *Proc. Natl. Acad. Sci. U.S.A.,* 78, 7124, 1981.
19. **Harman, D.,** Free radical theory of aging: history, in *Free Radicals and Aging,* Emerit, I. and Chance, B., Eds., Birkhauser, Basel, 1992, 1.
20. **Harman, D.,** Free radical theory of aging: the "free radical" diseases, *Age,* 7, 111, 1984.
21. **Halliwell, B. and Gutteridge, J. M. C.,** Eds., *Free Radicals in Biology and Medicine,* 2nd ed., Clarendon Press, Oxford, 1989.
22. **Slater, T. F. and Block, G.,** Eds., *Antioxidant vitamins and β- carotene in disease prevention, Am. J. Clin. Nutr.,* 53, (Suppl. 1), 189S, 1991.
23. **Pitot, H. C.,** The natural history of neoplastic development: the relation of experimental models to human cancer, *Cancer,* 49, 1206, 1982.
24. **Tubiana, M.,** Human carcinogenesis-introductory remarks, *Am. J. Clin. Nutr.,* 53 (Suppl. 1), 223S, 1991.
25. **Yunis, J. J.,** The chromosomal basis of human neoplasia, *Science,* 221, 227, 1983.
26. **Hamlyn, P. and Sikora, K.,** Oncogenes, *Lancet,* 1, 326, 1983.
27. **Land, H., Parada, L. F., and Weinberg, R. A.,** Cellular oncogenes and multistep carcinogenesis, *Science,* 222, 771, 1983.
28. **Totter, J. R.,** Spontaneous cancer and the possible relationship to oxygen metabolism, *Proc. Natl. Acad. Sci. U.S.A.,* 77, 1763, 1980.

29. **Harman, D.,** Free radical theory of aging: effect of the amount and degree of unsaturation of dietary fat on mortality rate, *J. Gerontol.,* 26, 451, 1971.

30. **Wald, N. J., Boreham, J., Hayward, J. L., and Bulbrook, R. D.,** Plasma retinol, β-carotene, and vitamin E levels in relation to the future risk of breast cancer, *Br. J. Cancer,* 49, 321, 1984.

31. **Diplock, A. T.,** Antioxidant nutrients and disease prevention: an overview, *Am. J. Clin. Nutr.,* 53 (Suppl. 1), 189S, 1991.

32. **Schrauzer, G. N. and White, D. A.,** Selenium in human nutrition: dietary intake and effects of supplementation, *Bioinorg. Chem.,* 8, 303, 1978.

33. **Willett, W. C., Polk, B. F., Morris, J. S., Stampfer, M. J., Pressel, S., Rosner, B., Taylor, J. D., Schneider, K., and Hames, C. G.,** Prediagnostic serum selenium and risk of cancer, *Lancet,* II, 130, 1983.

34. **Stadtman, E. R. and Oliver, C. N.,** Minireview: metal-catalyzed oxidation of proteins, *J. Biol. Chem.,* 266, 2005, 1991.

35. **Sagai, M. and Ichinose, T.,** Age-related changes in lipid peroxidation as measured by ethane, ethylene, butane and pentane in respired gases by rats, *Life Sci.,* 27, 731, 1980.

36. **Friend, S. H., Dryja, T. P., and Weinberg, R. H.,** Oncogenes and tumor-suppressing genes, *N. Engl. J. Med.,* 318, 618, 1988.

37. **Hollstein, M., Sidransky, O., Vogelstein, B., and Harris, C. C.,** p53 mutations in human cancers, *Science,* 253, 49, 1991.

38. **Kay, M. M. B. and Makinodan, T.,** Immunobiology of aging: evaluation of current status, *Clin. Immunol. Immunopathol.,* 6, 394, 1976.

39. **Harman, D.,** Atherosclerosis: effect of rate of growth, *Circ. Res.,* 10, 851, 1962.

40. **Harman, D.,** Atherosclerosis: inhibiting effect of an antihistaminic drug, chlorpheniramine, *Circ. Res.,* 11, 277, 1962.

41. **Texon, M.,** *Hemodynamic Basis of Atherosclerosis,* Hemisphere, New York, 1980.

42. **Minick, C. R.,** Synergy of arterial injury and hypercholesterolemia in atherosclerosis, in *Vascular Injury and Atherosclerosis,* Moore, S., Ed., Marcel Dekker, New York, 1981, 149.

43. **Fuster, V., Badimon, L., Badimon, J. J., and Chesebro, J. H.,** The pathogenesis of coronary artery disease and the acute coronary syndromes, *N. Engl. J. Med.,* 326, 242 and 310, 1992.

44. **Stenfanovich, V. and Gore, I.,** Cholesterol diet and permeability of rabbit aorta, *Exp. Mol. Pathol.,* 14, 20, 1971.

45. **Harman, D.,** Atherosclerosis: a hypothesis concerning initiating steps in pathogenesis, *J. Gerontol.,* 12, 199, 1957.

46. **Gerrity, R. G.,** The role of the monocyte in atherogenesis. I. Transition of blood-borne monocytes into foam cells in fatty lesions, *Am. J. Pathol.,* 103, 181, 1981.

47. **Cybulsky, M. I. and Gimbrone, M. A., Jr.,** Endothelial expression of a mononuclear leukocyte adhesion molecule during atherosclerosis, *Science,* 251, 788, 1991.

48. **Clarke, R. C., Daly, L., Robinson, K., Naughten, E., Cahalane, S., Fowler, B., and Graham, I.,** Hyperhomocysteinemia: an independent risk factor for vascular disease, *N. Engl. J. Med.,* 324, 1149, 1991.

49. **Harker, L. A., Ross, R., Slichter, S. J., and Scott, C. R.,** Homocystine-induced atherosclerosis: the role of endothelial cell injury and platelet response in its genesis, *J. Clin. Invest.,* 58, 731, 1976.

50. **Oster, K. A.,** Plasmalogen diseases: a new concept of the etiology of the atherosclerotic process, *Am. J. Clin. Res.,* 2, 30, 1971.

51. **McCord, J. M. and Fridovich, I.,** The reduction of cytochrome c by milk xanthine oxidase in lysosomes and erythrocyte membranes, *Lipids,* 17, 331, 1982.

52. **Linder, A., Charra, B., Sherrard, D. J., and Scribner, A. H.,** Accelerated atherosclerosis in prolonged maintenance hemodialysis, *N. Engl. J. Med.,* 209, 697, 1974.

53. **Jacob, H. S., Craddock, P. R., Hammerschmidt, D. E., and Moldow, C. F.,** Complement-induced granulocyte aggregation: an unsuspected mechanism of disease, *N. Engl. J. Med.,* 302, 789, 1980.

54. **McCready, R. A., Hyde, G. L., Bivins, B. A., Mattingly, S. S., and Griffen, W. O., Jr.,** Radiation-induced arterial injuries, *Surgery,* 93, 306, 1983.

55. **Selwign, A. P.,** The cardiovascular system and radiation, *Lancet,* 2, 152, 1983.

56. **Moore, J. A., Noiva, R., and Wells, L. C.,** Selenium concentrations in plasma of patients with arteriographically defined coronary atherosclerosis, *Clin. Chem.,* 30, 1171, 1984.

57. **Riemersma, R. A., Wood, D. A., MacIntyre, C. C. A., Elton, R. A., Gey, K. F., and Oliver, M. F.,** Risk of angina pectoris and plasma concentrations of vitamins A, C, and E, and carotene, *Lancet,* 337, 1, 1991.

58. **Gey, K. F., Pusha, P., Jordan, P., and Moser, U. K.,** Inverse correlation between vitamin E and mortality from ischemic heart disease in cross-cultural epidemiology, *Am. J. Clin. Nutr.,* 53 (Suppl. 1), 326S, 1991.

59. **Steinberg, D. and Witztum, J. L.,** Lipoproteins and atherogenesis, *JAMA,* 264, 3047, 1990.

60. **Editorial,** Atherosclerosis goes to the wall, *Lancet,* 339, 647, 1992.

61. **Luc, G. and Fruckart, J.-C.,** Oxidation of lipoproteins and atherosclerosis, *Am. J. Clin. Nutr.,* 53 (Suppl. 1), 206S, 1991.

62. **Reaven, P. D., Parthasarathy, S., Beltz, W. F., and Witztum, J. L.,** Effect of probucol dosage on plasma lipid and lipoprotein levels and on protection of low density lipoprotein against *in vitro* oxidation in humans, *Arterioscler. Thromb.,* 12, 318, 1992.

63. **Buchan, T. W., Henderson, W. K., Walker, D. E., Symington, T., and McNeil, I. H.,** Arterial blood pressure in men and women, *Health Bull. Edinburgh,* 18, 3, 1960.

64. **Zachariah, P. K., Sheps, S. G., Bailey, K. R., Wiltgen, C. M., and Moore, A. G.,** Age-related characteristics of ambulatory blood pressure load and mean blood pressure in normotensive subjects, *JAMA,* 265, 1414, 1991.

65. **Manger, W. M. and Page, I. H.,** An overview of current concepts regarding the pathogenesis and pathophysiology of hypertension, in *Arterial Hypertension,* Rosenthal, J., Ed., Springer-Verlag, New York, 1982, 1.

66. **Kaplan, N. M.,** *Clinical Hypertension,* 2nd ed., Williams & Wilkins, Baltimore, 1978, 7.

67. **Rajo-Ortega, J. M. and Hatt, P. Y.,** Histopathology of cardiovascular lesions in hypertension, in *Hypertension,* Genest, J., Koiw, E., and Kuchel, O., Eds., McGraw-Hill, New York, 1977, 910.

68. **Mulvany, M. J.,** Are vascular abnormalities a primary cause or a secondary consequence of hypertension?, *Hypertension,* 18 (Suppl. I), I-52, 1991.

69. **Krieger, J. E. and Dzau, V. J.,** Molecular biology of hypertension, *Hypertension,* 18 (Suppl. I), I-3, 1991.

70. **Katusic, Z. S. and Vanhoutte, P. M.,** Superoxide anion is an endothelium-derived contracting factor, *Am. J. Physiol.,* 297, H33, 1989.

71. **Nakazono, K., Watanabe, N., Matsumo, K., Sasaki, J., and Sato, T.,** Does superoxide underlie the pathogenesis of hypertension?, *Proc. Natl. Acad. Sci. U.S.A.,* 88, 10045, 1991.

72. **Selby, J. V., Friedman, G. D., and Quesenberry, C. P., Jr.,** Precursors of essential hypertension: pulmonary function, heart rate, uric acid, serum cholesterol, and other serum chemistries, *Am. J. Epidemiol.,* 131, 1017, 1990.

73. **Panza, J. A., Quyyumi, A. A., Brush, J. E., Jr., and Epstein, S. E.,** Abnormal endothelium-dependent vascular relaxation in patients with essential hypertension, *N. Engl. J. Med.,* 323, 22, 1990.

74. **Glenner, G. G.,** Amyloid deposits and amyloidosis: the β-fibriloses, *N. Engl. J. Med.,* 302, 1283 and 1333, 1980.

75. **Harman, D.,** Free radical theory of aging: effect of free radical inhibitors on the mortality rate of male LAF_1 mice, *J. Gerontol.,* 23, 476, 1968.

76. **Harman, D., Eddy, D. E., and Noffsinger, J.,** Free radical theory of aging: inhibition of amyloidosis in mice by antioxidants: possible mechanism, *J. Am. Geriatr. Soc.,* 24, 203, 1976.

77. **Harman, D., Heidrick, M. L., and Eddy, D. E.,** Free radical theory of aging: effect of free radical reaction inhibitors on the immune response, *J. Am. Geriatr. Soc.,* 251, 400, 1977.

78. **Harman, D.,** The free radical theory of aging: the effect of age on serum mercaptan levels, *J. Gerontol.,* 15, 38, 1960.

79. **Leto, S., Yiengst, M. J., and Barrows, C. H., Jr.,** The effect of aging and protein deprivation on the sulfhydryl content of serum albumin, *J. Gerontol.,* 25, 4, 1970.

80. **Katzman, R.,** Alzheimer's disease, *N. Engl. J. Med.,* 314, 964, 1986.

81. **St. George-Hyslop, P. H., Tanzi, R. E., Polinsky, R. J., et al.,** The genetic defect causing familial Alzheimer's disease maps on chromosome 21, *Science,* 235, 885, 1987.

82. **Murrell, J., Farlow, M., Ghetti, B., and Benson, M. D.,** A mutation in the amyloid precursor protein associated with hereditary Alzheimer's disease, *Science,* 254, 97, 1991.

83. **Levy, E., Carman, M. D., Fernandez-Madrid, I. J., et al.,** Mutation of the Alzheimer's disease amyloid gene in hereditary cerebral hemorrhage, Dutch type, *Science,* 248, 1124, 1990.

84. **Goate, A., Chartier-Harlin, M.-C., Mullan, M., et al.,** Segregation of a missense mutation in the amyloid precursor protein gene with familial Alzheimer's disease, *Nature,* 349, 704, 1991.

85. **Katzman, R. and Jackson, J. E.,** Alzheimer's disease: basic and clinical advances, *J. Am. Geriatr. Soc.,* 39, 516, 1991.

86. **Terry, R. D.,** Ultrastructural alterations in senile dementia, in *Alzheimer's Disease: Senile Dementia and Related Disorders,* Katzman, R., Terry, R. D., and Bick, K. L., Eds., Raven Press, New York, 1978, 375.

87. **Wisniewski, H. M. and Merz, G. S.,** Neuropathology of the aging brain and dementia of the Alzheimer type, in *Aging 2000: Our Health Care Destiny, Vol. 1: Biomedical Issues,* Springer-Verlag, New York, 1983, 231.

88. **Wisniewski, H. M. and Terry, R. D.,** Morphology of the aging brain, human and animal, *Progr. Brain Res.,* 49, 167, 1973.

89. **Masliah, E., Terry, R. D., DeTeresa, R. M., and Hansen, L. A.,** Immunohistochemical quantification of the synapse-related protein synaptophysin in Alzheimer's disease, *Neurosci. Lett.,* 103, 234, 1989.

90. **DeKosky, S. T. and Schaff, S. W.,** Synapse loss in frontal cortex biopsies in Alzheimer's disease: correlation with cognitive severity, *Ann. Neurol.,* 27, 457, 1990.

91. **Crystal, H., Dickson, D., Fuld, P., et al.,** Clinico-pathologic studies in dementia: nondemented subjects with pathologically confirmed Alzheimer's disease, *Neurology.,* 38, 1682, 1988.

92. **Mann, D. M. A., Yates, P. O., and Marcymick, B.,** Changes in nerve cells of the nucleus basalis of Meynert in Alzheimer's disease and their relationship to ageing and to the accumulation of lipofuscin pigment, *Mech. Ageing Dev.,* 25, 189, 1984.

93. **Mann, D. M. A.,** The locus coeruleus and its possible role in ageing and degenerative disease of the human central nervous system, *Mech. Ageing Dev.,* 23, 73, 1983.

94. **Mann, D. M. A. and Yates, P. O.,** Serotonin nerve cells in Alzheimer's disease, *J. Neurol. Neurosurg. Psychiatry,* 46, 96, 1983.

95. **Mann, D. M. A. and Yates, P. O.,** Possible role of neuromelanin in the pathogenesis of Parkinson's disease, *Mech. Ageing Dev.,* 21, 193, 1983.

96. **Boller, F., Mizutani, T., Roessmann, U., and Gambetti, P.,** Parkinson's disease, dementia, and Alzheimer's disease: clinicopathological correlations, *Ann. Neurol.,* 7, 329, 1980.

97. **Barden, B. and Brizzee, K. R.,** The histochemistry of lipofuscin and neuromelanin, in *Advances in Biochemistry, Vol. 64, Advances in Age Pigment Research,* Tatoro, E. H., Glees, P., and Pisanti, F. A., Eds., Pergamon Press, Oxford, 1987, 339.

98. **Friede, R. L.,** The relation of the formation of lipofuscin to the distribution of oxidative enzymes in the human brain, *Acta Neuropathol.,* 2, 113, 1962.

99. **Harman, D.,** Lipofuscin and ceroid formation: the cellular recycling system, in *Lipofuscin and Ceroid Pigments,* Plenum Press, New York, 1990, 3.

100. **Brizzee, K. R., Eddy, D. E., Harman, D., and Ordy, J. M.,** Free radical theory of aging: effect of dietary lipids on lipofuscin accumulation in the hippocampus of rats, *Age,* 7, 9, 1984.
101. **Eddy, D. E. and Harman, D.,** Free radical theory of aging: effect of age, sex and dietary precursors on rat brain docosahexanoic acid, *J. Am. Geriatr. Soc.,* 25, 220, 1977.
102. **Eddy, D. E. and Harman, D.,** Rat brain fatty acid composition: effect of dietary fat and age, *J. Gerontol.,* 30, 647, 1975.
103. **Tinoco, J., Williams, M. A., Hincenbergs, I., and Lyman, R. L.,** Evidence for nonessentiality of linolenic acid in the diet of the rat, *J. Nutr.,* 101, 937, 1971.
104. **Walker, R. L.,** Maternal diet and brain fatty acids in young rats, *Lipids* 2, 497, 1967.
105. **Tamai, Y., Matsukawa, S., and Satake, M.,** Lipid composition of nerve cell perikarya, *Brain Res.,* 26, 149, 1971.
106. **Cotman, C., Blank, M. L., Moehl, A., and Synder, F.,** Lipid composition of synaptic plasma membranes isolated from rat brain by zonal centrifugation, *Biochemistry,* 8, 4606, 1969.
107. **Sun, G. Y. and Sun, A. Y.,** Phospholipids and acyl groups of synaptosomal and myelin membranes isolated from the cerebral cortex of squirrel monkey *(Saimiri sciureus), Biochem. Biophys. Acta,* 28, 306, 1972.
108. **Breckenridge, W. C., Gombos, G., and Morgan, I. G.,** The docosahexanoic acid of the phospholipids of synaptic membranes, vesicles and mitochondria, *Brain Res.,* 33, 581, 1971.
109. **Hubbard, B. M. and Anderson, J. M.,** Sex difference in age-related brain atrophy, *Lancet,* I, 1447, 1983.
110. **Mann, D. M. A. and Yates, P. O.,** Lipoprotein pigments — their relationship to aging in the human nervous system. I. The lipofuscin content of nerve cells, *Brain,* 97, 481, 1974.
111. **Stadtman, E. R.,** Oxidation of protein by mixed-function oxidation systems: implication in protein turnover, ageing and neutrophil function, *Trends Biochem. Sci.,* 11, 11, 1986.
112. **Stadtman, E. R.,** Biochemical markers of ageing, *Exp. Gerontol.,* 23, 327, 1988.
113. **Starke-Reed, P. E. and Oliver, C. N.,** Protein oxidation and proteolysis during aging and oxidative stress, *Arch. Biochem. Biophys.,* 275, 559, 1989.
114. **Stadtman, E. R.,** Metal ion-catalyzed oxidation of proteins: biochemical mechanisms and biological consequences, *Free Radical Biol. Med.,* 9, 315, 1990.
115. **Rivett, A. J. and Hare, J. F.,** Mixed function oxidation of glutamine synthetase leads to its rapid degradation *in vitro* and after fusion-mediated injection into hepatoma cells, *Biochem. Soc. Trans.,* 14, 643, 1986.
116. **Parker, W. D., Jr., Filley, C. M., and Parks, J. K.,** Cytochrome oxidase deficiency in Alzheimer's disease, *Neurology,* 40, 1302, 1990.
117. **Grundke-Iqbal, I., Iqbal, K., Tung, Y.-C., Quinlan, M., Wisniewski, H. M., and Bindes, L. I.,** Abnormal phosphorylation of the microtubule-associated protein, tau in Alzheimer cytoskeletal pathology, *Proc. Natl. Acad. Sci. U.S.A.,* 83, 4913, 1986.
118. **Iqbal, K., Zaidi, T., Wen, G. Y., Grundke-Iqbal, I., et al.,** Defective brain microtubule assembly in Alzheimer's disease, *Lancet,* II, 421, 1986.
119. **Zemlan, F. P., Thienhaus, O. J., and Bosmann, H. B.,** Superoxide dismutase activity in Alzheimer's disease: possible mechanism for paired helical filament formation, *Brain Res.,* 476, 160, 1989.
120. **Mori, H., Kondo, J., and Ihara, I.,** Ubiquitin is a component of paired helical filaments in Alzheimer's disease, *Science,* 235, 1641, 1987.
121. **Lowe, J., Blanchard, A., Morrell, K., et al.,** Ubiquitin is a common factor in intermediate filament inclusion bodies of diverse types in man, including those of Parkinson's disease, Pick's disease, and Alzheimer's disease, as well as Rosenthal fibers in cerebellar astrocytomas, cytoplastic bodies in muscle, and Mallory bodies in alcoholic liver disease, *J. Pathol.,* 155, 9, 1988.
122. **Golde, T. E., Estus, S., Younkin, L. H., Selkoe, D. J., and Younkin, S. G.,** Processing of the amyloid protein precursor to potentially amyloidgenic derivatives, *Science,* 255, 728, 1992.

123. **Hind, C. R. K., Caspi, D., Collins, P. M., and Baltz, M. L.,** Specific chemical dissociation of fibrillar and non-fibrillar components of amyloid deposits, *Lancet,* II, 376, 1984.

124. **Scheibel, A. B., Pommier, E., and Duang, T.,** Immunodetection of human serum amyloid P component in Alzheimer's disease, *Soc. Neurosci. Abstr.* 13, 1152, 1987.

125. **Kalaria, R. N. and Grahovac, I.,** Serum amyloid P immunoreactivity in hippocampal tangles, plaques and vessels: implications for leakage across the blood-brain barrier in Alzheimer's disease, *Brain Res.,* 516, 349, 1990.

126. **Yanker, B. A. and Mesulam, M. M.,** β-amyloid and the pathogenesis of Alzheimer's disease, *N. Engl. J. Med.,* 325, 1849, 1991.

127. **Selkoe, D. J.,** Amyloid protein and Alzheimer's disease, *Sci. Am.,* 265, No. 5, 40, 1991.

128. **Kowall, N. W., Beal, M. F., Busciglio, J., Duffy, L. K., and Yanker, B. A.,** An *in vivo* model for the neurodegenerative effects of β-amyloid and protection by substance P., *Proc. Natl. Acad. Sci. U.S.A.,* 88, 7247, 1991.

129. **Bugiani, O., Giaccone, G., Frangione, B., Ghetti, B., and Taagliavini, F.,** Alzheimer patients: preamyloid deposits are more widely distributed than senile plaques throughout the central nervous system, *Neurosci. Lett.,* 103, 263, 1989.

130. **Mann, D. M. A. and Esiri, M. M.,** The pattern of acquisition of plaques and tangles in the brains of patients under 50 years of age with Down's syndrome, *J. Neurol. Sci.,* 89, 169, 1989.

Chapter 10

FREE RADICALS, THE AGING BRAIN, AND AGE-RELATED NEURODEGENERATIVE DISORDERS

Randy Strong, Michael B. Mattamal, and Anne C. Andorn

TABLE OF CONTENTS

I. INTRODUCTION

It has been suggested that oxygen free radical-induced damage contributes to aging.[1] Of all the tissues in the body, the central nervous system (CNS) may be particularly vulnerable to free radicals, in part because certain brain regions are highly enriched in nonheme iron, which is catalytically involved in the production of oxygen free radicals.[2-6] Furthermore, the brain has high concentrations of ascorbic acid, an antioxidant that has prooxidant properties in the presence of iron.[7] In addition, the brain contains relatively high levels of unsaturated fatty acids that are particularly good substrates for peroxidation reactions.[8] As compared to other tissues, the brain is also relatively less fortified with the enzymes catalase, superoxide dismutase, and glutathione peroxidase, which catalyze the removal of free-radicals.[9] In this chapter, we will discuss the evidence for free radicals as a cause and/or consequence of age-related changes in the central nervous system and their role in age-associated neurological disorders such as stroke, Parkinson's disease, and Alzheimer's disease.

II. EVIDENCE FOR INCREASED PEROXIDATION IN THE CNS DURING AGING

There is considerable evidence for an increase in peroxidative damage in the brain consequent to the aging process. Much of the evidence comes from studies on age-related alterations in brain lipid composition. Lipids are important components of the neurochemical environment of the brain. Lipids constitute approximately 50% of the dry weight of the brain and are importantly involved in cell structure and function.[8] Changes in lipids have been proposed to be an important factor in aging of the central nervous system.[10] Lipids are particularly good substrates for peroxidation reactions. Free radicals are formed from the interaction of polyunsaturated fatty acids with molecular oxygen, and these produce a chain reaction involving the formation of lipid peroxides. Age-related changes in the composition of phospholipids, consisting of increases in the proportion of saturated fatty acids, may result from increased peroxidation of unsaturated fatty acids.[11] Studies have not consistently found age-related changes in the proportions of saturated to unsaturated fatty acids. Some of this inconsistency may result from methodological considerations. For example, a recent study found no alterations in the degree of saturation of fatty acids from total lipids isolated from different brain regions.[12] On the other hand, the fatty acid composition of individual phospholipids may be altered by aging. For example, the acyl group composition of ethanolamine phosphoglyceride (EPG), which contains most of the unsaturated acyl groups found in myelin, was studied in myelin fractions from brains of three age groups of mice, rhesus monkeys, and humans.[13,14] The older age groups of all three species had a higher proportion of fatty acids with less than three double bonds (mainly 18:1 and 20:1) and a lower

TABLE 1
The Effect of Age on the Number of
Double Bonds in the Fatty Acids of
Individual Phospholipids

| Phospholipid | Double bond index (Age in months) | | |
	4	16	28
PC	73.0 ± 0.5	67.3 ± 0.9[a]	68.5 ± 0.9[a]
PE	261.5 ± 8.2	267.0 ± 5.2	257.4 ± 5.8
PS + PI	223.0 ± 9.0	229.8 ± 9.6	210.4 ± 10.7

Note: Values are the mean ± SEM of three animals per age group. Phosphotidylcholine (PC), Phosphotidylethanolamine (PE), Phosphotidylserine (PS), Phosphotidylinositol (PI).

[a] $p < 0.02$ as compared to 4 month age group.

Adapted from Wood, W. G., Strong, R., Williamson, L. S., and Wise, R. W., *Life Sci.,* 35, 1947, 1984.

proportion of acyl groups with three or more double bonds (mainly 20:4 and 22:4). A decrease with age also was noted in polyunsaturated acyl groups of EPG isolated from nonmyelin fractions of frontal grey matter.[15] The proportion of polyunsaturated fatty acids in individual phospholipids isolated from synaptosomes prepared from the cerebral cortex of mice 4 to 28 months of age has also been measured.[16] As shown in Table 1, there was a significant decrease in the proportion of fatty acids containing double bonds in phosphotidylcholine, which comprises nearly half of the phospholipid content, but not of phosphotidylethanolamine, phosphotidylserine, or phosphotidylinositol. The increase in saturation may be evidence of increased peroxidation during aging.

Attempts to obtain more direct evidence of lipid peroxidation during aging have utilized measurements of lipid peroxides. Lipid peroxide levels have been reported to increase,[17] decrease,[12] and not significantly change during aging.[18] Some of these reported inconsistencies may be due to the ages compared and to the species of animal chosen for study. On the other hand, differences in assay techniques may also contribute to the conflicting results. Most studies have employed the thiobarbituric acid assay as an index of lipid peroxidation. In this assay, the lipid peroxides are assessed indirectly by the measurement of the malondialdehyde reaction product. However, the malondialdehyde product accounts for less than 5% of the actual lipid peroxides.[12] Recently, direct measurement of lipid peroxide levels using more sensitive methods has been used to evaluate age-related changes in lipid peroxidation.[12] Peroxides in the cerebellum, cerebral cortex, and brainstem of Fischer 344 rats 2 to 39 months of age were increased 1.6- to 3-fold.

The fluorescent end-product of lipid peroxidation is lipofuscin age pigment.[19] It is well established that lipofuscin pigment accumulates in neurons during aging.[20] Some researchers[21,22] suggested that the pigmented material might damage cells by disturbing cell geometry, and that, if the distortion were severe, cellular activity might be disturbed. Other investigators maintained that the pigment is inert and not harmful to cells.[23,24] It is clear that there is no uniform opinion regarding the functional significance of lipofuscin pigment. However, pigment accumulation may provide a clue to the degree to which peroxidative activity takes place during aging. Siakotos and coworkers[25] were the first to isolate lipofuscin in sufficient quantities for chemical identification. Lysosomal enzymes are present in lipofuscin of the human brain, suggesting a lysosomal origin or association. Further studies by Taubold, Siakotos, and Perkins[26] showed that lipofuscin contains cholesterol (3%), cholesterol esters (9%), mixed lipids including some polymers (68%), a colorless polymer (8%), and a colored polymer (12%). Gas-liquid chromatographic analysis suggested the presence of a complex lipid whose unsaturated fatty acids had undergone oxidation and polymerization.[26,27] Further evidence for a role for lipid peroxidation in the accumulation of lipofuscin comes from studies in which a direct correlation was demonstrated between lipid peroxidation products, lipofuscin, and malondialdehyde. Vitamin E traps free radicals formed by the interaction of polyunsaturated fatty acids and oxygen. Numerous studies have documented that animals that are fed a vitamin E-deficient diet show evidence of increased tissue peroxides, as measured by malondialdehyde formation, accompanied by lipofuscin accumulation.[19] Moreover, vitamin E supplementation to diets of aging animals retards lipofuscin formation.[19,28] Thus, lipofuscin formation is accelerated by conditions which favor peroxidation reactions and is inhibited by conditions which prevent peroxide formation. Since intraneuronal lipofuscin accumulates in the brain with increasing age, free radicals appear to play a significant role in brain aging.

III. MECHANISMS CONTRIBUTING TO INCREASED AGE-RELATED FREE RADICAL DAMAGE

A number of factors may contribute to increased free radical induced damage in the central nervous system during aging. These factors may include changes in the brain uptake and storage of free-radical generating and scavenging compounds from the diet and alterations in the expression of genes that code for antioxidant enzymes.

The accumulation and storage of prooxidants and antioxidants that are present in the diet may influence the degree of peroxidation in the brain during aging. Massie et al.[18] measured brain tissue content of iron, which catalyzes lipid peroxidation, and measured the presence of lipid peroxides using the thiobarbiturate assay. Iron content was significantly increased by 33% in brains of C57B1/6J mice during aging. Although there was a trend for increases in lipid peroxides, as measured by assaying malondialdehyde, the age-differences were not significant. Vitamin E levels in the brain have been reported to either decrease[29] or increase.[30] However, it has been suggested that vitamin E concentrations may not be a reliable indicator of bioavailable vitamin E. For example, vitamin E found in adipose tissue is not readily available upon metabolic demand.[31] The metabolic availability of vitamin E may be better predicted by turnover rates than by steady state tissue concentrations. Thus, Vitassery and colleagues[30] measured the effect of age on both vitamin E concentrations and uptake of radioactive vitamin E in Fischer 344 rats. Vitamin E was increased with age in the medulla and spinal cord, while no age-related differences were observed in the frontal cortex, pons, thalamus, and cerebellum. In contrast to these results, there were significant decreases in the uptake of radioactive vitamin E into the frontal cortex, pons, medulla, and spinal cord. Thus, the turnover of vitamin E appears to be reduced with age, suggesting that there is less bioavailable vitamin E to detoxify free radicals. Although this issue clearly requires further study, the available evidence suggests that increased iron concentrations and alterations in vitamin E uptake during aging may be significant factors in the increased peroxidation that occurs in the brain during aging.

Research with superoxide dismutase, catalase, and glutathione peroxidase suggests that by catalyzing the removal of superoxide radicals, these enzymes may be major intracellular barriers against oxygen toxicity. Glutathione peroxidase is present in both mitochondria and cytosol. It reduces lipid peroxides by utilizing the reducing power of reduced glutathione (GSH). An age-related decline in glutathione peroxidase has not been consistently reported.[32,33] Rao et al.[32] reported that the expression of glutathione peroxidase is not altered by age in the brains of Fischer 344 rats. In contrast, Vitorica et al.[33] reported that glutathione peroxidase was increased with age in mitochondrial preparations from the brain of Wistar rats. Since no change was found in glutathione reductase, they suggested that this could result in less GSH content and affect the reducing potential of the cell. These alterations, coupled with the reported age-related decrease in brain levels of glutathione,[34] may lead to a decreased ability of the cell to prevent the accumulation of lipid peroxides.

Superoxide dismutase and catalase work in concert to remove oxygen free radicals. Superoxide dismutase has been found in all anatomical brain regions and subcellular fractions. This enzyme dismutates superoxide free radicals to form hydrogen peroxide and oxygen. Catalase is a peroxisomal enzyme. It reduces the hydrogen peroxide that is produced mainly by dismutation of superoxide to yield oxygen and water. The activity and gene expression of catalase has been reported to decrease by 38% in the brain between 6 and 26 months of age in Fischer 344 rats.[32,35] On the other hand, Vitorica et al.[33] reported that catalase activity was not altered in Wistar rats up to 29 months old. Results for superoxide dismutase have been similarly inconsistent. There are reports that the specific activity of superoxide dismutase in the brain of rats and mice remains unchanged with age,[36] decreases with age,[32,37] or increases with age.[38] Dahn et al.[38] measured differences in the activity of different types of superoxide dismutase, Cu/Zn superoxide dismutase, and Mn superoxide dismutase. They found no age-associated differences in Cu/Zn superoxide dismutase activity, but there was an increase in the mitochondrial enzyme Mn superoxide dismutase, in the whole brain, cerebral cortex, neostriatum, and hypothalamus. As a result of these inconsistent findings in the brain and similar inconsistencies with regard to other tissues, the relevance of changes in superoxide dismutase activity as a cause or consequence of aging is not certain. A more compelling role for superoxide dismutase in aging has been suggested by Tolmasoff, Ono, and Cutler,[39] who examined the possible role of the enzyme in determining the life-span of primate species. They found a significant positive correlation between the ratio of superoxide dismutase-specific activity to metabolic rate in the liver, brain, and heart and the maximum life-span potential for these species. This correlation suggests that longer-lived species, such as humans, have better protection against the by-products of oxygen metabolism than do those with shorter lives. Further evidence for this idea comes from studies on the effects of dietary restriction, a treatment which increases both the median and maximum life-span of rats. Dietary restriction prevented the age-related decrease in the activity and expression of both catalase and superoxide dismutase in Fischer 344 rats.[32]

IV. FUNCTIONAL CORRELATES OF FREE RADICAL DAMAGE

The role of peroxidative damage in age-related alterations in the central nervous system is largely circumstantial. There are many parallels between the effects of aging and the effects of experimentally induced peroxidation on neurochemical parameters in the brain. There are several reports on the fluidity of membranes from the brain and other organs among different age groups of animals.[40] Generally, it has been reported that membranes of aged animals are less fluid as compared to those of younger animals. Age-related changes in membrane fluidity may be related to changes in fatty acid composition that are associated with lipid peroxidation.[16] An age-related decrease in neuronal membrane fluidity, particularly in microdomains of the membrane surrounding integral proteins, may impair the functional capacity of the membrane. For example, brain Na^+, K^+-ATPase activity has been reported to be affected by both age[10] and iron-induced lipid peroxidation.[41] Decreases in membrane fluidity with age are also associated with decreased neurotransmitter receptor binding.[42,43] Moreover, treatment with s-adenosyl-L-methionine, which increased membrane fluidity in old animals to the values of young animals, restored the age-related loss of β-adrenergic receptor binding.[43] Furthermore, experimentally induced ischemia, which is associated with increased brain lipid peroxidation, produced decreases in muscarinic acetylcholine receptors,[44] receptors which are also reduced in the brain during aging.[45,46] Another example of a parallel between the effects of aging and peroxidation is found in the brain dopamine system. Aging is associated with a decline in the synthesis and levels of dopamine in the nigrostriatal pathway, a neurotransmitter pathway involved in Parkinson's disease.[8,40] Iron-induced peroxidation has been shown to impair high affinity dopamine uptake in cultured dopaminergic neurons.[47] Moreover, in nerve endings (synaptosomes) prepared from the neostriatum, iron-induced lipid peroxidation was associated with decreased membrane fluidity and reduced dopamine synthesis.[48] Although there is considerable circumstantial evidence for an involvement of free radicals in age-related changes in brain function, there is a notable lack of direct evidence. Recently, however, more direct evidence of a role for oxygen free radicals in decreased brain function during aging was found in a study in which a free radical trapping agent was administered chronically to gerbils 3 to 18 months of age.[49] Administration of the spin-trapping compound N-tert-butyl-α-phenylnitrone reversed the age-related loss of brain glutamine synthetase enzyme activity and deficits in temporal and spatial memory in the aged gerbils.

V. THE ROLE OF LIPID PEROXIDATION IN STROKE

Researchers generally agree that cerebral blood flow and cerebral metabolic rate of oxygen decline in healthy individuals during aging.[50-52] The decrease in cerebral blood flow with age is independent of changes in brain volume.[52] The relative lack of change in glucose metabolic rate in resting brain during aging[53,54] indicates that, under resting conditions, oxygen demand for glucose metabolism is adequately met. There is evidence, however, that the capacity of the brain to respond to ischemia and hypoxic conditions is severely impaired in aged animals.[55,56]

There is considerable evidence that neuronal damage consequent to hemorrhagic or ischemic cortical infarction may be at least partly due to free radicals and lipid peroxidation. For example, transient ischemia was associated with neuronal death, reduction in acetylcholine levels, decreases in N-methyl-d-aspartate (NMDA) and muscarinic cholinergic receptors, and increases in lipid peroxidation in the hippocampus of gerbils.[44] Moreover, peroxidative damage is not limited to ischemic infarction. In hemorrhagic stroke, hemoglobin-mediated damage is also associated with lipid peroxidation.[57] Evidence that lipid peroxidation is not simply a secondary consequence of ischemia comes from studies in which pretreatment with drugs to prevent peroxidation has been shown to prevent neuronal damage induced by ischemia. Prior treatment of ischemic gerbils with the lipid peroxidation inhibitor KB-5666 prevented morphological and biochemical changes in the hippocampus.[58] Furthermore, pretreatment of mongolian gerbils with pyran-conjugated superoxide dismutase also had protective effects against the neuronal damage produced by 5 min of ischemia.[59] Thus, free radicals and lipid peroxidation clearly play a role in the neurological damage produced by cerebral infarction.

In view of the increasing vulnerability of the brain to free radicals during aging, it is not surprising that age is one of the most important risk factors for mortality from brain infarction.[60,61]

VI. FREE RADICALS IN ALZHEIMER'S DISEASE

Alzheimer's disease (AD) is a neurodegenerative disorder that is characterized by a progressive loss of memory, ongoing decline of intellectual function, and, finally, a loss of all cognitive function. A definitive diagnosis may only be obtained by a postmortem pathological examination of brain tissue. The diagnosis of Alzheimer's disease is confirmed postmortem by the presence of numerous amyloid-containing plaques and the presence of neurofibrillary tangles in the neocortex and hippocampus. Other postmortem findings in Alzheimer's disease include decreased membrane fluidity, gliosis, increased protein cross-linking, reduced solubility of membrane proteins, and vacuolarization of neurons, changes which are also associated with lipid peroxidation.[62,63]

Recent reports indicate that lipid peroxides are increased in the Alzheimer's brain. Increased basal peroxidation, as measured by malondialdehyde levels (MDA), was reported to occur in the prefrontal and frontal cortical areas of the AD brain[64,65] as compared to age-matched controls. On the other hand, it has been reported that there was no increase in MDA levels in the temporal cortex from patients who had Alzheimer's disease.[66] A possible reason for the increase in basal lipid peroxidation is the reported increase in iron content.[64] Compared to age-matched controls, nonheme iron was increased in the brain of individuals who had AD, particularly in the prefrontal cortex.

The increases in lipid peroxidation may be related to alterations in neurochemical parameters associated with Alzheimer's disease. For example, experimentally induced lipid peroxidation is known to decrease the density of $5HT_2$ and dopamine$_2$, and cholinergic muscarinic receptors in rodent and human brain.[67,68] In general, neurotransmitter receptor density is also decreased in the cortex of brains of patients who had AD. Decreases in the density of serotonin $(5HT)_2$, α_2-adrenergic, and β_2 adrenergic receptors, and muscarinic receptor density have been reported.[68-71]

Taken together, the set of observations of increased basal lipid peroxidation and increased nonheme iron in areas pathologically affected by the disease supports the concept that lipid peroxidation plays a role in the expression of neurodegenerative disease pathology. Moreover, the changes in neurotransmitter receptors, changes that are sensitive to increased lipid peroxidation, suggest that the lipid peroxidation seen in Alzheimer's disease may be functionally important. Whether lipid peroxidation is a causative factor remains to be proven.

VII. FREE RADICALS AND PARKINSON'S DISEASE

Parkinson's disease, first described in 1817, is a progressive neurological disorder which affects about 10% of people over the age of 65. A consistent pathological finding in Parkinson's disease is the loss of dopaminergic neurons from the pars compacta of the substantia nigra.[72-74] The loss of the dopaminergic input to the caudate nucleus and putamen leads to the characteristic symptoms of Parkinson's disease, which are hypokinesia, resting tremor in the extremities, and muscular rigidity. The cause of the neurodegeneration that characterizes this disease remains unknown. Among the hypothesized causes of the progressive neuronal degeneration include compromised blood flow,[75] endogenous or environmental neurotoxins,[76,77] increased oxidative stress accompanying elevated dopamine turnover,[78,79] oxygen free radicals,[80] and increased lipid peroxidation.[81]

The role of free radicals in Parkinson's disease has recently received considerable attention.[82-84] Recent evidence indicates that, in Parkinson's disease, there is decreased glutathione content and reduced activity of glutathione peroxidase and catalase.[85,86] Evidence for the involvement of free radicals also comes, in part, from measurements of lipid peroxides in the substantia nigra of Parkinson's patients. For example, basal malondialdehyde levels were higher in the substantia nigra from patients who had Parkinson's as compared to age-matched controls.[87] Moreover, polyunsaturated fatty acids were also reduced, perhaps as a consequence of peroxidation. Much of the increase in lipid peroxidation may be due to the selective accumulation of iron by the substantia nigra. For example, a recent postmortem study on Parkinson's patients demonstrated an increase in iron content selectively in the substantia nigra pars compacta, the location of cell bodies of dopaminergic neurons that are affected in this disease.[88] Elevated iron content consisted mainly of an increase in iron (III). Thus, the ratio of iron (II) to iron (III) was 2:1 in controls, but 1:2 in the Parkinson's brain. This change in reducing potential favors the generation of free radicals. The selectivity of the increase in iron (III) by the dopaminergic neurons of the substantia nigra may relate to the fact that these neurons contain melanin pigment. There is evidence to suggest that the selective accumulation of iron by the substantia nigra pars compacta is related to the high affinity of melanin for iron (III).[89] Moreover, melanin may potentiate iron-induced lipid peroxidation.[89] Another, hypothesis is that abnormal iron handling by the transferrin receptor may contribute to the selective accumulation of iron and increased lipid peroxidation in the substantia nigra in Parkinson's disease. Mice treated with a neurotoxin selective for dopaminergic neurons showed a significant decrease in transferrin receptor binding associated with a decrease in dopamine uptake sites, a specific neurochemical marker of dopaminergic neurons.[90] Thus, dopaminergic neurons contain a high density of transferrin receptors. Moreover, transferrin receptors were significantly decreased in Parkinson's brain compared to controls.[90]

Another possible cause of increased H_2O_2 in the substantia nigra in Parkinson's disease is altered mitochondrial function. One reported difference in mitochondrial function in Parkinson's disease is a generalized defect in oxidative phosphorylation at the level of complex I.[91] For example, in one study, four out of six patients had a type I oxidative phosphorylation defect, while one of the six had a complex IV defect.[92] In 16 age-matched controls, no defect was detected. It was suggested by the authors of that study that energetic impairment associated with increased H_2O_2 production may be the cause of the cell death in this disorder. Another possible cause of the increase in hydrogen peroxide is the altered activity of monoamine oxidase B (MAO B). Monoamine oxidase is an enzyme present on the external mitochondrial wall and is present in neurons and glial cells. There are two forms of the enzyme, MAO A and MAO B, which are distinguished by their selective sensitivity to different types of monoamine oxidase inhibitors. The form of the enzyme that predominates in dopamine containing neurons is MAO B. It is relatively less sensitive to the MAO A inhibitor, clorgyline, and more sensitive to the MAO B inhibitor, deprenyl. Monoamine oxidase B catalyzes the metabolism of dopamine to an intermediate metabolite, dopaldehyde (DOPAL), and H_2O_2. The activity of MAO B is reportedly increased in Parkinson's disease; thus, the resulting increase in H_2O_2 production may contribute to increased lipid peroxidation.[80,83,85]

Alterations in MAO B activity may also contribute to the accumulation of abnormal metabolites that are neurotoxic. Much of this line of research was motivated by studies with 1-methyl-4-phenyl-1,2,3,6-tetrahydropyridine (MPTP), a contaminate formed during the synthesis of the opiate meperidine.[93,94] MPTP is transformed by MAO-B to the toxic metabolite MPP+ which interferes with mitochondrial respiratory activity and, in turn, leads to degeneration of dopaminergic neurons.[95] Interestingly, the effects of MPTP are greater in older mice than in younger mice.[96] The actions of MPP+ on mitochondrial respiratory function are strikingly similar to those found in Parkinson's disease.[97-99] Thus, it has been suggested that an environmental protoxin[100] or an endogenous neurotoxic metabolite of dopamine,[101-104] with inhibitory actions on mitochondrial respiratory function similar to those of MPP+, may be the cause of the neurodegeneration of Parkinson's disease. This hypothesis is supported by the results of clinical studies which have shown that the progression of the disease was slowed in Parkinson's disease patients treated with the monoamine oxidase B inhibitor, deprenyl.[105]

We have attempted to reconcile the peroxidation and endogenous neurotoxin hypotheses by combining them into a single model. Figure 1 shows a model which attempts to reconcile the lipid peroxidation hypothesis with the endogenous neurotoxin hypothesis by suggesting that the increased MAO B activity, increased peroxidation, and presence of endogenous neurotoxic metabolites are all components of the same mechanism. Figure 1 shows the pathway by which 3,4-dihydroxyphenylacetaldehyde (DOPAL; dopaldehyde) is formed by the oxidative deamination of dopamine, a reaction catalyzed by MAO (Figure 1, steps A and F). Another product of dopamine metabolism

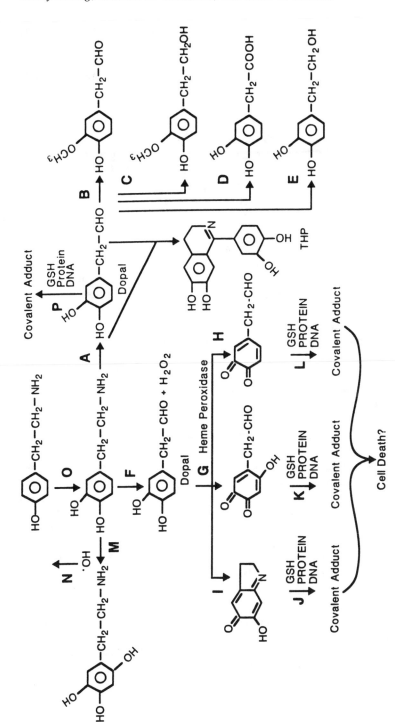

FIGURE 1. Possible metabolic pathways for dopamine that lead to the formation of potentially neurotoxic metabolites.

by MAO is the production of H_2O_2. The hydrogen peroxide thus formed may then contribute to another metabolic pathway which utilizes heme peroxidases (Figure 1, steps F to L). Based on this scheme, we have developed an approach utilizing *in vitro* systems that model the essential aspects of each of these two pathways. The first step in this strategy is to identify potentially toxic products produced by the two systems. We then test those compounds *in vitro* in cell culture and *in vivo* in rat brain to determine if the compounds are neurotoxic. Using this information, we then examine postmortem human brain tissue to determine if the products are present in the substantia nigra of Parkinson's brain and if they are elevated as compared to age-matched controls.

The first step in this approach is illustrated in Table 2. Dopamine was incubated in the presence of either the peroxidase system or the monoamine oxidase system, with the expectation that one or more of the aldehydes shown in Figure 1 would be generated. There is accumulating evidence to show that some biogenic aldehydes may be cytotoxic,[108] inhibit enzyme activity,[106,107,109] react with DNA to form adducts,[110] and damage microtubules.[111] To determine if there were potentially neurotoxic dopamine metabolites produced by the two systems, we took advantage of the fact that the suspected neurotoxic aldehydes will covalently bind to DNA and protein.

Table 2 illustrates that potentially neurotoxic metabolite(s) are generated from ^{3}H-dopamine in the model peroxidase system, as measured by their ability to covalently bind to DNA and tubulin. Hydrogen peroxide can serve as a cosubstrate for the heme peroxidases, tyrosine hydroxylase and prostaglandin H synthase. These enzymes coexist in the substantia nigra neurons.[112-114] The presence of heme-containing enzymes PHS and tyrosine hydroxylase and the intracellular availability H_2O_2 suggests that peroxidative metabolism of dopamine is possible in neurons. Studies from our laboratory[115] and others[116,117] have shown that the hydroperoxidase activity of PHS can utilize H_2O_2 in the hydroperoxidase-dependent oxidation of catecholamines, indoleamines, and aromatic amines. Horseradish peroxidase has been shown to be a valuable model for PHS and other mammalian peroxidases and has been successfully used to study the *in vitro* metabolism of various phenolic compounds.[115-119] We employed HRP/H_2O_2 as the model system to mimic *in vitro* the characteristics of brain dopamine neurons. Peroxidative metabolism of ^{3}H-dopamine resulted in covalent binding to DNA, microtubulin protein, and bovine serum albumin (BSA). MAO inhibitors did not affect binding. Thus, covalent binding was observed in the presence of the MAO inhibitors, pargyline and clorgyline. In contrast, ascorbate, glutathione, and *N*-acetylcysteine inhibited the peroxidatic metabolism of dopamine and/or prevented binding to DNA and tubulin.

Table 2 also shows the effect of incubation of ^{3}H-dopamine with an *in vitro* system containing adrenal MAO. Following incubation in the presence of MAO for 20 min, covalent binding to BSA, microtubulin protein, and DNA were detected. The MAO mediated metabolism and covalent binding to DNA, and tubulin was inhibited by heat treatment, *N*-acetylcysteine,

TABLE 2
Effects of Various Inhibitors on the Covalent Binding of (2,5,6-3H) Dopamine Metabolite(s) to Protein, DNA, and Tubulin in a Reconstituted Peroxidatic[a] (H_2O_2/HRP) and MAO System[b]

	Inhibitor conc (mM)	Covalent binding (%)		
		Protein	**Tubulin**	**DNA**
H_2O_2/HRP				
Complete system[a]		100 ± 3	100 ± 3	100 ± 22
−HRP + H_2O_2		ND[d]	ND	ND
+HRP − H_2O_2		ND	ND	ND
Pargyline	0.100	223 ± 2	111 ± 3	107 ± 2
Clorgyline	0.100	227 ± 2	113 ± 4	104 ± 3
Glutathione	0.500	2 + 1	2 + 2	1 + 1
Thiourea	0.200	1 + 1	2 + 1	1 + 1
N-Acetyl cysteine	0.100	2 + 1	1 + 1	1 + 1
Ascorbic acid	0.500	13 + 4	28 + 3	35 + 4
MAO				
Complete system[c]		100 + 11	100 + 11	100 + 9
−MAO		ND	ND	ND
Heat treated		ND	ND	ND
Hydralazine	0.100	90 + 10	91 + 11	106 + 8
Pargyline	0.100	1 + 1	2 + 2	1 + 1
Clorgyline	0.100	11 + 3	25 + 4	100 + 9
Glutathione	0.500	1 + 1	2 + 1	1 + 1
N-Acetyl cysteine	0.100	1 + 1	1 + 1	2 + 1
Ascorbic acid	0.100	96 + 4	91 + 8	93 + 7
	1.000	ND	ND	ND

[a]   Complete system consisted of 50 μM (2,5,6 – 3H) Dopamine, 1.0 mg/ml of either PSI or tubulin protein or DNA, 3 units of HRP, 100 μM of H_2O_2 in a total volume of 0.5 ml. All inhibitors were preincubated for 2 min at 25°C. The reaction was started by the addition of H_2O_2, and incubations were carried out for 3 min.

[b]   Mean of + SE (n = 3 to 6). 100% covalent binding values corresponds to BSA protein: 3.05 + 0.11 nmol/mg/min, Tubulin protein: 6.38 + 0.2 nmol/mg/min, and DNA: 5.82 + 0.18 nmol/mg. For MAO mediated covalent binding, protein: 0.62 + 0.11 nmol/mg/min, tubulin protein: 1.21 + 0.15 nmol/mg/min, and DNA: 1.31 + 0.12 mg/min.

[c]   Complete system consisted of 50 μM (2,5,6 – 3H) dopamine, 1.0 mg of adrenal monoamine oxidase, 1.0 mg of tubulin, protein or DNA in a total volume of 0.5 ml. All inhibitors were preincubated for 2 min at 25°C. The reaction was started by the addition of dopamine, and incubations were carried out for 20 min.

[d]   ND, not detected and corresponds to blank values.

glutathione, ascorbic acid, or the monoamine oxidase inhibitor pargyline. Clorgyline, a selective MAO A inhibitor, had less effect than did pargyline on binding to protein and no effect on the covalent binding to DNA. Thus, the two dopamine metabolic pathways, catalyzed by peroxidase or monoamine oxidase, are capable of generating potentially neurotoxic compounds.

Using mass spectroscopy, we have identified several potentially neurotoxic dopamine metabolites generated by the two systems. We have tested some of these compounds for neurotoxicity, using *in vivo* and *in vitro* experimental approaches. If a compound is neurotoxic in these experimental models, we then attempt to detect the suspected neurotoxins in the brains of individuals who had Parkinson's disease. To illustrate the utility of this approach, we will discuss findings from studies with one of the dopamine metabolites identified using this strategy.

The structure of DOPAL, isolated from incubations of dopamine in an enzymatic system containing adrenal MAO, was firmly established by high resolution, metastable mass spectrometry. To determine if this compound was a neurotoxin, we employed both *in vitro* and *in vivo* systems. *In vitro* studies were carried out with PC12 cells. PC12 cells were chosen because of their ability to synthesize and store a large amount of dopamine and norepinephrine and to release these neurotransmitter substances when depolarized. PC12 cells can be induced to stop proliferating and to acquire a neuron-like morphology when exposed to nerve growth factor (NGF). PC12 cells (2 × 105 cells per well) were differentiated in the presence of NGF and exposed to three different concentrations (1, 3, and 5 µg) of DOPAL. The lowest concentration of DOPAL produced no effect. The next highest concentration (3 µg) produced a 20% reduction of cell number after 18 h. The highest concentration tested (5 µg) caused a decrease in the number of neurites after 8 h and nearly complete cell death after 18 h (Figure 2).

In vivo studies of the neurotoxicity of DOPAL were carried out using rats. Stereotaxic injection (1 µl) of DOPAL (5 µg/µl) into substantia nigra (SN) of two-month-old rats caused a loss of tyrosine hydroxylase immunoreactive neurons. No neuronal damage was seen when phosphate buffered saline and dopamine were used as controls. Neuronal damage occurred only in the presence of DOPAL. Notably, the concentration of DOPAL that was toxic *in vitro* was also toxic *in vivo*.

Having determined that this compound is neurotoxic, we then developed methods to determine if DOPAL is present in the substantia nigra in Parkinson's disease. The trimethylsilyl-gas chromatography-mass spectrometry-selected ion method (TMS-GC-MS-SIM) was developed to identify DOPAL in postmortem human brain tissue. Postmortem tissue was obtained from the St. Louis University Brain Bank. We used tissue obtained at autopsy from individuals who were identified pathologically and from patient records as having a primary diagnosis of Alzheimer's disease with a secondary diagnosis of Parkinson's disease (AD/PD). We chose to use tissue from individuals with this mixed diagnosis because they were less likely to have received

L-DOPA therapy. Studies were thus carried out with cases in which the patient records indicated that there was no clinical history of L-DOPA therapy. As shown in Table 3, the GC-MS-SIM of samples prepared from the substantia nigra of AD/PD cases revealed the presence of DOPAL. DOPAL was absent from substantia nigra of the control brains. Moreover, DOPAL was absent from the hippocampus of AD/PD patients, an area not affected in Parkinson's disease (Table 3).

Using this approach, we have also identified dopamine metabolites generated in the peroxidase system and can now determine which of these potentially neurotoxic compounds are elevated in Parkinson's disease. Moreover, the results of these preliminary studies support the idea that the increased peroxides, elevated MAO B activity, and accumulation of endogenous neurotoxin(s) may all be a part of the same process, and together contribute to neurodegeneration during Parkinson's disease. Further elucidating these mechanisms may enable us to devise treatments to slow or halt the neurodegenerative process.

VIII. SUMMARY

There are numerous conflicting reports in the literature regarding the role that free radicals play in age-associated alterations in the central nervous system. The reasons for the disagreements may be due to the ages compared, differences in the types of organisms studied, the tissues examined, and the assay methods employed. Many of the methods available are relatively insensitive, and the age differences, when found, may be relatively small and thus easily missed with some of the less sensitive assays. Despite these problems, there is a breadth of evidence supporting the idea that free radicals play a significant part in aging of the postmitotic cells of the central nervous system. Moreover, the occurrence of diseases late in life may add yet another echelon of challenges to the already accelerating accumulation of free radical-induced damage in the brain. Thus, age-related increases in vulnerability to free radicals may be especially important in relation to the capacity to respond to disease states where increased free radical formation is fundamentally involved, such as in stroke, Parkinson's disease, and Alzheimer's disease.

ACKNOWLEDGMENTS

This work was supported by the Geriatric Research, Education and Clinical Center of the St. Louis Department of Veterans Affairs Medical Centers (Strong, M. B. Mattamal), by a grant from the Merit Review Research Program of the Department of Veterans Affairs Medical Research Service (R. Strong), and by National Institutes of Health Grant AG09557 (R. Strong). We thank the St. Louis University brain bank for supplying autopsy specimens.

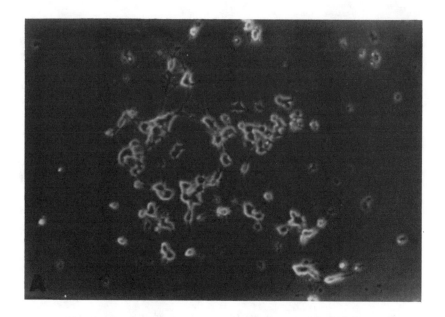

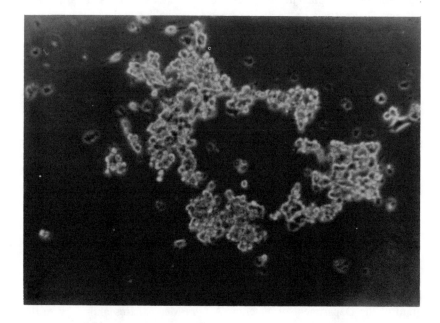

FIGURE 2.   The toxic effects of DOPAL on PC12 cells treated with nerve growth factor. (A) No DOPAL treatment; (B) treatment with 5 μg of DOPAL for 8 h; (C) treatment with 5μg of DOPAL for 18 h.

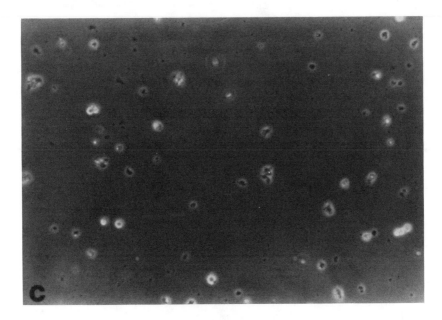

FIGURE 2C (continued).

TABLE 3
Concentrations of DOPAL in Brain of
Parkinson's Disease Patients

	Concentration of DOPAL (μg/g wet weight)	
	Parkinson's	Control
Substantia nigra	7 ± 0.5[a]	ND[b]
Hippocampus	ND[b]	—
Number of samples	3	2

Note: Tissue samples (250 to 500 mg) from three Parkinson's brains and two age-matched control brains were individually homogenized in 25 ml of acetone containing 1.0 ml of 0.01 N hydrochloric acid and extracted with acetone:ethyl acetate (1:1) and evaporated to dryness. The TMS derivative was prepared in a final volume of 20 μl, and GC-MS-SIM was carried out on 5 μl of the extracted sample.

[a] Estimated from an external standard calibration curve using undeuterated DOPAL. The estimated concentrations of DOPAL in the substantia nigra from brains of individuals who had Parkinson's disease ranged from 7 to 8 μg/g wet weight of tissue.
[b] ND, not detectable.

REFERENCES

1. **Harman, D.**, Prolongation of life: role of free radicals in aging, *J. Am. Geriatr. Soc.*, 17, 721, 1969.
2. **Zaleska, M. M. and Floyd, R. A.**, Regional lipid peroxidation in rat brain *in vitro:* possible role of endogenous iron, *Neurochem. Res.*, 10, 397, 1985.
3. **Wilmore, L. J., Hiramatsu, M., Kochi, H., and Mori, A.**, Formation of superoxide radicals after FeCl₃ injection into rat isocortex, *Brain Res.*, 277, 393, 1983.
4. **Triggs, W. J. and Wilmore, L. J.**, *In vivo* lipid peroxidation following intracortical Fe²⁺ injection, *J. Neurochem.*, 42, 967, 1984.
5. **Ciuffi, M., Gentillini, G., Franchi-Micheli, S., and Zilletti, L.**, Lipid peroxidation induced "*in vivo*" by iron carbohydrate complex in the rat brain cortex, *Neurochem. Res.*, 16, 43, 1991.
6. **Subbarao, K. V. and Richardson, J. S.**, Iron dependent peroxidation of rat brain: a regional study, *J. Neurosci. Res.*, 26, 224, 1990.
7. **Sadrzadeh, S. M. H. and Eaton, J. W.**, Hemoglobin-mediated oxidant damage to the central nervous system requires endogenous ascorbate, *J. Clin. Invest.*, 82, 1510, 1988.
8. **Strong, R., Wood, W. G., and Samorajski, T.**, Neurochemistry of ageing, in *Principles and Practice of Geriatric Medicine*, 2nd ed., Pathy, M. S. J., Ed., John Wiley & Sons, New York, 1991, 69.
9. **Halliwell, B. and Gutteridge, J. M. C.**, Oxygen radicals and the nervous system, *Trend Neurosci.*, 8, 22, 1985.
10. **Sun, A. Y. and Sun, G. Y.**, Neurochemical aspects of the membrane hypothesis of aging, in *Interdisciplinary Topics on Gerontology*, Vol. 15, von Hahn, H. P., Ed., S. Karger, Basel, 1979, 34.
11. **Hegner, D.**, Age-dependence of molecular and functional changes in biological membrane properties, *Mech. Ageing Dev.*, 14, 101, 1980.
12. **Ando, S., Kon, K., Aino, K. and Totani, Y.**, Increased levels of lipid peroxides in aged rat brain as revealed by direct assay of peroxide values, *Neurosci. Lett.*, 113, 199, 1990.
13. **Samorajski, T. and Rolsten, C.**, Age and regional differences in the chemical composition of brains of mice, monkeys and humans, in *Progress in Brain Research, Vol. 40, Neurobiological Aspects of Maturation and Ageing*, Ford, D. H., Ed., Elsevier, New York, 1973, 253.
14. **Sun, G. Y. and Samorajski, T.**, Age differences in the acyl group composition of phosphoglycerides in myelin isolated from the brain of the rhesus monkey, *Biochim. Biophys. Acta*, 316, 19, 1973.
15. **Bowen, D. M., Smith, C. B., and Davison, A. N.**, Molecular changes in senile dementia, *Brain*, 96, 849, 1973.
16. **Wood, W. G., Strong, R., Williamson, L. S., and Wise, R. W.**, Changes in lipid composition of cortical synaptosomes from different age groups of mice, *Life Sci.*, 35, 1947, 1984.
17. **Yoshikawa, M. and Hirai, S.**, Lipid peroxide formation in the brain of aging rats, *J. Gerontol.*, 22, 162, 1967.
18. **Massie, H. R., Aiello, V. R., and Banzinger, V.**, Iron accumulation and lipid peroxidation in aging C57BL/6J mice, *Exp. Gerontol.*, 18, 277, 1983.
19. **Nandy, K.**, Lipofuscin as a marker of impaired homeostasis in aging organisms, in *Homeostatic Function and Aging*, Davis, B. B. and Wood, W. G., Eds., Raven Press, New York, 1985, 139.
20. **Brizzee, K. and Ordy, J. M.**, Age pigments cell loss and functional implications in the brain, in *Age Pigments*, Sohal, R., Ed., Elsevier/North Holland, 1981, 317.
21. **Samorajski, T., Ordy, J. M., and Keefe, J. R.**, The fine structure of lipofuscin age pigment in the nervous system of aged mice, *J. Cell. Biol.*, 26, 779, 1965.

22. **Zeman, W.,** The neuronal ceroid-lipofuscinosis Batten-Vogt syndrome. A model for human ageing, *Adv. Geront. Res.,* 3, 147, 1971.
23. **Hyden, H. and Lindstrom, B.,** Microspectographic studies on the yellow pigment in nerve cells, *Discuss. Faraday Soc.,* 9, 436, 1950.
24. **Tscheng, K. T.,** Some observations on the lipofuscin pigments in the pyramidal and Purkinje cells of the monkey, *J. Hirnforsch.,* 6, 323, 1964.
25. **Siakotos, A. N., Watanabe, I., Saito, A. L., and Fleischer, S.,** Procedures for the isolation of two distinct lipopigments from human brain lipofuscin and ceroid, *Biochem. Med.,* 4, 361, 1970.
26. **Taubold, R. D., Siakotos, A. N., and Perkins, E. G.,** Studies on chemical nature of lipofuscin (age pigment) isolated from normal human brain, *Lipids,* 10, 383, 1975.
27. **Siakotos, A. N. and Armstrong, D.,** Age pigment, a biochemical indicator of intra-cellular ageing, in *Advances in Behavioral Biology, Vol. 16, Neurobiology of Ageing,* Ordy, J. M. and Brizzee, K. R., Eds., Plenum Press, New York., 1975, 369.
28. **Nelson, J. S., Fitch, C. D., Fischer, V. W., Broun, G. O., and Chou A. C.,** Progressive neuropathological lesions in vitamin E-deficient rhesus monkeys, *J. Neuropathol. Exp. Neurol.,* 40, 166, 1981.
29. **Noda, Y., McGeer, P. L., and McGeer, E. G.,** Lipid peroxides in brain during aging and vitamin E deficiency: possible relationship to changes in neurotransmitter indices, *Neurobiol. Aging,* 3, 173, 1982.
30. **Vatassery, G. T., Angerhofer, C. K., and Knox, C. A.,** Effect of age on vitamin E concentrations in various regions of the brain and a few selected peripheral tissues of the rat, and on the uptake of radioactive vitamin E by various regions of the rat brain, *J. Neurochem.,* 43, 409, 1984.
31. **Machlin, L. J., Keating, J., Nelson, J., Brin, M., Filipski, R., and Miller, O. N.,** Availability of adipose tissue tocopherol in the guinea pig, *J. Nutr.,* 109, 105, 1979.
32. **Rao, G., Xia, E., and Richardson, A.,** Effect of dietary restriction and aging on the expression of antioxidant enzymes, in *Molecular Biology of Aging,* Alan R. Liss, New Yrk, 1990, 391.
33. **Vitorica, J., Machado, A., and Satrustegui, J.,** Age-dependent variations in peroxide-utilizing enzymes from rat brain mitochondria and cytoplasm, *J. Neurochem.,* 42, 351, 1984.
34. **Ravindranath, V., Shivakumar, B. R., and Anandatheerthavarada, H. K.,** Low glutathione levels in brains of aged rats, *Neurosci. Lett.,* 101, 187, 1989.
35. **Semsei, I., Rao, G., and Richardson, A.,** Expression of superoxide dismutase and catalase in rat brain as a function of aging, *Mech. Ageing Dev.,* 1991.
36. **Reiss, V. and Gershon, D.,** Comparison of cytoplasmic superoxide dismutase in liver, heart, and brain of ageing rats and mice, *Biochem. Biophys. Res. Commun.,* 73, 255, 1976.
37. **Massie, H. R., Aiello, V. R., and Iodice, A. A.,** Changes with age in copper and superoxide dismutase levels in brains of C57BL/6J mice, *Mech. Ageing Dev.,* 10, 93, 1979.
38. **Dahn, H. C., Benedetti, M. S., and Dostert, P.,** Differential changes in superoxide dismutase in brain and liver of old rats, *J. Neurochem.,* 40, 1003, 1983.
39. **Tolmasoff, J. M., Ono, T., and Cutler, R. G.,** Superoxide dismutase: correlations with life-span and specific metabolic rate in primate species, *Proc. Natl. Acad. Sci. U.S.A.,* 77, 2777, 1980.
40. **Strong, R.,** Neurochemistry of aging: 1982–1984, in *Review of Biological Research in Aging,* Rothstein, M., Ed., Alan R. Liss, New York, 1985, 181.
41. **Domanska-Janik, K. and Bourre, J. M.,** Effect of lipid peroxidation on Na^+, K^+-ATPase, 5'-nucleotidase and CNPase in mouse brain myelin, *Biochem. Biophys. Acta,* 1034, 200, 1990.

42. **Samuel, D., Heron, D. S., Hershkowitz, M., and Shinitsky, M.**, Aging, receptor binding, and membrane microviscosity, in *The Aging Brain: Cellular and Molecular Mechanisms of Aging in the Nervous System*, Giacobini, E., Filogamma, G., and Vernakakis, A., Eds., Raven Press, New York, 1982, 93.

43. **Cimino, M., Vantini, G., Algeri, S., Curotola, G., Pezzoli, C., and Stramentinoli, G.**, Age-related modification of dopaminergic and β-adrenergic receptor system: restoration to normal activity by modification of membrane fluidity with s-adenosyl methionine, *Life Sci.*, 34, 2029, 1984.

44. **Haba, K., Ogawa, N., Mizukawa, K., and Myori, A.**, Time course of changes in lipid peroxidation, pre- and postsynaptic cholinergic indices, NMDA receptor binding and neuronal death in the gerbil hippocampus following transient ischemia, *Brain Res.*, 540, 116, 1991.

45. **Strong, R., Samorajski, T., and Gottesfeld, Z.**, Regional mapping of neostriatal neurotransmitter systems as a function of aging, *J. Neurochem.*, 39, 831, 1982.

46. **Strong, R., Samorajski, T., and Gottesfeld, Z.**, High-affinity uptake of neurotransmitters in rat neostriatum: effects of aging, *J. Neurochem.*, 43, 1766, 1984.

47. **Michel, P. P., Vyas, S., and Agid, Y.**, Toxic effects of iron for cultured mesencephalic dopaminergic neurons derived from embryonic rat brains, *J. Neurochem.*, 59, 118, 1992.

48. **Zaleska, M. M., Nagy, K., and Floyd, R. A.**, Iron-induced lipid peroxidation and inhibition of dopamine synthesis in striatum synaptosomes, *Neurochem. Res.*, 14, 597, 1989.

49. **Carney, J. M., Starke-Reed, P. E., Oliver, C. N., Landum, R. W., Cheng, M. S., Wu, J. F., and Floyd, R. A.**, Reversal of age-related increase in brain protein oxidation, decrease in enzyme activity, and loss in temporal and spatial memory by chronic administration of the spin-trapping compound N-tert-butyl-α-phenylnitrone, *Proc. Natl. Acad. Sci. U.S.A.*, 88, 3633, 1991.

50. **Pantano, P., Baron, J.-C., Lebrun-Grandie, P., Duquesnoy, N., Bousser, M.-G., and Comar, D.**, Regional cerebral blood flow and oxygen consumption in human aging, *Stroke*, 15, 635, 1984.

51. **Marshall, J.**, Clinical approach to the aged brain, *Gerontology*, 33, 125, 1987.

52. **Takeda, S., Matsuzawa, T., and Hiroshige, M.**, Age-related changes in regional cerebral blood flow and brain volume in healthy subjects, *J. Am. Geriatr. Soc.*, 36, 293, 1988.

53. **DeLeon, M. J., George, A. E., Tomanelli, J., Christman, D., Kluger, A., Miller, J., Ferris, S. H., Fowler, J., Brodie, J. D., Van Gelder, P., Klinger, A., and Wolf, A. P.**, Positron emission tomography studies of normal aging: a replication of PET III and 18-FDG using PET VI and 11-CDG, *Neurobiol. Aging*, 8, 319, 1987.

54. **Schlageter, N. L., Horwitz, B., Creasey, H., Carson, R., Duara, R., Berg, G. W., and Rapoport, S. I.**, Relation of measured brain glucose utilization and cerebral atrophy in man, *J. Neurol. Neurosurg. Psychiat.*, 50, 779, 1987.

55. **Hoyer, S.**, Ischemia in aged brain, *Gerontology*, 33, 203, 1987.

56. **Benzi, G., Pastoris, O., Vercesi, L., Gorini, A., Viganotti, C., and Villa, R. F.**, Energetic states of aged brain during hypoxia, *Gerontology*, 33, 207, 1987.

57. **Sadrzadeh, S. M. H., Anderson, D. K., Panter, S. S., Hallaway, P. E., and Eaton, J. W.**, Hemoglobin potentiates central nervous system damage, *J. Clin. Inv.*, 79, 662, 1987.

58. **Hara, H. and Kogure, K.**, Prevention of hippocampus neuronal damage in ischemic gerbils by a novel lipid peroxidation inhibitor (quinazoline derivative), *J. Pharmacol. Exp. Ther.*, 255, 906, 1990.

59. **Kitagawa, K., Matsumoto, M., Oda, T., Niinobe, M., Hata, R., Handa, N., Fukunaga, R., Isaka, Y., Kimura, K., Maeda, H., Mikoshiba, K., and Kamada, T.**, Free radical generation during brief period of cerebral ischemia may trigger delayed neuronal death, *Neuroscience*, 35, 551, 1990.

60. **Fuller, J. H., Shipley, M. J., Rose, G., Jarrett, J. R., and Keen, H.,** Mortality from coronary heart disease and stroke in relation to degree of glycaemia: the Whitehall study, *Br. Med. J.*, 2, 867, 1985.

61. **Hubert, H. B., Feinlab, M., McNamara, P. M., and Castelli, W. P.,** Obesity as an independent risk factor for cardiovascular disease: a 26 year follow-up of participants in the Framingham heart study, *Circulation*, 67, 968, 1983.

62. **Nagy, I. Z. and Nagy, K.,** On the role of cross-linking of cellular proteins in aging, *Mech. Ageing Dev.*, 14, 245, 1980.

63. **Willmore, L. J. and Rubin, J. J.,** Antiperoxidant pretreatment and iron induced epileptiform discharges in the rat EEG and histopathological studies, *Neurology*, 31, 63, 1981.

64. **Andorn, A. C., Britton, R. S., Bacon, B. R., Franko, M., Hamazaki, N., and Kalaria, R. N.,** Non-heme iron is increased and ascorbate-stimulated lipid peroxidation is reduced in postmortem prefrontal cortex in Alzheimer's disease (AD): a comparison of findings in AD and normal age matched controls, *Neurosci. Abstr.*, 16, 462, 1990.

65. **Subbarao, K. V., Richardson, J. S., and Ang, L. C.,** Autopsy samples of Alzheimer's cortex show increased peroxidation *in vitro*, *J. Neurochem.*, 55, 342, 1990.

66. **Hajimohammadreza, I. and Brammer, M.,** Brain membrane fluidity and lipid peroxidation in Alzheimer's disease, *Neurosci. Lett.*, 112, 333, 1990.

67. **Heikkila, R. E. and Cabbato, F. S.,** Ascorbate-induced lipid peroxidation and inhibition of [³H]spiroperidol binding in neostriatal membrane preparations, *J. Neurochem.*, 41, 1384, 1983.

68. **Andorn, A. C., Bacon, B. R., Nguyen-Hunh, A. T., Parloato, S. J., and Stitts, J. A.,** Guanyl nucleotide interactions with dopaminergic binding sites labeled by [³H]spiroperidol in human caudate and putamen: guanyl nucleotides enhance ascorbate-induced lipid peroxidation and cause an apparent loss of high affinity binding sites, *Mol. Pharmacol.*, 33, 155, 1988.

69. **Kalaria, R. N. and Andorn, A. C.,** Adrenergic receptors in aging and Alzheimer's disease: decreased α_2-receptors demonstrated by [³H]*p*-aminoclonidine binding in prefrontal cortex, *Neurobiol. Aging*, 12, 131, 1991.

70. **Bowen, D. M., Allen, S. J., Benton, J. S., Goodhardt, J. J., Haan, A. E., Palmer, A. M., Sims, N. R., Smith, C. C. T., Spilane, J. A., Esirir, M. M., Neary, D., Snowdon, J. S., Wilcock, G. K., and Davison, G. K.,** Biochemical assessment of serotonergic and cholinergic dysfunction and cerebral atrophy in Alzheimer's disease, *J. Neurochem.*, 41, 266, 1983.

71. **Mash, D. C., Flynn, D. D., and Poetter, L. T.,** Loss of M2 muscarine receptors in the cerebral cortex in Alzheimer's disease and experimental cholinergic denervation, *Science*, 238, 1115, 1985.

72. **Hornykiez, O. and Kish, S. J.,** Biochemical pathophysiology of Parkinson's disease, in *Advances in Neurology*, Yahr, M. D. and Bergman, K. I., Eds., Raven Press, New York, 1986, 19.

73. **Gibbs, W. R. G.,** *The Neuropathology of Parkinson's Disorder, in Parkinson's Disease and Movement Disorders*, Jankovic, J. and Tolosa, E., Eds., Urban & Schwarzenberg, Baltimore, 1988, 205.

74. **Weiner, W. J. and Lang, A. E.,** Parkinson's disease, in *Movement Disorders: A Comprehensive Survey*, Futura Publishing, Mount Kisco, New York, 1989, 23.

75. **Melamed, E. and Mildworf, B.,** Regional cerebral blood flow reduction in patients with Parkinsons disease: correlation with normal aging, cognitive functions, and dopaminergic mechanism, in *Parkinsonism and Aging*, Calne, D. B., Crippa, D., Trabucchi, M., Comi, G., and Horowaski, R., Eds., Raven Press, New York, 1989, 221.

76. **Markey, S. P., Johannessen, J. W., Chiueh, C. C., Burns, R. S., and Herkenham, M. A.,** Intraneuronal generation of a pyridium metabolite may cause drug-induced Parkinsonism, *Nature*, 311, 464, 1984.

77. **Langston, J. W., Ballard, P., Tetrud, J. W., and Irwin, I.,** Chronic Parkinsonism in humans due to a product of meperidine-analog synthesis, *Science,* 219, 979, 1983.

78. **Spina, M. B. and Cohen, G.,** Dopamine turnover and glutathione oxidation: implications for Parkinson's disease, *Proc. Natl. Acad. Sci. U.S.A.,* 86, 1398, 1989.

79. **Tatton, W. G., Greenwood, G. E., Salo, P. T., and Seniuk, N. A.,** Transmitter synthesis increases in substantia nigra neurons of aged mouse, *Neurosci. Lett.,* 131, 179, 1991.

80. **Adams, J. D. and Odunze, I. N.,** Oxygen free radicals and Parkinson's disease, *Free Radical Biol. Aging,* 10, 161, 1991.

81. **Dexter, D., Carter, C., Agid, Y., Lees, A. J., Jenner, P., and Marsden, C. D.,** Lipid peroxidation as cause of nigral cell death in Parkinson's disease, *Lancet,* 2, 639, 1986.

82. **Marttila, R. J., Lorentz, H., and Rinne, U. K.,** Oxygen toxicity protecting enzymes in Parkinson's disease, *J. Neurol. Sci.,* 86, 321, 1988.

83. **Gotz, M. E., Freyberger, A., and Riederer, P.,** Oxidative stress: a role in the pathogenesis of Parkinson's disease, *J. Neural Transm. Suppl.,* 29, 241, 1990.

84. **Olanow, C. W.,** Oxidation reactions in Parkinson's disease, *Neurology,* 40, 32, 1990.

85. **Youdim, M. B., Ben-Shachar, D., and Riederer, P.,** The role of monoamine oxidase, iron-melanin interaction, and intracellular calcium in Parkinson's disease, *J. Neural Transm. Suppl.,* 32, 239, 1990.

86. **Kilinc, A., Yalcin, A. S., Yalcin, D., Taga, Y., and Emerk, K.,** Increased erythrocyte susceptibility to lipid peroxidation in human Parkinson's disease, *Neurosci. Lett.,* 87, 307, 1988.

87. **Dexter, D. T., Carter, C. J., Wells, F. R., Javoy-Agid, F., Agid, Y., Lees, A., Jenner, P., and Marsden, C. D.,** Basal lipid peroxidation in substantia nigra is increased in Parkinson's disease, *J. Neurochem.,* 52, 381, 1989.

88. **Sofic, E., Paulus, W., Jellinger, K., Riederer, P., and Youdim, M. B.,** Selective increase of iron in substantia nigra zona compacta of Parkinsonian brains, *J. Neurochem.,* 56, 978, 1991.

89. **Ben-Shachar, D. and Youdim, M. B.,** Selectivity of melanized nigra-striatal dopamine neurons to degeneration in Parkinson's disease may depend on iron-melanin interaction, *J. Neural Transm. Suppl.,* 29, 251, 1990.

90. **Mash, D. C., Pablo, J., Buck, B. E., Sanchez-Ramos, J., and Weiner, W. J.,** Distribution and number of transferrin receptors in Parkinson's disease and in MPTP-treated mice, *Exp. Neurol.,* 114, 73, 1991.

91. **Jenner, P.,** Oxidative stress as a cause of Parkinson's disease, *Acta Neurol. Scand. Suppl.,* 136, 6, 1991.

92. **Shoffner, J. M., Watts, R. L., Juncos, J. L., Torroni, A., and Wallace, D. C.,** Mitochondrial oxidative phosphorylation defects in Parkinson's disease, *Ann. Neurol.,* 30, 332, 1991.

93. **Davis, G. C., Williams, A. C., Markey, S. P., Ebert, M. H., Caine, E. D., Reichert, C. M., and Kopin, I. J.,** Chronic parkinsonism secondary to intravenous injection of meperidine analogues, *Psychiat. Res.,* 1, 249, 1979.

94. **Javitch, J. A. and Snyder, S. H.,** Utake of MPP (+) by dopamine neurons explains selectivity of parkinsonism-inducing neurotoxin, MPTP, *Eur. J. Pharmacol.,* 106, 455, 1985.

95. **Heikkila, R. E., Nicklas, W. J., Vyas, I., and Duvoisin, R. C.,** Dopaminergic toxicity of rotenone and the 1-methyl-4-phenylpyridinium ion after their stereotaxic administration to rats: implication for the mechanism of 1-methyl-4-phenyl-1,2,3,6-tetrahydropyridine toxicity, *Neurosci. Lett.,* 62, 389, 1985.

96. **Saitoh, T., Niijima, K., and Mizuno, Y.,** Long-term effect of 1-methyl-4-phenyl-1,2,3,6-tetrahydropyridine (MPTP) on striatal dopamine content in young and mature mice, *J. Neurol. Sci.,* 77, 229, 1987.

97. **Ramsay, R. R., Mehlhorn, R. J., and Singer, T. P.**, Enhancement by tetraphenylboron of the interaction of the 1-methyl-4-phenylpyridinium ion (MPP+) with mitochondria, *Biochem. Biophys. Res. Commun.*, 159, 983, 1989.

98. **Hollinden, G. E., Sanchez-Ramos, J. R., Sick, T. J., and Rosenthal, M.**, Mpp+-induced increases in extracellular potassium ion activity in rat striatal slices suggest that consequences of MPP+ neurotoxicity are spread beyond dopaminergic terminals, *Brain Res.*, 475, 283, 1988.

99. **Kopin, I. J.**, MPTP: an industrial chemical and contaminant of illicit narcotics stimulates a new era of research on Parkinson's disease, *Environ. Health Perspect.*, 75, 45, 1987.

100. **Pinsky, C. and Bose, R.**, Pyridine and other coal tar constituents as free-radical generating environmental neurotoxicants, *Mol. Cell. Biochem.*, 84, 217, 1988.

101. **Suzuki, K., Mizuno, Y., and Yoshida, M.**, Inhibition of mitochondrial NADH-ubiquinone oxidoreductase activity and ATP synthesis by tetrahydroisoquinoline, *Neurosci. Lett.*, 86, 105, 1988.

102. **Sayre, L. M., Wang, F. J., Arora, P. K., Riachi, N. J., Harik, S. I., and Hoppel, C. L.**, Dopaminergic neurotoxicity *in vivo* and inhibition of mitochondrial respiration *in vitro* by possible pyridinium-like substances, *J. Neurochem.*, 57, 2106, 1991.

103. **Suzuki, K., Mizuno, Y., and Yoshida, M.**, Effects of 1-methyl-4-phenyl-1,2,3,6-tetrahydropyridine (MPTP)-like compounds on mitochondrial respiration, *Adv. Neurol.*, 53, 215, 1990.

104. **Suzuki, K., Mizuno, Y., and Yoshida, M.**, Inhibition of mitochondrial respiration by 1-methyl-4-phenyl-1,2,3,6-tetrahydropyridine-like endogenous alkaloids in mouse brain, *Neurochem. Res.*, 15, 705, 1990.

105. **LeWitt, P. A.**, Deprenyl's effect at slowing progression of parkinsonian disability: the DATATOP study, *Acta Neurolog. Scand. Suppl.*, 136, 79, 1991.

106. **Tipton, K. F., Houslay, M. D., and Turner, A. J.**, Metabolism of aldehydes in brain, in *Essays in Neurochemistry and Neuropharmacology*, Youdim, M. B. H., Lovenberg, W. D., Sharman, F., and Lagdo, J. R., Eds., John Wiley & Sons, New York, 1977, 103.

107. **Schsuenstein, E., Esterbauer, H., and Zollner, H.**, *Aldehydes in Biological Systems*, Lagnado, J. R., Ed., Pion Limited, London, 1977, 1.

108. **Lieber, C. S.**, Biochemical and molecular basis of alcohol-induced injury to liver and other tissues, *N. Engl. J. Med.*, 319, 1639, 1988.

109. **Dianazani, M. U.**, Biochemical effects of saturated and unsaturated aldehydes, in *Free Radicals, Lipid Peroxidation and Cancer*, McBrien, D. C. H. and Slater, T. F., Eds., Academic Press, New York, 1982, 129.

110. **Sodum, S. S. and Chung, F. L.**, Sterioselective formation of *in vitro* nucleic acid adducts by 2,3-epoxy-4-hydroxy nonal, *Cancer Res.*, 51, 137, 1991.

111. **Miglietta, M., Olivero, A., Gadoni, E., and Gabriel, L.**, Effects of some aldehydes on brain microtubular protein, *Chem. Biol. Interact.*, 78, 183, 1991.

112. **Msacchio, J. N.**, Enzymes involved in the biosynthesis and degradation of catecholamines, in *Handbook of Psychopharmacology*, Vol. 3, Iversen, L. L., Iversen, S. D., and Snyder, S. H., Eds., Plenum Press, New York, 1975, 1.

113. **Ogorochi, T., Narumiya, S., Mizuno, N., Yamashita, K., Miyazaki, H., and Hayaishi, O.**, Regional distribution of prostaglandins D2, E2, and F2 and related enzymes in postmortem human brain, *J. Neurochem.*, 43, 71, 1984.

114. **Anggard, E.**, Essential fatty acids, prostaglandins and the brain in Alzhemier's disease: a report of progress, in *Research Aging*, Vol. 19, Gorkin, S., Davis, K. L., Growdon, J. H., and Usdin, E., Eds., Raven Press, New York, 1982, 295.

115. **Mattammal, M. B., Lakshmi, V. M., Zenser, T. V., and Davis, B. B.**, Metabolism of aromatic and heterocyclic amine bladder carcinogens, *J. Pharm. Biomed. Anal.*, 8, 151, 1990.

116. **Kalayanaraman, B., Felix, C. C., and Sealy, R. C.,** Peroxidatic oxidation of catecholamines: a kinetic electron spin resonance investigation using the spin stabilization, *J. Biol. Chem.,* 259, 7584, 1984.
117. **Nakatani, H. and Dunford, H. B.,** Binding of indole to horseradish peroxidase, *Arch. Biochem. Biophys.,* 204, 413, 1980.
118. **Smith, B. J., Curtis, J. F., and Eling, T. E.,** Bioactivation of xenobiotics by prostaglandin H synthase, *Chem. Biol. Interact.,* 79, 245, 1991.
119. **Josephy, P. D., Eling, T. E., and Mason, R. P.,** Cooxidation of benzidine by prostaglandin synthase: comparison with the action of horseradish peroxidase, *J. Biol. Chem.,* 258, 5561, 1983.

Chapter 11

OXYGEN RADICALS AND CANCER

Terry D. Oberley and Larry W. Oberley

TABLE OF CONTENTS

0-8493-4518-9/93/$0.00 + $.50

I. INTRODUCTION

A. GENERAL

Reactive oxygen species (ROS) are formed as incomplete reduction products of molecular oxygen during aerobic cellular metabolism. The relationship between ROS and cancer has been the subject of much speculation and controversy. Because the possible role(s) of ROS in radiation and chemical carcinogenesis has been reviewed frequently, the present chapter will focus primarily on a model of hormone-induced cancer, the estrogen-induced renal cancer in the Syrian hamster. We chose this model both because of our familiarity with it and because recent results using this model suggest an important role for ROS in hormone-induced neoplasia, a concept only recently developed. Studies of this system allow us to postulate a generalized model of cancer, whether the etiologic agent be radiation or a chemical, virus, or hormone.

B. OXYGEN RADICALS AND ANTIOXIDANT ENZYMES

Reactive oxygen species, which include superoxide anion radical (O_2^-), hydroxyl radical ($\cdot OH$), hydrogen peroxide (H_2O_2), organic peroxide radicals ($ROO\cdot$), and singlet molecular oxygen ($^1O_2$), are constantly generated intracellularly in aerobic organisms[1-12] and released extracellularly during the respiratory burst of phagocytes.[2] They are thought to be the major mediators of oxygen cytotoxicity.[4-6] The discovery of an intracellular system that detoxifies ROS in aerobic cells suggested that an oxidant-antioxidant equilibrium exists in these cells.[7,8] Major constituents of the antioxidant system include: (1) certain enzyme systems (superoxide dismutase-catalase-peroxidase and glutathione peroxidase-glutathione reductase-glucose-6-phosphate dehydrogenase), (2) certain vitamins (E, C, and A), (3) low-molecular-weight reducing agents (glutathione and other thiols), and (4) polyunsaturated fatty acids.[7-11]

The primary antioxidant enzyme (AE) system consists of three enzymes: (1) the superoxide dismutases (SOD), (2) catalases (CAT), and (3) peroxidases, of which glutathione peroxidase is the most common in mammalian cells. Each of these occurs in several forms and is highly compartmentalized. For instance, a copper- and zinc-containing superoxide dismutase (CuZnSOD) is found in the cytoplasm, whereas a manganese-containing superoxide dismutase (MnSOD) is found primarily in mitochondria. Glutathione peroxidase has at least two distinct isozymes: one found in the cytosol and the other in mitochondria. There are also several forms of catalase, the predominant one being found in peroxisomes.

The basic function of these enzymes is to convert superoxide radical (O_2^-) produced during metabolism into water, as shown in the following scheme:

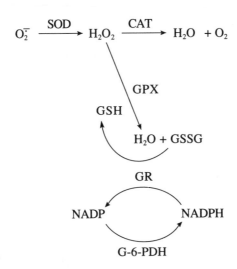

where GSH is reduced glutathione, GSSG is oxidized glutathione, GR is glutathione reductase, G-6-PDH is glucose-6-phosphate dehydrogenase, GPX is glutathione peroxidase, and NADP and NADPH are oxidized and reduced nicotinamide adenine dinucleotide phosphate, respectively.

Removal of H_2O_2 and O_2^- from biological systems prevents the iron-catalyzed Haber-Weiss reaction from occurring:

$$O_2^- + Fe^{3+} \rightarrow O_2 + Fe^{2+}$$

$$H_2O_2 + Fe^{2+} \rightarrow \cdot OH + OH^- + Fe^{3+}$$

$$O_2^- + H_2O_2 \xrightarrow{Fe^{2+}} \cdot OH + OH^- + O_2$$

Any of the active oxygen species can be damaging or lethal to cells under certain circumstances. However, $\cdot OH$ is by far the most reactive, and most damage in biological systems is probably due to its formation. Thus, the AE system is important in preventing $\cdot OH$ formation.

C. OXYGEN RADICALS, ANTIOXIDANT ENZYMES, AND MALIGNANCY

We reviewed this area in 1986.[13] In general, at least one antioxidant enzyme is lower in tumor cells than in their normal cell counterparts. It is not clear whether the lack of AE is a cause or an effect of cancer. Nor is the role of oxygen radicals in cancer completely understood, although it is known that oxygen radicals are mutagenic[14-16] and may contribute to the carcinogenic process.[17,18]

In experimental animals, the known causes of cancer include radiation, chemicals, hormones, and viruses. Radiation directly generates ROS in biological systems, and these ROS are thought to cause cancer by directly or indirectly altering DNA.[19]

Although ROS are thought to be involved in many models of chemical carcinogenesis, we shall restrict our introductory discussion to experimental models of skin cancer in mice. Papillomas can be induced in SENCAR mice by topical application of a single nontumorigenic dose of carcinogen (initiation), followed by repetitive treatments with the noncarcinogenic tumor promoter *12-O-tetradecanoylphorbol-13-acetate* (TPA). With time, some of the papillomas arising from this protocol progress to squamous cell carcinomas, irrespective of continuing TPA treatment. The following lines of evidence suggest a role for ROS in this model of chemical carcinogenesis:

1. The rate of progression and the percentage of papillomas that progress to squamous cell carcinomas can be enhanced by treating the papillomas with oxidants.[20]
2. Long-term treatment of initiated skin with 5 or 10% solutions of hydrogen peroxide weakly promotes papilloma development.[21]
3. Topical application of the SOD biomimetic CuII [3,5-diisopropylsalicylate]$_2$ inhibits TPA-dependent promotion.[22]
4. Topical or intraperitoneal administration of several agents that possess antioxidant activity or are capable of enhancing the cellular antioxidant system also inhibit TPA-dependent promotion.[23-26]
5. ROS-generating systems mimic several of the effects of TPA in a variety of *in vitro* cellular systems.[27-29]
6. ROS levels are elevated in epidermal cells prepared from TPA-treated mice.[30]
7. SOD and CAT activities are reduced in TPA-treated skin, while xanthine oxidase (XO) activities are increased.[31] Similarly, SOD and CAT activities are decreased in papillomas and squamous cell carcinomas, while XO activity is increased.

The finding of lowered AE activity in the presence of oxygen free radicals suggests that a prooxidant state exists during development of neoplasia.[32]

D. CANCER AS A DEFECT IN DIFFERENTIATION

It is generally accepted that cancerous growth depends on derangements of cell differentiation.[33] At least three pathways to a tumor could be (1) stem cells fail to produce one nonstem cell daughter in each division, thereby proliferating to form a tumor; (2) daughter cells fail to differentiate normally; or (3) cells die at a slower rate than normal. Whether tumors arise from stem cells or from differentiated cells is hotly debated. However, evidence from chemical carcinogenesis suggests that, while both origins are possible, most tumors arise from stem cells.[34] Recently, it has become evident that cancer may also arise by inhibition of apoptosis or programmed cell death.[35]

E. HORMONES AND CANCER

It is well established that chemical carcinogens, usually after their intracellular metabolism, modify nuclear DNA and thus produce mutations. However, the concept of hormones altering DNA has not been widely accepted. Instead, two major mechanisms have been proposed for hormone-induced malignant neoplasia.[36] One hypothesis states that hormones cause cancer by increasing cell proliferation in a target organ. Since DNA repair is not 100% efficient, this increases the chance of mutation, and hence, of cancer. The second hypothesis deals specifically with human vaginal neoplasia induced by the synthetic estrogen diethylstilbestrol (DES).[37] Daughters whose mothers were treated with DES during pregnancy may develop vaginal cancer. Pathologic studies demonstrated that DES causes retention of columnar estrogen-responsive epithelium in the vagina. Normally, this epithelium is converted to nonestrogen-responsive squamous epithelium during development. In the case of DES-induced cancer, the release of estrogens at puberty causes the estrogen-responsive columnar epithelium to proliferate and form cancer.[38,39]

In neither of these hypotheses are hormones postulated to cause DNA alterations or mutations. The question of hormone interaction with DNA is now being re-evaluated (see below).

II. ESTROGEN-INDUCED KIDNEY CANCER IN THE SYRIAN HAMSTER

A. GENERAL

For more than 30 years, natural (steroid) and synthetic (stilbene) estrogens have been known to be potent carcinogens in the Syrian golden hamster.[40] Malignant renal neoplasms develop after long-term hormonal treatment.[41-43] The mechanism by which estrogens cause cancer in this model is the subject of intense investigation. It seems most likely that both the hormonal properties of estrogens and their intracellular metabolites are involved. The renal cortex of the hamster is a bona fide estrogen-sensitive target,[44-47] as was ascertained by the presence of a specific estrogen receptor, its increase after prolonged estrogen stimulation, and a 13-fold increase in progesterone receptors after estrogen treatment. While it has been suggested that the hormonal property of estrogens is essential in causing *in vivo* neoplastic transformation of the hamster renal cortex, other studies suggest an important role for estrogen metabolites in DES-induced carcinogenesis.[47-48]

B. MORPHOLOGY

Morphological and immunohistochemical studies were performed in our laboratory to characterize DES-induced renal tumors.[49] The neoplasms were composed of two distinct cell populations: a large-cell component that appeared highly epithelial (i.e., possessing cell polarity) and a poorly differentiated small-cell component. Both cell types contained desmosomes at their surfaces, an epithelial characteristic. However, only the large-cell component possessed additional epithelial features (microvilli, intracytoplasmic lumens, and cilia). One explanation for this may be that the distinctly epithelial large-cell component is derived from the small-cell component by cell differentiation. Comparative studies of renal tumors and developing normal renal tissue from fetal and newborn hamsters revealed remarkable histological similarities. The earliest tumor foci were found after 4.5 months of treatment with DES. They occurred consistently in the kidney interstitium (the area between tubules) in proximity to large arteries. Estrogen-induced renal tumor cells showed immunostaining with antibodies to keratin; vimentin; and desmin, markers of epithelial; mesenchymal; and smooth muscle cells, respectively. Kidney differentiation is unusual in that mesenchymal tissue (metanephric mesenchyme) is converted to epithelium after induction by the ureteric bud. Therefore, developing kidney shows morphologic and biochemical features of both mesenchyme and epithelium. Based on the tumors' morphological resemblance to embryonic kidney cells and the presence of epithelial and mesenchymal intermediate filaments, **our findings provide strong evidence that the cell of origin of this malignant tumor is a precursor cell (presumably mesenchymal) that is committed to a tubular epithelial differentiation pathway.**

C. ANALYSIS OF EARLY LESIONS

Although most investigators would accept the concept that cancer arises from a single cell (i.e., is clonal), precisely which cell is the subject of considerable controversy. While some investigators feel that cancer arises from differentiated cells that subsequently dedifferentiate, others feel that cancer arises in stem cells. While the latter concept is easy to accept in an organ such as bone marrow in which cells are constantly renewed, in an adult parenchymal organ such as the liver, cells rarely divide, and many investigators do not accept the notion of a stem cell being present. However, recent studies using a variety of antibodies, tissue culture, and molecular probe techniques all suggest the presence of relatively primitive precursor cells in the adult liver.[50-52]

The issue of the cell of origin of neoplasia is of paramount importance in understanding the process of carcinogenesis. Most studies of mechanisms of carcinogenesis involve studies of whole organ or tissue homogenates. The parameters measured thus reflect the carcinogenic process only if the tissue is comprised largely of cells with the potential to become cancerous. On the other hand, if the cell of origin represents a minority population, these measurements may not reflect processes in the carcinogenic mechanism at all.

With this principle in mind, we felt it was important to try to identify the cell of origin of the estrogen-induced kidney tumor in the hamster. To do this, we studied early lesions induced by estrogens.[53]

Syrian hamsters were treated with DES, a potent estrogen and carcinogen, or with ethinyl estradiol (EE), a strong estrogen but weak carcinogen, for one to nine months. At monthly intervals, their kidneys were studied using light, immunoperoxidase, and electron microscopic techniques. At 5 months, DES-treated animals showed interstitial (between tubules) lesions composed of clusters of small round cells with a high nuclear-cytoplasmic ratio (Figure 1); normally the renal interstitium is populated by a sparse number of elongated fibroblast-like (spindle) cells. Immunoperoxidase and ultrastructural studies showed these cells to be identical to cells in fully formed tumors at nine months. Early lesions in EE-treated animals (as early as 1 month) were very different. In the deep cortex adjacent to the renal pelvis, proximal tubules underwent hyperplastic changes (increases in cell number per unit area), showing columnar cells with large nuclei, occasional mitoses, and sloughing of apical cytoplasm (Figure 1). These cells did not resemble the fully developed tumor in either immunoperoxidase or ultrastructural features. With longer treatment, the lesions progressed to dysplasia (3 to 5 months) and carcinoma *in situ* (7 months). However, EE-induced lesions did not form grossly visible tumors during the 9-month study, suggesting that the EE-induced hyperplastic lesion was not the precursor of the renal tumor. Both early lesions were specific, since controls and hamsters treated with β-dienestrol or 17α-estradiol (noncarcinogenic estrogens) did not show them. Animals given a combination of DES and EE showed tubular hyperplasia, but not interstitial lesions. This finding was of particular interest because hamsters given this combination of estrogens do not develop gross tumors; thus, EE was able to block both DES-induced interstitial foci and tumor formation. Neither interstitial foci nor tubular hyperplastic lesions stained with antibodies to MnSOD. Since recent studies in our laboratory suggested that MnSOD is a marker of terminal differentiation, we interpreted these findings to mean that both early lesions are composed of precursor cells (see Section III.B). Immunoperoxidase studies using antibodies to proliferating cell nuclear antigen (anti-PCNA, anticyclin) demonstrated immunostaining of a large number of cells in interstitial lesions and fully developed tumors, but only occasional immunostaining of nuclei of cells in tubular hyperplastic lesions. Since only the interstitial cell stained like the tumor, this cell is strongly implicated as the cell of origin of the DES-induced neoplasm.

These studies reveal the complexity of cellular events in the kidney, and underscore the difficulty of interpreting biochemical studies using homogenates containing multiple cell types, when kidney cell populations are constantly changing and the DES-induced tumor originates from a minority cell type.

D. EFFECT OF ESTROGENS ON KIDNEY CELL PROLIFERATION *IN VITRO*

Since light microscopy demonstrated estrogen effects on proximal tubules *in vivo*, i.e., hyperplasia, we decided to study the effects of estrogens on proximal tubules in culture.[54] Renal tubular cells were grown on a PF-HR-9 basement membrane in chemically defined medium. Cells in explant outgrowths exhibited ultrastructural features typical of proximal tubules,

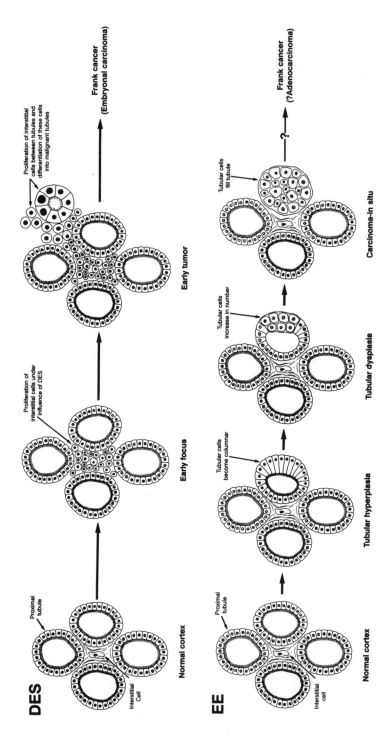

FIGURE 1. Morphological events in development of early lesions. Animals treated with DES develop early lesions in the renal interstitium, while animals treated with EE develop intratubular lesions. (From Oberley, T. D., Gonzalez, A., Lauchner, L. J., Oberley, L. W., and Li, J. J., *Cancer Res.*, 51, 1922, 1991. With permission.)

including junctional complexes, numerous mitochondria, peroxisomes, and microvilli. After 7 to 14 d in culture, cell number had increased threefold in the presence of 17β-estradiol or DES. Maximal proliferative response occurred at hormone concentrations of 0.6 to 1.0 nM. A similar threefold increase in cell number was seen with 1 nM 17β-estradiol in subcultures of **dissociated** tubular cells (proximal tubules were disrupted by EDTA to form single cells). Neither progesterone, 5α-dihydrotestosterone, nor the inactive DES metabolite β-dienestrol elicited this mitogenic effect. Concomitant exposure of cultures to a threefold molar excess of the antiestrogen tamoxifen completely prevented the increase in cell number seen with 17β-estradiol. The proliferative effect of estrogens on proximal tubular cells was species-specific: 17β-estradiol did not alter the growth of either rat or guinea pig proximal tubules in culture. In addition, after 7 to 10 d in culture in the presence of 17β-estradiol, [³H]thymidine labeling of hamster tubular cells was enhanced threefold. A similar increase in mitoses occurred in cultures containing these potent estrogens during the same interval of exposure.

These results indicated that estrogens at physiologic concentrations can directly induce proliferation of primary epithelial cells. However, autoradiographic studies after labeling with [³H]thymidine showed the situation to be more complex than that. While label did appear in cultured proximal tubular cells, significant label was observed in interstitial cells attached to the outside of the tubular basement membranes of the isolated proximal tubules.[101] Therefore, it seems that both the proximal tubule and the interstitial cell undergo cell division in response to estrogens. Administration of bromodeoxyuridine (BrdU) to hamsters that had been treated with estrogens for 5 to 9 months allowed *in vivo* analysis of cell proliferation. Very little anti-BrdU immunostaining was observed in proximal tubules, but strong immunostaining was observed in interstitial early lesions.[101] Therefore, it is possible that estrogens cause proliferation of both the tubular cell and interstitial cell, but much more proliferation occurs in the latter case.

E. OXYGEN RADICALS ALSO CAUSE CELL PROLIFERATION *IN VITRO*

Recent studies have demonstrated a direct effect of oxygen radicals on cell proliferation *in vitro*.[55-61] To test whether ROS affect proliferation of tubular cells, we studied the effects of liposome-packaged antioxidant enzymes on DES-induced cell proliferation.[62] DES initiated proliferation of Syrian hamster renal proximal tubular cells. By counting the number of cells in culture, we showed that liposomes containing CuZnSOD or CAT suppressed DES-induced proliferation, whereas empty liposomes or liposomes containing inactivated SOD did not. Liposomes containing AE did not suppress proliferation of cells in control media or of cells treated with ethinyl estradiol. In the absence of liposomes, exogenous SOD did not suppress DES-induced proliferation. The decrease in cell number when DES-treated cells were treated with AE-containing liposomes was not due to decreased cell viability. Results were confirmed by measuring a correlate of cell proliferation immunohistochemically using an antibody to proliferating cell nuclear antigen, a marker of cell proliferation. A larger proportion of DES-treated cells than of control cells showed nuclear immunostaining with this antibody. The number of cells immunostained in DES-treated cultures was sharply decreased by the addition of SOD- or CAT-containing liposomes. These studies suggest a prominent role for active oxygen species in DES-induced proliferation of cultured kidney cells.

F. METABOLISM OF ESTROGENS

DES is metabolically oxidized to DES-4′,4″quinone (DES Q)[63] by cytochrome P450 and is extremely reactive chemically. It binds to small peptides,[63] cellular proteins,[64] and DNA.[65] Roy and Liehr[66] found DES Q in tissues of hamsters given DES for a prolonged period. Because DES Q was found in organs other than kidney — in which DES does not induce cancer — these authors conclude that oxidation of DES to DES Q and the genotoxicity of DES Q may be necessary, but not sufficient, for tumor development. They hypothesized that hormone-dependent growth of initiated cells may also be necessary for the occurrence of cancer.[66]

Of particular interest in relation to the role of oxygen radicals is recent work on the metabolism of DES. Redox cycling occurs between DES and DES Q, catalyzed by microsomal drug-metabolizing enzymes.[66,67] Such redox cycling generates free radicals[68] that have been postulated to damage DNA or other cellular macromolecules.[69,70] Recently, it was directly demonstrated that peroxidative metabolism of DES induces formation of 8-hydroxy-2′-deoxyguanosine,[71] a marker of oxidative DNA damage.

G. EVIDENCE FOR A PROOXIDANT STATE

Antioxidant enzyme activities were determined in Syrian hamster kidney tumors and kidney cortex from immature and adult estrogenized and untreated male hamsters.[72] SOD (both CuZn and Mn forms) and CAT activities were significantly lower in primary tumors than in renal cortex from untreated and DES-treated male hamsters. Primary tumors were serially passaged in the ascites form in DES-treated castrated hamsters. CAT, CuZnSOD, and MnSOD were lower in passaged autonomous (hormone-independent) renal tumors than in primary tumors. Quantitative Western blot analysis of immunoreactive protein(s) confirmed that MnSOD, CuZnSOD, and CAT levels were lower in both primary tumors and passaged autonomous tumors than in normal adult renal cortex. Similar levels of antioxidant enzymes were found in tumor and newborn kidney, and these values were much lower than those in normal adult kidney cortex or isolated proximal tubules. These results suggest that the lack of SOD and CAT may serve as a marker for hormonally induced renal neoplasia in this species, and immunoperoxidase studies confirmed this hypothesis by demonstrating that **the earliest neoplastic lesions observed (4.5 months) had no detectable immunostaining with antibodies to**

CuZnSOD, MnSOD, or CAT. The absence of AE suggested the presence of a prooxidant state in both early lesions and tumor cells.

Roy and Liehr[73] recently demonstrated increases in glutathione, activity of glutathione peroxidase, and products of lipid peroxidation in kidneys of hamsters given prolonged estrogen treatment. **These authors concluded that such estrogen treatment results in "elevated levels of oxidative stress."**

Additional evidence of oxidative stress was recently demonstrated in a study of oxidative damage to proteins in hormone-treated animals.[74] Oxidative damage to proteins occurs via conversion of side-chain amino groups to carbonyl derivatives. Such damage to enzymes and purified proteins has been quantified previously by reduction with tritium-labeled sodium boro[^{3}H]hydride (NaB^{3}H$_4$) and subsequent measurement of the incorporation of ^{3}H into amino acid fractions. In this study, the NaB^{3}H$_4$ reduction assay was modified to permit the quantitation of free radical-mediated oxidative damage to proteins obtained from animals. Modifications included additional extractions of protein isolates with organic solvents to remove lipids and with nitric acid to remove metal ions. The modified assay was first validated *in vitro* by measuring changes in levels of oxidative damage to bovine serum albumin (BSA) exposed to xanthine plus xanthine oxidase (2-fold increase), hydrogen peroxide and iron (II) sulfate (5-fold increase), or γ radiation (30-fold increase over controls). γ Radiation of isolated hamster kidney protein also raised the carbonyl content in a dose-dependent manner.

The modified assay was validated *in vivo* by measuring the changes in oxidative damage to lung tissue in animals exposed to approximately 85% oxygen (twofold increase) or paraquat (fivefold increase over controls). The assay was then used to examine free radical-mediated oxidation introduced by acute or long-term treatment of hamsters with estrogens. Oxidative damage to kidney proteins was assayed in hamsters treated with estradiol implants for up to seven months, a regimen known to induce kidney tumors. Significant increases in covalent oxidative modification to renal proteins over values in age-matched controls (up to fivefold increase over controls) were detected after 1, 2, and 7 months of continuous estradiol exposure.

A final piece of evidence that suggests a prooxidant state in this model of carcinogenesis was inhibition of tumor formation by vitamin C.[75] Vitamin C decreased the tumor incidence by approximately 50%, but did not influence hormone-dependent growth of kidney tumors. Moreover, vitamin C lowered the concentration of DES Q, the genotoxic metabolite of DES *in vitro*, and in Syrian hamsters treated with DES *in vivo*. Vitamin C also decreased the levels of DES-DNA adducts formed by the quinone metabolite in hamsters. The authors concluded that estrogens may thus initiate tumors by their metabolic oxidation to quinones, which bind covalently to cellular macromolecules. Vitamin C may inhibit tumorigenesis by decreasing concentrations of quinone metabolites and their DNA adducts. Lowering the quinone metabolite concentrations may also inhibit free radical generation by decreasing redox cycling between estrogens and their corresponding quinones.

H. EVIDENCE FOR DNA ALTERATIONS

Liehr[76] has suggested that DNA alterations occur via the following mechanisms: (1) Steroid estrogens are metabolized by estrogen 2- and 4-hydroxylases to catecholestrogens. (2) The catecholestrogens or DES are oxidized to semiquinones and quinones by the peroxidative activity of cytochrome P450. (3) The quinones may be reduced to catecholestrogens and DES, and redox cycling may ensue. Redox cycling of estrogens generates free radicals which may react to form the organic hydroperoxides needed as cofactors for oxidation to quinones. (4) DES Q and the quinone metabolites of catechol estrogens bind covalently to DNA *in vitro,* whereas DNA binding *in vivo* has only been examined for DES. When DES is administered to hamsters, the resulting DES-DNA adduct profile in liver, kidney, or other organs closely matches that of DES Q-DNA adducts *in vitro. In vitro,* DES-DNA adducts are chemically unstable and are generated in incubations with organic hydroperoxide as cofactor. It is proposed that the instability of adducts and the lower sensitivity of previous assay methods contributed to previously reported failures to detect adducts. (5) Tumors are postulated to arise in cells that are rapidly proliferating due to the growth stimulus provided by estrogens. The covalent modification of DNA in these cells is temporary because of the chemical instability of adducts and will result in altered genetic messages only in proliferating daughter cells, whereas in nonproliferating cells there will be no lasting genetic damage.

Roy et al.[77] recently detected oxidative damage to DNA. The reaction of guanine bases of DNA with hydroxyl radicals to form 8-hydroxydeoxyguanosine was used to monitor free radical generation in the kidney and liver of Syrian hamsters. In the kidney, but not the liver, DNA of hamsters treated with DES implants for 15 days, 8-hydroxydeoxyguanosine levels more than doubled from control values. This finding was of interest, since hamsters develop kidney, but not liver, tumors in response to long-term administration of DES. It was concluded that *in vitro* and *in vivo* redox cycling of DES caused hydroxylation of guanine bases in DNA.

I. ROLE OF ANEUPLOIDY

DES can directly induce morphologic transformation of Syrian hamster embryonic fibroblasts in culture.[78,79] This property appears to be distinct from the estrogenic ability of DES because cell transformation in culture occurs in the absence of any measurable induction of cell proliferation, and the ability of DES and related analogs to transform cells in culture does not correlate with the reported estrogenic potency of the compounds *in vivo.*[79] DES can induce transformation in the absence of measurable gene mutation.[78]

DES causes aneuploidy (possessing a chromosome number other than an exact multiple of the haploid number) in many cell systems,[80-83] possibly due to its effects on microtubules.[84-88] It has been proposed that the resulting

II. ROLE OF ANTIOXIDANT ENZYMES IN CELL DIFFERENTIATION

ITRO

and Balin[94] have proposed that oxidant stress causes cell differ-
A corollary of this hypothesis is that since MnSOD and CAT are
by their substrates (reactive oxygen species), these enzymes should
during cell differentiation. We studied SOD levels in the X-REF-23
onic fibroblast cell line.[95] X-REF-23 is an immortal cell line that
a nontransformed phenotype throughout its known life-span. Low-
-REF-23 cells undergo spontaneous differentiation into muscle and
ells, whereas high-passage X-REF-23 cells undergo little or no
ation. SOD activities were measured in subclones of X-REF-23,
ferentiate into muscle (AMC subclone) or adipose (AMB-J) cells,
the parental nondifferentiating high-passage X-REF-23 cells. Total
vity increased with time in culture in all three cell lines. CuZnSOD
ced in AMB-J and X-REF-23 cells with time in culture, whereas
ls showed no induction. MnSOD activity was induced during the
n differentiation occurred in the two differentiating clones. In con-
SOD was not induced in the nondifferentiating X-REF-23 cell line
s time. Levels of immunoreactive MnSOD correlated quite well
OD activity in all three cell lines. The nondifferentiating X-REF-
howed a large increase in cell organelles with time in culture, but
ifferentiating cell lines did not. In particular, an increase in very
ochondria was observed. These mitochondria often showed evidence
nization. **These observations are consistent with our hypothesis
of Allen and Balin[94] that oxidant stress, in this case presumably
by culture conditions, can stimulate cell differentiation; MnSOD,
ucible by its substrate, is thus induced during differentiation.**
cannot induce MnSOD during oxidant stress show sublethal damage,
ly to mitochondria. This has led us to hypothesize that, in these
uction of MnSOD is a necessary, but not sufficient, condition for
ation. Beckman et al.[96] demonstrated that liposomes containing SOD
ferentiation of Friend erythroleukemia cells. However, differentia-
lue to H_2O_2 production by SOD, since low-molecular-weight oxi-
induced differentiation. Thus, normal, immortal, and malignant
ow a relationship between oxidant stress, antioxidant enzymes, and
entiation.

VO

es from adult Syrian hamsters were studied with immunoperoxidase
using polyclonal antibodies to antioxidant enzymes (CuZnSOD,
CAT).[97] Tissues from labile organs, in which cell renewal is prom-
sitional epithelium of the genitourinary tract, uterus, intestine) showed
ioxidant enzyme immunostaining in differentiated cells, but not in

chromosome nondisjunction is important in
DES.[81,82] Treatment of Syrian hamster em
aneuploid cells with a near-diploid chromoso
lated that numerical chromosome changes are
transformation.[82] In fact, a recent study pro
chromosome changes (trisomy 11 and/or 19)
escape from cellular senescence (immortali
embryo cells.[89] However, additional structu
curred during acquisition of tumorigenicity,[89]
of neoplastic progression suggested for these

The major criticisms of these studies we
culture, not *in vivo,* and (2) embryonic fibro
of cancer in animals. To circumvent these diff
of DES-induced hamster kidney tumors.[92] Th
karyotypic changes, including loss of specific
translocations. Therefore, there is a strong
chromosome changes *in vivo.*

J. ROLE OF CELL DEATH

Although both estrogens and oxygen radi
by affecting cell proliferation, estrogens als
cell death (apoptosis).[93] The role of cell de
growth and regression was studied by Burs
dependent, transplantable kidney tumor cell l
line was originally derived from an estroge
tumor. When H301 cells were injected subcu
Syrian hamsters, they developed into solid
3 weeks. Upon withdrawal of estrogen, the
within four days. Mitoses, necrotic areas, a
indicated by small condensed cell residues,
tions of the tumors stained with hematoxylin a
regression after DES withdrawal, mitotic act
imately 90%, and single cell death increase
of necrotic areas was not affected by DES
reduced single cell death by 80% within 8 h
within 24 h to the level observed before DES
of necrotic areas did not change. As a result,
size within 2 d after resumption of DES tre
following conclusions: (1) DES treatment in
hances single cell death of H301 tumor cells.
and its morphology characterize single cell d
(3) Estrogen-dependent cell death, along with
the growth rate of H301 tumors.

A. *IN*

Alle
entiatio
inducib
increase
rat emb
maintai
passage
adipose
differen
which d
as well
SOD ac
was ind
AMC c
time wh
trast, M
during
with M
23 cells
the two
small mi
of disor
**and tha
triggere
being i**
Cells tha
particula
cells, in
differen
induce c
tion was
dants a
cells all
cell diff

B. *IN*

Tiss
techniqu
MnSOD
inent (tra
strong a

stem cells. Germ cells of the testis resembled cell renewal systems in their antioxidant enzyme immunostaining pattern; spermatogonia were negative, whereas spermatozoa were strongly positive. The tubules of the kidney showed no antioxidant enzyme immunostaining until after birth. **These *in vivo* results suggest a prominent role for antioxidant enzymes in cell differentiation during development and cell renewal. They further suggest the possibility that AE are markers of cell differentiation *in vivo*.**

We also studied glutathione-dependent enzymes.[98] Tissues from adult Syrian hamsters were studied with immunoperoxidase techniques using polyclonal antibodies to glutathione-*S*-transferase (rat liver and human placental enzymes) and human erythrocyte glutathione peroxidase. The role of these enzymes in cell differentiation of a stable organ was studied by immunostaining the kidney during its development. Early stroma of the kidney (metanephric mesenchyme) from 13- and 15-d-old fetuses showed strong cell-surface staining for glutathione transferases and moderate staining for glutathione peroxidase. At this stage, renal tubules (which are epithelial cells) were negative for these markers. As renal tubules differentiated, first cytoplasm and then nuclei stained moderately, suggesting that glutathione-*S*-transferases and glutathione peroxidase are markers both for mesenchymal cells, including embryonic mesenchyme, and for terminal differentiation of at least some epithelial cells, e.g., kidney tubule.

IV. MODEL OF NEOPLASIA

Our proposed model for neoplasia is similar to that proposed by Ames and Gold.[99] In summary, our results suggest that the cell of origin of the estrogen-induced hamster cancer is an embryologic cell located in the renal interstitium. This cell type may be stimulated to proliferate by both hormonal influences and reactive oxygen species. There is considerable evidence for a prooxidant state in the hamster model. However, it is not certain what the consequences of the prooxidant state are, although DNA alterations have been demonstrated. Our laboratory has demonstrated aneuploidy in hamster renal tumors. The relationship between malignancy and DNA alterations, including DNA-DES adducts, oxidative DNA alterations, and aneuploidy, remains to be elucidated. It is not certain whether one or all of these alterations are necessary for carcinogenesis in the hamster system.

The first prerequisite for neoplasia is mutation, possibly by DNA adducts or induction of aneuploidy, in a cell capable of cell division. This postulate has some important corollaries. First, since we believe that most cancers arise in precursor cells and not in terminally differentiated cells, and since precursor cells have lowered antioxidant enzymes, then tumor cells should have low AEs. Second, although the nature of the mutation varies, most mutations that lead to cancer must involve growth regulation or inhibition of terminal differentiation.

The role of oxygen radicals is certainly not understood, but stimulation of cell proliferation must be important. As Ames and Gold have emphasized, proliferation is crucial for "fixing" genetic damage. A second important role of oxygen radicals is oxidative DNA damage, which could conceivably cause further DNA changes in promotion or progression.

Our laboratories are attempting to test these hypotheses. As an example, we have recently demonstrated that human fibroblasts transfected with the gene for MnSOD *in vitro* are resistant to radiation-induced transformation.[100] It seems certain that ROS can cause cancer, but what proportion of all malignancies are attributable to them? In a similar vein, changes in AEs are associated with cancer, but are these cause or effect? We are currently transfecting genes for antioxidant enzymes into tumor cells to determine their effects on the tumor cell phenotype. Our research should provide insights into these questions.

REFERENCES

1. **Freeman, B. A.**, Biological sites and mechanisms of free radical production, in *Molecular Biology, Aging, and Disease,* Armstrong, R. S., Cutler, R. G., and Slater, T. F., Eds., Raven Press, New York, 1984, 43.
2. **Fridovich, I.**, The biology of oxygen radicals, *Science,* 201, 875, 1978.
3. **Mason, R. P. and Chignell, C. F.**, Free radicals in pharmacology and toxicology, *Pharmacol. Rev.,* 33, 189, 1983.
4. **Beauchamp, C. and Fridovich, I.**, A mechanism for the production of ethylene from methional: the generation of hydroxyl radicals by xanthine oxidase, *J. Biol. Chem.,* 245, 4641, 1970.
5. **Frank, L.**, Oxygen toxicity in eukaryotes, in *Superoxide Dismutase,* Vol. 3, Oberley, L. W., Ed., CRC Press, Boca Raton, FL, 1985, 1.
6. **Sies, H. and Cadenas, E.**, Oxidative stress: damage to intact cells and organs, *Philos. Trans. R. Soc. Lond.,* 311, 617, 1985.
7. **Brawn, K. and Fridovich, I.**, Superoxide radical and superoxide dismutase: threat and defense, *Acta Physiol. Scand. Suppl.,* 492, 9, 1980.
8. **Fridovich, I.**, Superoxide dismutase, in *Molecular Mechanism of Oxygen Activation,* Hayaishi, O., Ed., Academic Press, New York, 1974, 453.
9. **Freeman, B. A. and Crapo, J. D.**, Biology of disease: free radicals and tissue injury, *Lab. Invest.,* 47, 412, 1982.
10. **Meister, A.**, Selective modification of glutathione metabolism, *Science,* 220, 472, 1963.
11. **Witting, L. A.**, Vitamin E and lipid peroxidation in free radical-initiated reactions, in *Free Radicals in Biology,* Vol. 4, Pryor, W. A., Ed., Academic Press, New York, 1980, 295.
12. **Oberley, L. W., Ed.,** *Superoxide Dismutase,* Vol. 3, CRC Press, Boca Raton, FL, 1985, 266.
13. **Oberley, L. W. and Oberley, T. D.**, Free radicals, cancer, and aging, in *Free Radicals, Aging, and Degenerative Diseases,* Johnson, J. E., Ed., Alan R. Liss, New York, 1986, 325.
14. **Farr, S. B., D'Ari, R., and Touati, D.**, Oxygen-dependent mutagenesis in *Escherichia coli* lacking superoxide dismutase, *Proc. Natl. Acad. Sci. U.S.A.,* 83, 8268, 1986.

15. **Storz, G., Christman, M. F., Sies, H., and Ames, B.**, Spontaneous mutagenesis and oxidative damage to DNA in *Salmonella typhimurium*, *Proc. Natl. Acad. Sci. U.S.A.,* 84, 8917, 1987.

16. **Moraes, E. C., Keyse, S. M., and Tyrell, R. M.**, Mutagenesis by hydrogen peroxide treatment in mammalian cells: a molecular analysis, *Carcinogenesis*, 11, 263, 1990.

17. **Borek, L.**, Free radical processes in multistage carcinogenesis, *Free Radical Res. Commun.,* 12–13, 745, 1991.

18. **Floyd, R. A.**, Role of oxygen free radicals in carcinogenesis and brain ischemia, *FASEB J.,* 4, 2587, 1990.

19. **Kennedy, A. R., Troll, W., and Little, J. B.**, Role of free radicals in the initiation and promotion of radiation transformation *in vitro, Carcinogenesis,* 5, 1213, 1984.

20. **O'Connell, J. F., Klein-Szanto, A. J. P., DiGiovanni, D. M., Fries, J. W., and Slaga, T. J.**, Enhanced malignant progression of mouse skin tumors by the free-radical generator benzoyl peroxide, *Cancer Res.,* 46, 2863, 1986.

21. **Klein-Szanto, A. J. P. and Slaga, T. J.**, Effects of peroxides in rodent skin: epidermal hyperplasia and tumor promotion, *J. Invest. Dermatol.,* 79, 30, 1982.

22. **Egner, P. A. and Kensler, T. W.**, Effects of a biomimetic superoxide dismutase on complete and multistage carcinogenesis in mouse skin, *Carcinogenesis,* 6, 1167, 1985.

23. **Perchelet, E. M., Maata, E. C., Abney, N. L., and Perchelet, J. P.**, Effects of diverse intracellular thiol delivery agents on glutathione peroxidase activity, the ratio of reduced/oxidized glutathione, and ornithine decarboxylase induction in isolated mouse epidermal cells treated with 12-O-tetradecanoylphorbol-13-acetate, *J. Cell. Physiol.,* 131, 64, 1987.

24. **Perchelet, J. P., Perchelet, E. M., Orten, D. K., and Schneider, B. A.**, Inhibition of the effects of 12-O-tetradecanoylphorbol-13-acetate on mouse epidermal glutathione peroxidase and ornithine decarboxylase activities by glutathione level-raising agents and selenium-containing compounds, *Cancer Lett.,* 26, 283, 1985.

25. **Perchelet, J. P., Abney, N. L., Thomas, R. M., Guislain, Y. L., and Perchelet, E. M.**, Effects of combined treatments with selenium, glutathione and vitamin E on glutathione peroxidase activity, ornithine decarboxylase induction and complete and multistage carcinogenesis in mouse skin, *Cancer Res.,* 47, 477, 1987.

26. **Perchelet, J. P., Abney, N. L., Thomas, R. M., Perchelet, E. M., and Maata, E. A.**, Inhibition of multistage tumor promotion in mouse skin by diethyldithiocarbamate, *Cancer Res.,* 47, 6302, 1987.

27. **Zimmerman, R. and Cerutti, P.**, Active oxygen acts as a promoter of transformation in mouse embryo C3H/10T1/2C18 fibroblasts, *Proc. Natl. Acad. Sci. U.S.A.,* 81, 2085, 1980.

28. **Fischer, S. M., Reiners, J. J., Jr., Pence, B. L., Aldaz, C. M., Conti, C. J., Morris, R. J., and Slaga, T. J.**, Mechanisms of carcinogenesis using mouse skin: the multistage assay revisited, in *Tumor Promoters: Biological Approaches for Mechanistic Studies and Assay Systems,* Langenbach, R., Barrett, J. L., and Elmore, E., Eds., Raven Press, New York, 1988, 11.

29. **Kensler, T. W., Egner, P. A., Jaffe, B. G., and Trush, M. A.**, Role of free radicals in tumor promotion and progression, in *Skin Carcinogenesis: Mechanisms and Human Relevance,* Slaga, T. J., Klein-Szanto, A. J. P., Boutwell, R. K., Stevenson, D. E., Spitzer, H. L., and D'Motto, B., Eds., Alan R. Liss, New York, 1989, 233.

30. **Robertson, F. M., Bearis, A. J., Oberyszyn, T. M., O'Connell, S. M., Dokidos, A., Laskin, D. L., Laskin, J. D., and Reiners, J. J., Jr.**, Production of hydrogen peroxide by murine epidermal keratinocytes following treatment with the tumor promoter 12-O-tetradecanoylphorbol-13-acetate, *Cancer Res.,* 58, 6062, 1990.

31. **Reiners, J. J., Jr., Thai, G., Rupp, T., and Cantu, A. R.**, Assessment of the antioxidant/prooxidant status of murine skin following topical treatment with 12-O-tetradecanoylphorbol-13-acetate and throughout the ontogeny of skin cancer. Quantitation of superoxide dismutase, catalase, glutathione peroxidase and xanthine oxidase, *Carcinogenesis,* 12, 2337, 1991.

32. **Cerutti, P.**, Prooxidant states and tumor promotion, *Science*, 227, 375, 1975.
33. **Sachs, L.**, Growth, differentiation, and the reversal of malignancy, *Sci. Am.*, 254, 40, 1986.
34. **Sell, S. and Dunsford, H. A.**, Evidence for the stem cell origin of hepatocellular carcinoma and cholangiocarcinoma, *Am. J. Pathol.*, 134, 1347, 1989.
35. **Hockenbery, D., Nunez, G., Millimen, C., Schreiber, R. D., and Korsmoyer, S. J.**, Bcl-2 is an inner mitochondrial membrane protein that blocks programmed cell death, *Nature*, 348, 334, 1990.
36. **Henderson, B. E., Ross, R., and Bernstein, L.**, Estrogens as a cause of human cancer, *Cancer Res.*, 48, 246, 1988.
37. **Herbst, A. L., Aubhy, M. M., and Anderson, D.**, Neoplastic changes in the human female genital tract following intrauterine exposure to diethyl stilbestrol, *Prog. Cancer Res. Ther.*, 31, 389, 1984.
38. **Forsberg, J. G.**, Estrogen, vaginal cancer, and vaginal development, *Am. J. Obstet. Gynecol.*, 113, 83, 1977.
39. **Forsberg, J. G.**, Neonatal estrogen treatment and epithelial abnormalities in the cervicovaginal epithelium of adult mice, *Cancer Res.*, 41, 721, 1981.
40. **Matthews, V. S., Kirkman, H., and Bacon, R. L.**, Kidney damage in the golden hamster following chronic administration of diethylstilbestrol and sesame oil, *Proc. Soc. Exp. Biol. Med.*, 66, 195, 1947.
41. **Kirkman, H. and Bacon, R. L.**, Malignant renal tumors in male hamsters (*Cricetus auratus*) treated with estrogen, *Cancer Res.*, 10, 122, 1950.
42. **Horning, E. S. and Whittick, J. W.**, The histogenesis of stilboestrol-induced renal tumors in the male golden hamster, *Br. J. Cancer*, 8, 451, 1954.
43. **Kirkman, H. and Robbins, M.**, Estrogen-induced tumors of the kidney. V. Histology and histogenesis in the Syrian hamster, *Natl. Cancer Inst. Monogr.*, 1, 93, 1959.
44. **Li, J. J., Talley, K. J., Li, S. A., and Villee, C. A.**, An estrogen binding protein in the renal cytosol of the intact, castrated, and estrogenized golden hamster, *Endocrinology*, 96, 1106, 1974.
45. **Li, S. A. and Li, J. J.**, Estrogen-induced progesterone receptor in the Syrian hamster kidney. I. Modulation by antiestrogens and androgens, *Endocrinology*, 193, 2119, 1978.
46. **Li, J. J., Cuthbertson, T. L., and Li, S. A.**, Inhibition of estrogen carcinogenesis in the Syrian golden hamster kidney by antiestrogens, *J. Natl. Cancer Inst.*, 64, 795, 1980.
47. **Li, J. J. and Li, S. A.**, Estrogen-induced tumorigenesis in the Syrian hamster: roles for hormonal and carcinogenic activities, *Arch. Toxicol.*, 55, 110, 1984.
48. **Li, J. J. and Li, S. A.**, Estrogen carcinogenesis in hamster tissues: role of metabolism, *Fed. Proc.*, 46, 1858, 1987.
49. **Gonzalez, A., Oberley, T. D., and Li, J. J.**, Morphological and immunohistochemical studies of the estrogen-induced Syrian hamster renal tumor: probable cell of origin, *Cancer Res.*, 49, 1020, 1989.
50. **Sell, S. and Dunsford, H. H.**, Evidence for the stem cell origin of hepatocellular carcinoma and cholangiocarcinoma, *Am. J. Pathol.*, 134, 1347, 1989.
51. **Germain, L., Blouin, M. J., and Marceau, N.**, Biliary epithelial and hepatocytic cell lineage relationships in embryonic rat liver as determined by the differential expression of cytokeratins, α-fetoprotein, albumin, and cell surface-expressed components. *Cancer Res.*, 48, 4909, 1988.
52. **Marceau, N., Blouin, M. J., and Noel, M.**, Role of different epithelial cell types in liver ontogenesis, regeneration and neoplasia, *In Vitro Cell. Dev. Biol.*, 25, 336, 1989.
53. **Oberley, T. D., Gonzalez, A., Lauchner, L. J., Oberley, L. W., and Li, J. J.**, Characterization of early kidney lesions in estrogen-induced tumors in the Syrian hamster, *Cancer Res.*, 51, 1922, 1991.
54. **Oberley, T. D., Lauchner, L. J., Pugh, T. D., Gonzalez, A., Goldfarb, S., Li, S. A., and Li, J. J.**, Specific estrogen-induced cell proliferation of cultured Syrian hamster renal proximal tubular cells in serum-free chemically defined media, *Proc. Natl. Acad. Sci. U.S.A.*, 86, 2107, 1989.

55. **Burdon, R. H. and Rice-Evans, C.,** Free radicals and the regulation of mammalian cell proliferation, *Free Radical Res. Commun.,* 6, 345, 1989.

56. **Morgan, M., Dettmer, R., Liuzzo, J., Johnson, R., Safirstein, R., and Goligorsky, M. S.,** Mechanisms of oxidative stress-induced proliferative response in renal tubular cells, *Am. Soc. Nephrol.,* (Abstr.), 302A, 1989.

57. **Murrell, G. A. L., Francis, M. J. O., and Bromley, L.,** Modulation of fibroblast proliferation by oxygen free radicals, *Biochem. J.,* 265, 659, 1990.

58. **Craven, P. A., Pfanstiel, J., and DeRubertis, F. R.,** Role of reactive oxygen in bile salt stimulation of colonic epithelial proliferation, *J. Clin. Invest.,* 77, 850, 1986.

59. **Armato, U., Andreis, P. G., and Romano, F.,** Exogenous Cu,Zn-superoxide dismutase suppresses the stimulation of neonatal rat hepatocytes' growth by tumor promoters, *Carcinogenesis,* 5, 1547, 1984.

60. **Shibanuma, M., Koroki, T., and Nose, K.,** Induction of DNA replication and expression of proto-oncogene c-myc and c-fos in quiescent Balb/3T3 cells by xanthine/xanthine oxidase, *Oncogene* 3, 17, 1988.

61. **Oberley, T.,** The possible role of reactive oxygen metabolism in cell division, in *Superoxide Dismutase,* Vol. 3, Oberley, L. W., Ed., CRC Press, Boca Raton, FL, 1985, 83.

62. **Oberley, T. D., Allen, R. G., Schultz, J. L., and Lauchner, L. J.,** Antioxidant enzymes and steroid-induced proliferation of kidney tubular cells, *Free Radical Biol. Med.,* 10, 79, 1991.

63. **Liehr, J. G., DaGue, B. B., and Ballatore, A. M.,** Reactivity of 4′,4″-diethylstilbestrol quinone, a metabolic intermediate of diethylstilbestrol, *Carcinogenesis,* 6, 829, 1985.

64. **Metzler, M. and McLachlan, J. A.,** Peroxide-mediated oxidation, a possible pathway for metabolic activation of diethylstilbestrol, *Biochem. Biophys. Res. Commun.,* 85, 874, 1978.

65. **Liehr, J. G., DaGue, B. B., Ballatore, A. M., and Henkin, J.,** Diethylstilbestrol (DES) quinone: a reactive intermediate in DES metabolism, *Biochem. Pharmacol.,* 16, 3711, 1983.

66. **Roy, D. and Liehr, J. G.,** Metabolic oxidation of diethylstilbestrol to diethylstilbestrol-4′,4″-quinone in Syrian hamsters, *Carcinogenesis,* 10, 1241, 1989.

67. **Liehr, J. G., Ulubelen, A. A., and Strobel, H. W.,** Cytochrome P-450-mediated redox cycling of estrogens, *J. Biol. Chem.,* 261, 16865, 1986.

68. **Roy, D. and Liehr, J. G.,** Temporary decrease in renal quinone reductase activity induced by chronic administration of estradiol to male Syrian hamsters. Increased superoxide formation by redox cycling of estrogen, *J. Biol. Chem.,* 263, 3646, 1988.

69. **Liehr, J. G., Avitts, T. A., Randerath, E., and Randerath, K.,** Estrogen-induced endogenous DNA adduction: possible mechanism of hormonal cancer, *Proc. Natl. Acad. Sci. U.S.A.,* 83, 5301, 1986.

70. **Lesko, S. A., Ts'o, P. O. P., Yang, S. U., and Zhang, R.,** Benzo[a]pyrene radicals and oxygen radical involvement in DNA damage, cellular toxicity and carcinogenesis, in *Free Radicals, Lipid Peroxidation and Cancer,* McBrien, D. C. H. and Slater, T. F., Eds., Academic Press, New York, 1982, 401.

71. **Rosier, J. A. and Van Peteghem, C. H.,** Peroxidative *in vitro* metabolism of diethylstilbestrol induces formation of 8-hydroxy-2′deoxyguanosine, *Carcinogenesis,* 10, 405, 1989.

72. **McCormick, M. L., Oberley, T. D., Elwell, J. H., Oberley, L. W., Sun, Y., and Li, J. J.,** Superoxide dismutase and catalase levels during estrogen-induced renal tumorigenesis, in renal tumors and their autonomous variants in the Syrian hamster, *Carcinogenesis,* 12, 977, 1991.

73. **Roy, D. and Liehr, J. G.,** Changes in activities of free radical detoxifying enzymes in kidneys of male Syrian hamsters with estradiol, *Cancer Res.,* 49, 1475, 1989.

74. **Winter, M. L. and Liehr, J. G.,** Free radical-induced carbonyl content in protein of estrogen-treated hamsters assayed by sodium boro[^{3}H]hydride reduction, *J. Biol. Chem.,* 266, 14446, 1991.

75. **Liehr, J. G.**, Vitamin C reduces the incidence and severity of renal tumors induced by estradiol or diethylstilbestrol, *Am. J. Clin. Nutr.*, 54, 12565, 1991.

76. **Liehr, J. G.**, Genotoxic effects of estrogens, *Mutat. Res.*, 238, 269, 1990.

77. **Roy, D., Floyd, R. A., and Liehr, J. G.**, Elevated 8-hydroxydeoxyguanosine levels in DNA of diethylstilbestrol-treated Syrian hamsters: covalent DNA damage by free radicals generated by redox cycling of diethylstilbestrol, *Cancer Res.*, 51, 3882, 1991.

78. **Barrett, J. C., Wong, A., and McLachlan, J. A.**, Diethylstilbestrol induces neoplasia transformation without measurable gene mutation at two loci, *Science*, 212, 1402, 1981.

79. **McLachlan, J. A., Wong, A., Dejen, G. H., and Barrett, J. L.**, Morphological and neoplastic transformation of Syrian hamster embryo fibroblasts by diethylstilbestrol and its analogs, *Cancer Res.*, 42, 3040, 1982.

80. **Ishidate, M. and Odashima, S.**, Chromosome tests with 134 compounds on Chinese hamster cells *in vitro* — a screening for chemical carcinogens, *Mutat. Res.*, 48, 337, 1977.

81. **Barrett, J. C.**, Cell transformation, mutation, and cancer, *Gann Monogr.*, 27, 195, 1981.

82. **Tsutsui, T., Maizumi, H., McLachlan, J. A., and Barrett, J. C.**, Aneuploidy induction and cell transformation by diethylstilbestrol: a possible mechanism in carcinogenesis, *Cancer Res.*, 43, 3814, 1983.

83. **Danford, N. and Parry, J. M.**, Abnormal cell division in cultured human fibroblasts after exposure to diethylstilbestrol, *Mutat. Res.*, 103, 379, 1982.

84. **Tucker, R. W. and Barrett, J. C.**, Decreased numbers of spindle and cytoplasmic microtubules in hamster embryo cells treated with diethylstilbestrol, *Cancer Res.*, 46, 2088, 1986.

85. **Sato, Y., Murai, T., Tsumuraya, M., Saito, M., and Kodama, M.**, Disruptive effects of diethylstilbestrol in microtubules, *Gann*, 75, 1046, 1984.

86. **Sharp, K. L. and Parry, J. M.**, Diethylstilbestrol: the binding and effects of diethylstilbestrol upon the polymerization of purified microtubule protein *in vivo*, *Carcinogenesis*, 6, 865, 1985.

87. **Epe, B., Harttig, U., Stopper, H., and Metzler, M.**, Covalent binding of reactive estrogen metabolites to microtubular protein as a possible mechanism of aneuploidy induction and neoplastic cell transformation, *Environ. Health Perspect.*, 88, 123, 1990.

88. **Hartley-Asp, B., Deinum, J., and Wallin, M.**, Diethylstilbestrol induces metaphase arrest and inhibits microtubule assembly, *Mutat. Res.*, 143, 231, 1985.

89. **Ozawa, N., Oshimura, M., McLachlan, J. A., and Barrett, J. C.**, Nonrandom karyotypic changes in immortal and tumorigenic Syrian hamster cells induced by diethylstilbestrol, *Cancer Genet. Cytogenet.*, 38, 271, 1989.

90. **Oshimura, M., Gilmer, T. M., and Barrett, J. C.**, Nonrandom loss of chromosome 15 in Syrian hamster tumors induced by *v-Ha-ras* plus *v-myc* oncogenes, *Nature*, 316, 636, 1985.

91. **Barrett, J. C. and Tso, P. O. P.**, Evidence for the progressive nature of neoplastic transformation *in vitro*, *Proc. Natl. Acad. Sci. U.S.A.*, 75, 3761, 1978.

92. **Gonzalez, A., Oberley, T. D., Schultz, J. L., Ostrom, J., and Li, J. J.**, *In vitro* characterization of estrogen-induced Syrian hamster renal tumors: comparison with an immortalized cell line derived from diethylstilbestrol-treated adult hamster kidney, *In Vitro Cell. Devel. Biol.*, submitted.

93. **Bursch, W., Liehr, J. G., Sirbasku, D. A., Patz, B., Taper, H., and Schulte-Herman, R.**, Control of cell death (apoptosis) by diethylstilbestrol in an estrogen-dependent kidney tumor, *Carcinogenesis*, 12, 855, 1991.

94. **Allen, R. G. and Balin, A. K.**, Oxidative influence on development and differentiation: an overview of a free radical theory of development, *Free Radical Biol. Med.*, 6, 631, 1989.

95. **Oberley, L. W., Ridnour, L. A., Sierra-Rivera, E., Oberley, T. D., and Guernsey, D. L.**, Superoxide dismutase activities of differentiating clones from an immortal cell line, *J. Cell. Physiol.*, 138, 50, 1989.

96. **Beckman, B. S., Balin, A. K., and Allen, R. G.,** Superoxide dismutase induces differentiation of Friend erythroleukemia cells, *J. Cell. Physiol.,* 139, 370, 1989.

97. **Oberley, T. D., Oberley, L. W., Slattery, A. F., Lauchner, L. J., and Elwell, J. H.,** Immunohistochemical localization of antioxidant enzymes in adult Syrian hamster tissues and during kidney development, *Am. J. Pathol.,* 137, 199, 1990.

98. **Oberley, T. D., Oberley, L. W., Slattery, A. F., and Elwell, J. H.,** Immunohistochemical localization of glutathione-*S*-transferase and glutathione peroxidase in adult Syrian hamster tissues and during kidney development, *Am. J. Pathol.,* 139, 355, 1991.

99. **Ames, B. W. and Gold, L. S.,** Endogenous mutagens and the causes of aging and cancer, *Mutat. Res.,* 250, 3, 1991.

100. **St. Clair, D., Wan, S. X., Oberley, T. D., Muse, K. E., and St. Clair, W. H.,** Overexpression of mitochondrial superoxide dismutase suppresses radiation-induced neoplastic transformation, *Molec. Carcinog.,* in press.

101. **Oberley, T. D.,** unpublished observation.

Chapter 12

FUTURE DIRECTIONS OF FREE RADICAL RESEARCH IN AGING

Richard Weindruch, Huber R. Warner, and Pamela E. Starke-Reed

TABLE OF CONTENTS

0-8493-4518-9/93/$0.00 + $.50
© 1993 by CRC Press, Inc.

I. INTRODUCTION

As this book amply demonstrates, the possibility that free radicals play a significant role in aging processes and in the pathogenesis of late-life diseases continues to intrigue many gerontologists and other investigators. The number of scientists interested in "free radicals and aging" appears to be growing in stride with the broadening appreciation of the prominent physiologic and pathologic actions of free radicals. However, present information is inconclusive as to the extent to which these reactive oxygen species (ROS) contribute to the processes of aging. An important and obvious future challenge is to resolve this central issue.

In this chapter, we speculate first on the possible role of ROS in aging from the standpoints of free radical *generation, removal,* and *repair of radical-inflicted damage.* Next, the assessment of *outcomes* of free radical damage is discussed. We assume that the balance between the rate of generation and that of removal plus repair results in some net level of ROS exposure which then produces an outcome. Such outcomes have overwhelmingly related to cellular damage; however, recent suggestions indicate other more physiological possibilities, such as oxidative stress causing alterations in gene expression by mechanisms not involving cellular damage.[1] Another example is nitric oxide which appears to be a neurotransmitter utilizing ROS reactions to convey its messages, not all of which involve neurotoxicity.[2] Throughout this chapter, we have identified areas which appear worthy of increased attention. We do so knowing that predicting the future course of two rapidly evolving and complex fields (gerontology and free radical biology) is a risky undertaking.

II. FREE RADICAL GENERATION

Perhaps the most crucial need with regard to understanding the role of ROS in aging is to obtain reliable quantitative data on the balance between ROS generation and antioxidant defense mechanisms in various tissues. While it is relatively easy to assay for the activities of the major antioxidant enzymes such as catalase (CAT), superoxide dismutase (SOD), and glutathione peroxidase (GSH-Px), and to measure levels of low molecular weight antioxidants such as ascorbate, vitamin E, β-carotene, uric acid, glutathione (GSH), and other essential cofactors such as NADPH, it is far more difficult to obtain absolute values for the rates of free radical generation which have relevance *in vivo.*

The difficulty in measuring the endogenous rate of free radical production stems from several factors. Free radicals, by nature, are highly reactive and rather nonselective with regard to what they attack. Furthermore, they are generated in the presence of antioxidant defense systems which, unless they are inactivated, will destroy some of the ROS before they can be detected by the assay system chosen. Finally, ROS can be generated in such a way that they may be unable to react with any of the traditional assay systems. For example, significant generation of ROS may occur as "caged" reactions on the very surface of a macromolecule, at or very near to a metal binding site.[3] These difficulties suggest that most measurements of the rate of generation of ROS are likely to be underestimates.

Although previous chapters have discussed various aspects of free radical generation and antioxidant defense mechanisms, it is worth covering selected aspects briefly here.

A. SOURCES OF FREE RADICALS IN LIVING TISSUE

Chance et al.[4] have reviewed the metabolism of hydrogen peroxide (H_2O_2) in mammalian systems. H_2O_2 may be produced directly as a product of biological oxidations, or it may be produced by the dismutation of superoxide. These authors have made relative estimates of the subcellular sources of H_2O_2, and these are as follows:

- Endoplasmic reticulum (mixed function oxidations)   45%
- Peroxisomes (metal-catalyzed oxidations)   35%
- Mitochondria (oxidative phosphorylation)   15%
- Cytosol (xanthine oxidation)   5%

However, because of the conversion of superoxide to H_2O_2 by SOD, it is not clear whether the above figures represent only the direct production of H_2O_2 or whether they also include that produced from superoxide as well. For example, Chance et al.[4] estimate that rat liver microsomes produce 6 to 15 nmol H_2O_2 and 2 to 10 nmol superoxide per min/mg protein, mostly from autooxidation of reduced cytochromes C and P-450. Thus, some of the 6 to 15 nmol H_2O_2 may have come from the superoxide produced.

There are more than 20 metal-catalyzed oxidation (MCO) systems which have been shown to oxidize proteins.[5] Perhaps the most physiologically relevant of these are as follows:[3]

1. NAD(P)H oxidase/NAD(P)H/O_2/Fe(III)
2. Xanthine oxidase/xanthine/Fe(III)/O_2
3. Cytochrome P-450/cytochrome P-450 reductase/Fe(III)/O_2
4. Ascorbate/O_2/Fe(III)
5. Fe(III)/O_2 (or H_2O_2)
6. RSH/Fe(III)/O_2

The relative contributions of these systems to protein oxidation *in vivo* are currently unknown. Jesaitis et al.[6] have pointed out that NADPH-oxidase is the main source of superoxide radicals in human phagocytes, producing up to 15 fmol per cell per minute for the explicit purpose of destroying the biological activity of foreign organisms. Unfortunately, some damage to host material in the vicinity of the invading organism also occurs.

Based on the measure of 8-hydroxy-2'-deoxyguanosine (8-OH-dG), a very high level of oxidative damage was found in rat liver mitochondrial DNA (mtDNA) (1 per 8000 bases) as compared to nuclear DNA (1 per 130,000 bases).[7] Wallace[8] concludes that oxidative phosphorylation may be responsible for the high rate of mtDNA mutation due to the generation of superoxide and H_2O_2 by direct transfer of electrons from reduced flavins, cytochromes, and coenzyme Q to oxygen. He states (but does not provide a reference thereto) that 1 to 4% of oxygen uptake is converted to these oxidizing species, and that age-related declines in oxidative phosphorylation (discussed below) may be one result of this self-inflicted mitochondrial damage. Among the observations to support this thought is that the mitochondrial electron transport chain components and ATPase are inactivated following *in vitro* exposure to ROS.[9] Clearly, the abundance of mitochondrial ROS production is a critical figure to investigate gerontologically. It may well be that production rates do not change with age, and that damage accumulates due to the chronicity of a steady level of exposure which slightly exceeds defense capacities.

From the above, it is clear that oxidative damage is inescapable in cells capable of aerobic metabolism. Whereas superoxide itself may not be particularly reactive and has limited ability to penetrate membranes, H_2O_2 can readily cross membranes and, in the presence of metal ions, e.g., Fe^{2+}, is converted to the highly reactive hydroxyl radical. An example of one such reaction of potential importance is as follows: the *in vitro* exposure of mitochondrial F_1 ATPase to H_2O_2 resulted in a major loss of ATP hydrolytic activity in a reaction mediated by iron ions.[10] Minotti and Aust[11] find that lipid peroxidation is mediated by an Fe^{2+}/Fe^{3+} complex which can be formed by Fe^{2+} oxidation or Fe^{3+} reduction. The role of metal ions such as Fe^{2+} and Fe^{3+} in oxidative damage suggests the wisdom of considering interventions which will reduce the amount of free heavy metal ions in living systems.[12]

It is important to improve our knowledge of where ROS are generated in the body, how many, and what kind. Such information can then be correlated with data on levels of antioxidant defense mechanisms, location and extent of oxidative damage, and epidemiological data on diseases whose etiology may include oxidative damage (see Section V., below). However, the acquisition of such data depends on the yet unacquired capacities to accurately measure rates of ROS production and to identify which antioxidant defense mechanisms are critical in preventing damage due to the ROS produced. Pryor and Godber[13] have stated that they " . . . believe one of the greatest needs in the field of free radical biology to be the development of reliable measures of oxidative stress status." An improved understanding of the possible role ROS play in aging awaits the development of such measures.

B. ASSAYS FOR HYDROGEN PEROXIDE AND OXYRADICALS

Whereas techniques are available to measure superoxide, H_2O_2, and hydroxyl radical in purified systems, in some cases these assays are less effective in biological material. H_2O_2 can be readily assayed spectrophotometrically by measuring the amount of hydrogen donor consumed or product formed, and these assays can be performed in biological samples. H_2O_2 can also be measured fluorometrically by following its enzymatic reduction by horseradish peroxidase. Sohal et al.[14] studied liver mitochondrial H_2O_2 production in various species and found that the production rate was inversely correlated with species life-span. In contrast, the assay for superoxide is much more difficult in biological material where spontaneous decay is a problem. One possible technique is to convert the superoxide to H_2O_2 using SOD and then assay the amount of H_2O_2 produced. Hydroxyl radical can be assayed by spin trapping with a nitroso compound to detect the signal this produced. However, because free radicals are so reactive, they are, in fact, difficult to measure directly.[13]

Free radical generation can be estimated indirectly in biological systems by measuring the amount of oxidized product formed. For example, free radical attack on DNA can be estimated from its content of 8-OH-dG or thymine glycol, protein oxidation can be estimated from its carbonyl content, and fatty acid oxidation can be estimated from the amount of malondialdehyde (MDA) produced. However, such assays are obviously only useful for determining relative values, as the products being measured represent only a fraction of the total oxidation which has occurred. Furthermore, because oxidation and repair are dynamic processes, the levels that are detected reflect only the steady state concentrations at the time of sampling.

Research in the area of free radical damage and aging would clearly be facilitated by technical improvements in the measurements of the rate of endogenous generation of ROS, the rate of oxidative damage actually occurring, and the rate of repair of damaged molecules. New techniques are particularly needed to trap oxidation products in a nonrepairable form so that radical generation and/or damage can be integrated over a specific time period.

III. PRIMARY DEFENSE SYSTEMS: FREE RADICAL REMOVAL

A. EXPERIMENTAL APPROACHES

As discussed and tabulated by Matsuo in Chapter 7 of this volume, many studies have examined the influences of aging on antioxidant defenses. Most of what is known concerns liver and brain activities of the enzymes CAT, GSH-Px, and SOD, as well as changes in levels of GSH in many tissues. Nonetheless, these seemingly abundant data contain many contradictions which together underscore the need to examine multiple animal models, to include both genders, and to study more than one tissue whenever possible. As is typical for most aging studies, rodent models have been used most often. There appears to be an imbalance heavily favoring rats over mice in frequency of study. Also, there exists a gender imbalance, with more known about males than females. The work of Rikans and co-workers[15-17] clearly demonstrates major influences of gender on the direction of age-related influences on hepatic antioxidant and GSH-synthesizing enzymes. For example, the cytosolic activity of liver CAT fell sharply in late life in male Fischer rats, but rose in old females.

The tissue specificity of the direction of change conferred by aging on antioxidant defenses is quite striking. For example, Ji et al.[18] found that aging was generally accompanied with an elevation of antioxidant enzyme activities and lipid peroxidation in skeletal muscle, but not in the liver of male Wistar-Furth rats. The design employed was advantageous (and gerontologically atypical) because it allowed comparison of more than one tissue. Although antioxidant enzyme status as a function of aging has been investigated predominately in the liver, two reports describe age-related increases in skeletal muscle antioxidant enzyme activities in mice[19] and rats.[20] The relative lack of study of muscle represents a significant gap in knowledge in view of the fact that skeletal muscle accounts for about 20% to 30% of the total resting oxygen uptake.[21]

Adding further complexity to the situation, cardiac muscle shows yet another pattern of age-related change in aging male Wistar-Furth rats.[22] Here, the cytosolic antioxidant enzymes decrease in activity with aging, while those in the mitochondria increase. In this study, the MDA content of both whole homogenates and mitochondrial fractions increases with aging, while activities of enzymes of energy production (e.g., citrate synthase, malate dehydrogenase, lactate dehydrogenase) decline. This investigation provided an extensive view of the oxidative status of the aging heart in a way that "enzyme only" studies cannot approach. Compensatory increases in mitochondrial antioxidant defenses appear to occur with aging in muscle.

Sensitive methods have also indicated that rat brain and human cerebrospinal fluid SOD activities increase with aging.[23] Interestingly, the relative increase in rat brain SOD was much more exaggerated in mitochondrial than in cytosolic isolates. Another group also found increases with aging in brain SOD activity in rodents (de Haan et al.).[24] Although contradictory data exist,[25,26] it may be that tissues such as muscle or brain, which have low capacities of cell proliferation and high requirements for oxidative metabolism, will show increases in antioxidant defense activities with aging in response to increases in free radical production and/or damage.

Another area requiring further investigation concerns the subcellular distribution of antioxidant enzymes and metabolites. Recent findings indicate the presence of SOD in peroxisomes,[27] but, to our knowledge, isolated peroxisomes have received scant gerontologic attention, despite this organelle's important role in cellular ROS metabolism. In addition, only recently has CAT been reproducibly detectable in rat heart mitochondria, where it may provide a primary antioxidant defense.[28] These new insights on the cellular localization of relevant activities require exploration in the context of aging.

B. PIECING TOGETHER THE "BIG PICTURE"

All of the above information underscores the fact that current understanding of the extent and significance of age-related influences on ROS removal capacities is not great. What is encouraging is that much has been learned in the past few years, and that the pace of advances appears to be accelerating. The challenge now is to carry out the necessary experiments so that the "big picture" in this area of inquiry becomes evident.

Research is critically needed to define the *physiological* effects of changes in levels of antioxidant enzyme activities or in associated metabolites. To increase our understanding, it will be necessary to measure free radical-influenced outcomes in addition to evaluating defense status. Several questions need to be kept in mind such as: (1) What does it mean to the organism to have a high or low liver, brain or muscle CAT or SOD activity? (2) What is the physiological importance of an age or treatment group difference in maximal enzyme activity, as measured at substrate concentrations which exceed *in vivo* reality? (3) Are there other aspects of an enzyme's behavior (e.g., rate constants, Michaelis-Menton parameters, susceptibility to inhibitors) which, in addition to peak activity, also require study? (4) To what extent do age-related alterations in enzyme activities depend on the levels of essential cofactors (e.g., NADPH, GSH) used to neutralize ROS? (5) Which enzyme activities or cofactor levels are rate-limiting in physiologically germane tests of ROS defense?

More thought is required on the interdependence of the individual detoxification steps. A design similar to that of Simmons and Jamall[29] might be employed productively in an aging study. These workers modulated the activities of rat liver GSH-Px and CAT and measured lipid peroxidation as an outcome. It was observed that GSH-Px played a more important role than CAT in preventing lipid peroxidation. Another recent approach begging gerontologic application is the use of SOD-transgenic mice which show elevated CuZn-SOD activities (2.0- to 3.5-fold higher in various brain regions) and increased resistance to certain paradigms of oxidative stress.[30-32] In these transgenic mice, the elevations in brain SOD are associated with increases in CAT activity, whereas GSH-Px is unaltered. One can also alter cellular enzyme levels by lysing and resealing red blood cells (RBCs) in the presence of exogenous enzyme, as was described for SOD.[33] Five- or ninefold increases in SOD activity achieved in human RBCs yielded no additional protection against superoxide-generating drugs, superoxide-induced methemaglobin formation, or generation of TBA-reactive substances.

Another gap in the "big picture" concerns the physiologic importance of circulating antioxidant defense molecules contained in serum, RBCs, or other circulating cells. Do circulating defenses serve to keep our milieu safely balanced with respect to oxidative stress, or are the intracellularly generated and acting radicals of dominant importance? What are the relationships among aging, circulating levels of antioxidant agents in plasma and cells, and the resistance to oxidative stress? At present, there exists a limited gerontologic literature on these topics. Góth[34] finds that serum CAT activity (the main sources of which are RBCs) increased with age in 742 healthy people between the ages of 14 and 60. Values in males were 18% higher than those of females.

A study from Poland found that RBC activities of GSH-Px and total peroxidase rose by about 30% in 60- to 85-year-old persons as compared to persons 25- to 50-years-old.[35] The activity of SOD decreased marginally ($\sim$10%), and that of CAT was uninfluenced by aging in these two groups. An even different picture emerged from the study of Guemouri et al.,[36] who observed that specific activities of RBC and plasma antioxidant enzymes tend to decrease in older persons. In line with this is other evidence for a marginal age-related decrease in RBC antioxidant enzyme activities in very old (average = 88 years) as compared to middle age (average = 55 years) people.[37] These RBC and serum-based measures hold added potential significance, as these are easy to monitor longitudinally and are, therefore, potential biomarkers of aging and oxidative stress.

IV. SECONDARY DEFENSE SYSTEMS: MACROMOLECULAR REPAIR

Although living organisms have defense systems capable of neutralizing most of the oxyradicals produced *in vivo* (Chapter 7, this volume), it is unreasonable to expect that these systems can be 100% effective. The very nature of free radicals as highly reactive molecules precludes this possibility. Thus, some small portion of the endogenously produced ROS can inflict damage to cellular components before they can be neutralized. The targets of oxidative damage most likely to have serious implications for cellular structure and function are DNA, proteins, and membranes. The bases in DNA,[38] the sidechains of the amino acids in proteins,[3,5,39,40] and the unsaturated fatty acids in membranes[41] can all be oxidized, resulting in altered structure and function.

In the following examples, it is not always clear whether or how much these processes actually occur *in vivo*, even though the reactions have been demonstrated *in vitro*. Because damage and repair *in vivo* are dynamic processes, it is not easy to determine the actual rate of either process. Furthermore, little is known definitely about: (1) how efficient these repair systems are, (2) what alternative pathways exist, (3) how these repair systems change during aging, and (4) species and tissue differences in damage and repair. These knowledge gaps describe some of the important future directions of free radical research in aging.

A. DNA DAMAGE AND REPAIR

The bases in both RNA and DNA are subject to attack by ROS, but because RNA is routinely degraded and resynthesized, RNA damage is probably of limited importance. However, if bases in DNA are damaged, it is essential to remove the damaged bases and to restore the original base if the genetic information is to be retained unchanged. Although oxygen can damage DNA in a variety of ways, the oxidation of thymine to thymine glycol and/or urea,[42] and guanine to 8-OH-dG[43] are common events. A typical repair path-

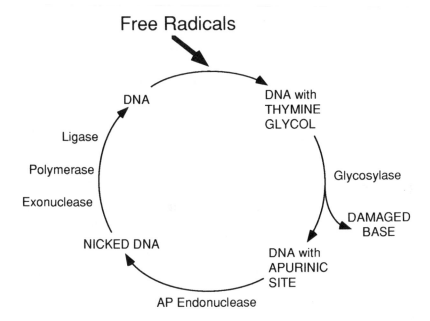

FIGURE 1. Oxidative damage to DNA. The reaction of DNA with free radicals leads to the formation of DNA with thymine glycol.

way is shown in Figure 1. The enzymes required for this repair have all been demonstrated in *Escherichia coli*[44] and are assumed to be present in most, if not all, mammalian cells.[45] The important point is whether repair of the damaged base can be accomplished before the damaged region is replicated. If it cannot, there is a high probability of mutations arising from mispairing during replication.

Although Hart and Setlow[46] have published data to suggest that species life-span directly correlates with capacity for unscheduled DNA synthesis in fibroblasts, the role of DNA damage and repair in aging remains intriguing, but ambiguous.[47] A recent approach is to look specifically at the natural levels of damaged bases in DNA to determine whether they may play a role in aging. That they do is suggested by the results of Cutler[48] and Fraga and co-workers.[38] Cutler showed that the level of 8-OH-dG in liver DNA is inversely proportional to species life-span, suggesting that the ability to prevent and/or remove damaged bases in DNA is related to longevity. Fraga et al.[38] found that the level of 8-OH-dG in DNA from various rat organs varied from 10 to 70 residues per 10^6 deoxyguanosine residues. From the knowledge that 8-OH-dG is only one of many oxidized products formed and that about 6.4×10^{10} oxygen radicals are estimated to be produced per rat cell each day, they calculated that one oxidized DNA residue is produced for every 7.6×10^5 oxygen radicals generated, or about 9×10^4 oxidized DNA bases are formed per cell per day. This is not a trivial amount of DNA damage to repair, and it is not surprising that cellular DNA contains oxidized bases. What is not clear is why the levels differ in various organs and why the levels increase with age in some tissues, e.g., the liver, kidney, and intestine, but not in others, e.g., the brain and testes. Fraga et al.[38] also observed that the urine content of 8-OH-dG decreases with age, suggesting that the increasing levels in organ DNA could be due either to a decreasing ability to initiate repair of the oxidized DNA, or to an increased rate of oxidative damage with increasing age. Thus, it would be useful to know whether DNA repair efficiency does decrease with age, what factors regulate the reparability of damaged DNA, and whether the rate of endogenous production of ROS increases with age.

B. PROTEIN DAMAGE AND REPAIR

Much of the work on ROS-mediated damage has concentrated on alterations of nucleic acids and lipids. Only recently have investigators focused on radical-mediated damage to proteins and the potential role these alterations may play in aging. The argument against ROS-mediated damage to proteins during aging has been heretofore based on the inability to show age-related defects in the protein synthesizing machinery or in the *in vivo* production of oxidatively modified proteins.[49] It had been argued that damaged proteins would not accumulate due to their rapid turnover; however, with the introduction of very sensitive measurement procedures it has been shown that oxidatively modified proteins do accumulate with aging. This accumulation could be due to an increase in ROS generation in a tissue, a decrease in the levels of antioxidants, or both.

Stadtman[3,5,39,50] has provided several excellent reviews on the subject of "protein oxidation and aging"; under mild oxidation conditions, histidine, proline, and arginine residues are oxidized to aspartyl, glutamyl, and glutamyl semialdehyde residues, respectively. Furthermore, side chains, such as those in histidine and lysine, can be oxidized to carbonyl derivatives,[51] and the carbonyl content of cultured human fibroblasts increases significantly with age of the donor. It is noteworthy that, in progeroid syndromes, e.g., Werner's syndrome and Hutchison-Guilford disease, protein is more subject to oxidation than in normal cells,[3] and that, in cultured rat hepatocytes, the accumulation of oxidized protein occurs at a rate roughly 40 times faster than it does in cultured human cells.[50] These data are consistent with the hypothesis that protein oxidation contributes to aging, but they do not clarify whether the increased levels of protein oxidation are due to increased oxyradical production or to decreased proteolytic degradation of oxidized protein.

Most amino acid oxidation is thought to occur via the Fenton reaction of Fe^{2+} and H_2O_2 generated by mixed function oxidases. The Fe^{2+} binds to an enzyme at a metal binding site and reacts with the H_2O_2 to yield a ROS which immediately attacks the side chains of amino acid residues in a site-specific manner at the metal binding sites of the proteins. During this MCO reaction, it is thought that the H_2O_2 and Fe^{2+} react to form the hydroxyl radical; however, other ROS may be formed, such as the ferryl ion, perferryl ion, or other peroxyradicals. The site-specific "caged" nature of this metal ion-catalyzed reaction is suggested by the findings that: (1) the reactions are only slightly sensitive to inhibition by ROS scavengers, indicating that the radicals are not formed in free solution; (2) only one or a few amino acid residues in a given protein are modified by MCO reactions; and (3) only amino acid residues at metal binding sites of the protein are readily oxidized. For example, the oxidation of glutamine synthetase leads to modification of two histidine and one arginine residues, which are situated at the metal binding sites of the enzyme.[52,53]

These oxidized proteins are highly susceptible to proteolytic degradation. In fact, the only known general pathway of repair of oxidatively damaged proteins is by complete degradation to amino acids. This may be accomplished in hepatocytes by a large, multicomponent protease which declines markedly with increasing age.[40] Although this protease may itself be susceptible to oxidative inactivation, and oxidized proteins accumulate with age,[40,54] there is no direct evidence that this protease actually plays a major role in the turnover of oxidized proteins *in vivo*.

Dice[55] reviewed the known pathways of protein degradation in eukaryotes, and only a few of these are known to decrease with aging. He has shown that two lysosomal pathways decrease with aging. One of these appears to be a general protease, whereas the other only degrades proteins containing the sequence lys-phe-glu-arg-gln. This latter protease requires the participation of an hsp-70 protein to promote delivery of these proteins to the lysosome, but induction of this protein is reduced in senescent fibroblasts. Finally, Dice has suggested that a short-lived protein is required for lysosomal proteolysis, and that, if this protein is degraded by ubiquitin-dependent pathways, the two pathways will be interactive if altered (e.g., oxidized) proteins induce the ubiquitin-dependent pathways. Thus, if altered proteins accumulate in senescent cells, the degradation of the short-lived control protein will be increased, leading to further reduction in lysosomal proteolysis. Clearly, more information is needed about this putative short-lived protein and its role in lysosomal degradation of altered proteins.

The most important unanswered question is whether accumulation of oxidized protein plays a major role in aging. Several lines of evidence suggest that it does, but more research is needed to clarify exactly how. Another important question is whether critical proteins exist which are particularly sensitive to oxidation, or whether deficits due to protein oxidation are more global in nature. Glutamine synthetase activity in glial cells may be one such critical protein because it is important in controlling the extracellular levels of ammonia and glutamate in the brain. Oliver et al.[56] and Carney et al.[54] have shown that reversal of protein oxidation in the brain with N-tert-butyl-α-phenylnitrone (PBN), a free radical spin trap, is accompanied by comparable increases in the activity of glutamine synthetase and the large multi-component protease and by an increased resistance to ischemia/reperfusion injury in gerbil brain. However, how PBN accomplishes this is unclear because it is unlikely

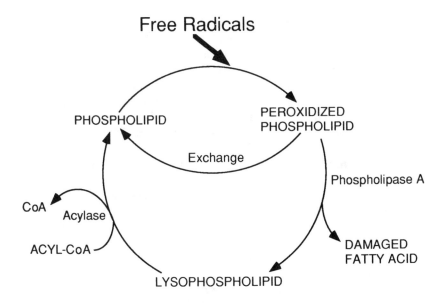

FIGURE 2.   Free radical-induced peroxidation of double bonds in membrane phospholipids.

that the amount of PBN required is sufficient to stoichiometrically neutralize
the ROS produced following reperfusion.

C. MEMBRANE DAMAGE AND REPAIR

In addition to membrane proteins, the double bonds of fatty acids in
membrane lipids are sites of oxidative damage leading to formation of lipid
peroxyl radicals and ultimately of lipid hydroperoxides which can decompose
into a variety of products.[41] Peroxidized membranes display altered structure
and function and have been implicated in a variety of pathological conditions.[57]
Repair might simply occur by exchange of the intact damaged lipid for an
undamaged one (Figure 2). Although GSH-Px and GSH can reduce a fatty
acid hydroperoxide to a hydroxy fatty acid, it may be necessary to first remove
the fatty acid from the phospholipid with phospholipase A_2,[58] although a more
recent report has identified a new GSH-Px apparently able to reduce phospholipid hydroperoxides *in situ*.[59] This new enzyme has not been investigated
gerontologically. Any lysophospholipid formed by the action of phospholipase
A_2 can be reacylated with the appropriate acyl-CoA,[60] but it is not clear
whether this can actually happen *in situ* in the membrane. However, it is
clear that complete repair of membrane lipid does occur following peroxidation,[61] whether through exchange or repair *in situ,* or both.

Several other questions remain. What is the fate of hydroxy fatty acids
produced by *in situ* reduction of oxidized fatty acids by GSH and GSH-Px?
The replacement of an unsaturated fatty acid by a hydroxy fatty acid will
certainly alter both the structure and function of the membrane. What defense

system is available if a polyunsaturated fatty acid is oxidized and proceeds to break down to dialdehydes, such as MDA? Such dialdehydes can not only react nonenzymatically with the amino groups of proteins to alter their structure and function, but can also have the potential to induce cross-linking. This potential could be related to the possible health benefits of replacing dietary polyunsaturated fatty acids with monounsaturated fatty acids.

V. ASSESSING THE OUTCOMES OF FREE RADICAL EXPOSURE

Following the ongoing events of free radical production, removal, damage, and repair, some net level of exposure must then result which produces biological consequences. Certain of the acute molecular outcomes have just been discussed in Section IV., above ("Secondary Defense Systems: Macromolecular Repair"). These (and many other) ROS-influenced changes likely interact with other important aging processes and produce the biological modifications and diseases of aging. This section provides commentary on selected outcomes which show promise for understanding the extent to which ROS drive aging processes.

A. MOLECULAR AND SUBCELLULAR OUTCOMES
1. Mitochondria

A major area of inquiry concerns the possible involvement of mitochondria in aging. Although a careful appraisal[62] of the influences of aging on mitochondria published in 1983 found it difficult to see major mitochondrial problems, more recent reviews of a rapidly growing literature argue otherwise.[63,64] The latter reviewers discuss and provide references for many mitochondrial changes found in old as compared to young mammals, including decreases in mitochondrial recovery, state 3 O_2 uptake, enzyme activities, substrate uptake rates, protein synthesis, membrane fluidity, and water content. Most of these studies involved either the brain, liver or heart of rats.

Very recent publications continue to document age-related mitochondrial changes of great potential physiological significance. For example, the buoyant density profile of liver mitochondrial DNA from old rats was quite different from that of young rats, and the difference was reduced by treatment with a proteinase.[65] The authors suggested the likelihood that mtDNA of old rat liver contains firmly bound protein(s) or peptides. Using nonradioactive DNA probes, this group next reported that rat liver mtDNA content is greatly decreased in old age with 30-month-old rats having only ~20% the amount found in 2-month-old rats.[66] Another intriguing observation is that the rate of mitochondrial RNA synthesis in isolated brain mitochondria from old rats is about 50% of that observed in adults.[67]

An emerging theme is that the mtDNA mutations which accumulate over the life-span contribute to aging, cancer, and other degenerative diseases.[8,64,68-79] All of these investigators emphasize that the assembly of functional mitochondria requires the joint expression of both mitochondrial and nuclear genes. Furthermore, the mutation rate for mtDNA is much higher than for most nuclear genes, leading to the view that aging and certain major degenerative diseases (e.g., Parkinson's and Alzheimer's diseases, ischemic heart disease, diabetes) may be due in part to mtDNA mutations leading to deficits in oxidative phosphorylation.

2. Regulation of Gene Expression

A major question is how the balance is maintained between oxidative damage and antioxidant defense. Although oxidative damage per se is undesirable, ROS are known to be essential for certain cellular processes, such as signal transduction.[2] An attractive possibility is that proteins necessary for repression of genes coding for antioxidant defense proteins (e.g., SOD) have easily oxidizable groups, and that the repressor activity is lost when these groups are oxidized. Conversely, an inducer active only in an oxidized state could promote transcription of these genes. The latter appears to be the case in bacteria, as the OxyR protein (when oxidized by H_2O_2?) promotes transcription of the OxyR regulon, which includes genes for CAT and an alkyl hydroperoxide reductase.[71,72] The nature of the putative oxidizable group in the OxyR protein remains unknown. Bacteria contain a second regulon, called soxRS, which is activated by superoxide ion and controls the expression of Mn-SOD, as well as a variety of other proteins, mostly of unknown function.

Comparable regulatory systems have not been described in mammalian systems, but examples of changing the regulatory properties of proteins by oxidation have been reported. For example, the NF-κB transcription factor is activated directly by H_2O_2, apparently by the oxidation of an associated inhibitor.[73] Oxidants such as H_2O_2 and superoxide have also been shown to induce CAT and Mn-SOD, but not GSH-Px or CuZnSOD, in lung epithelial cells.[74] Finally, while extracellular oxidants are known to induce the expression of the protooncogenes *c-fos* and *c-myc* in serum-starved mouse cells,[75] it is not clear whether these genes are specifically induced or are part of a general induction of proteins necessary for initiation at DNA synthesis. Clearly, we have a long way to go to understand the role(s) and mechanisms of ROS in enzyme induction in eukaryotic cells.

3. Molecular Epidemiology

A recent study[76] suggests a strong inverse correlation between ascorbic acid levels in seminal fluid and oxidized bases in sperm DNA. When the ascorbic acid levels fall below ~50 μmol, the levels of 8-OH-dG in DNA rose dramatically. The ascorbic acid levels in seminal fluid could be influenced by dietary intake, and it was suggested that because smoking reduces serum ascorbic acid levels, smoking may indirectly increase the levels of oxidized bases in sperm DNA. Nothing is currently known about relationships between these parameters and age, but it is clear that increased oxidative damage to sperm DNA may contribute to the increased incidence of cancer in offspring of smokers.[77]

Other epidemiological correlations involving antioxidants and their relationship to ischemic heart disease[78] and Alzheimer's disease[79] have been reported. Heart disease was strongly correlated with low plasma vitamin E levels, whereas there were only slight inverse correlations between plasma antioxidant levels, including vitamin E, and the incidence of Alzheimer's disease. However, Diplock[80] has pointed out the difficulty of interpreting much of the epidemiologic work because of the inadequate assay procedures often used and the failure to take into account interactions between various antioxidant defense systems. Nevertheless, there is substantial evidence that high intake of ascorbic acid through leafy vegetables and fruits has a protective effect against cardiovascular disease and cancer.

Even though studies and correlations such as these are bound to be improved through the use of more reliable techniques for assaying antioxidant levels in plasma, what is really required is a better understanding of the balance between generation of ROS and antioxidant defense in the actual tissues and of how this relates to pathological changes.

B. GERIATRIC DISORDERS AND DISEASES AS OUTCOMES

A need exists to define rigorously the possible role of ROS in the dominant diseases/disorders of old age. The diversity of plausible influences of ROS allows one to speculate logically in broad vistas about age-associated diseases induced by ROS-mediated damage, altered gene expression, and changed cell growth. We comment on these possibilities as they relate to cancer, muscle weakness, Alzheimer's and Parkinson's diseases, and osteoporosis. Wallace[8] points out that the main late-onset degenerative diseases affect the central nervous system and heart, and both of these have a strong reliance on mitochondrial oxidative phosphorylation for ATP production. Skeletal muscle also requires attention due to its high requirement for ATP and its contribution to geriatric physical frailty and associated immobility, injury, and dependence.

1. Cancer

Although not mainstream in current cancer research, free radicals may play a role in carcinogenesis. Pryor[81] suggests that ROS are involved in carcinogen activation and in the binding of activated species to DNA. Cerutti[82] discusses how cellular "prooxidant states", i.e., increased levels of ROS, may promote neoplastic growth in initiated cells. According to Pitot,[83] with the exception of the role hormones may play in certain cancers, the role of other endogenous factors (e.g., ROS) in tumor promotion is little investigated.

As noted, much recent emphasis is on mitochondrial mutations occurring due to a combination of high exposure of mtDNA to oxidants and poor intramitochondrial DNA repair capacities. Richter[68] proposed that transformation results from oxidatively generated DNA fragments escaping from mitochondria and integrating into the nuclear genome. Bandy and Davison[70] extensively developed a similar hypothesis with the predicted end result being aberrant mitochondria, aging, and cancer. Although ROS are being studied for their actions in experimental models of induced cancer, we are unaware of such studies in spontaneously arising late-life cancers. Experiments in appropriate models might prove informative. Another provocative approach would be to compare the mitochondrial status of persons from cancer-prone and cancer-resistant family histories.

2. Muscle Weakness

A recent literature builds a good case for a mitochondrially-driven etiology for the highly dependable age-related changes in skeletal and cardiac muscular strength and performance. Although not a large study (N = 29), skeletal muscle samples from persons ages 16 to 92 years showed a negative correlation between respiration rate and age, as well as age-associated decreases in respiratory enzyme activities.[84] Wallace[8] cites other studies which also reported age-related decreases in muscle oxidative metabolism. Most intriguing are findings on mtDNA, and these include the following observations:

- Using polymerase chain reaction (PCR) amplification of DNA, two groups[85,86] reported in 1990 that a specific 4989 base pair deletion of the mitochondrial genome (between positions 8470 and 13,459) occurs in a wide variety of tissues (including heart) of autopsied persons. The deletion occurs more frequently in tissues from older persons. One study[86] provided an estimate of the percent of mtDNA molecules with the deletion to be 0.1%. Linnane et al.[85] concluded " . . . that such deletions are not necessarily associated with particular mitochondrial diseases but occur naturally, and with increasing frequency with age." Importantly, a very recent study[87] presented evidence against the possibility that these mtDNA deletions are artifacts of PCR technology.

- Wallace's group studied hearts from persons dying with ischemic heart disease and from controls (i.e., dead from other causes or tissue from a cardiac implant biopsy specimen).[88] They found that a 4977 base pair deletion (essentially the same as just discussed) was observed in all control hearts from persons over age 40 and reached a maximum deletion of 0.0035% (note: % = deleted mtDNA to normal mtDNA). Ischemic hearts had higher levels (0.02% to 0.85%). Diseased hearts also showed an increase in the mRNA levels for oxidative phosphorylation genes. It was suggested that mtDNA damage is associated with oxidative phosphorylation deficiency.

- Ozawa's group has made major contributions in this area. They studied a 7.4 kb (from positions 8649 to 16,084) base-pair deletion in human myocardial mtDNA. This was found in all subjects studied who were over age 70.[89,90] This mtDNA population increased exponentially with aging and was estimated at ~5% of the total mitochondrial DNA in hearts from 80- to 90-year-old people.[90] The deletion is not benign, as it codes for seven subunits of the ATP production system.

Ozawa's group also studied mtDNA from human diaphragms and discovered age-related increases in deletions[91] and 8-OH-dG concentration.[92] The deletion was found in no one under age 30, in 20% of those in their 40s, in 73% of those in their 70s, and in all over age 80. The deleted region contained information coding for five electron transport system subunit molecules and five tRNA genes. For 8-OH-dG, the level was less than 0.02% of total deoxyguanosine in the two people studied who were under 55 years old, whereas it was 0.3% for a 77-year-old (who died of cancer) and 0.5% for an 85-year-old suicide victim. The possibility was discussed that conversion of guanine to 8-OH-dG may be an important cause of point mutations which could contribute to causing the deletions. Thus, a reasonable molecular explanation for the respiratory declines of aging is now forming.

These age-associated mitochondrial deletions are not confined to muscular tissues, but have been found in other human tissues. For example, an age-associated increase in the 4977 base pair deletion was seen in liver mtDNA (the deletion was found in all 34 subjects over 50 years old), but not in blood cells from Chinese subjects.[93] As is discussed below, very recent evidence links mtDNA deletions to major neurologic diseases of old age.

3. Neurodegenerative Diseases: Alzheimer's and Parkinson's Diseases

Excitotoxicity and ROS have been suggested as risk factors for both Alzheimer's disease and Parkinson's disease,[94,95] especially the latter. The metabolism of dopamine in neurons produces ROS, which may damage the neuron and subsequently kill it. In both diseases, high levels of excitatory amino acids, such as glutamate, may lead to excessive production of ROS. Although oxidative damage in any tissue can lead to dysfunction, the brain may be particularly vulnerable to such damage. One of the enzymes most sensitive to oxidation is glutamine synthetase,[56] the enzyme which converts glutamic acid and ammonia into glutamine. Both glutamic acid and ammonia are toxic if present in high levels, whereas glutamine is not. It is thought that one of the roles of the glial cells in the brain is to convert glutamate to glutamine when the former reaches neurotoxic levels. Therefore, if glutamine synthetase in these cells is inactivated by oxidation, the levels of glutamate and ammonia may both rise above acceptable levels.

The findings show an association between oxidative phosphorylation defects and these diseases, and these were recently reviewed by Wallace.[8] He points out that these are genetically and biochemically heterogeneous disorders. Nonetheless, five of six Alzheimer's patients studied showed complex IV (electron transport) defects in platelet mitochondria. In Parkinson's, complex I defects were found in the brain, platelet, and muscle mitochondria. Evidence of age-related and Parkinson's-related increases in mtDNA deletions exists. For example, the percentage of striatal mtDNA with the 4977 base pair deletion was 5% in a Parkinson's victim and 0.3% in a 38-year-old accident fatality.[96]

Whereas generation of ROS is an unavoidable by-product of normal metabolism, damage resulting from head trauma and ischemia leads to excessive production of ROS. Head trauma is a risk factor for Alzheimer's disease,[97] but damage due to head trauma is reduced in transgenic mice containing extra copies of the human gene for CuZn-SOD.[31] This is only one neuroprotective strategy which has been tried with some success. Others include administration of deprenyl and PBN. Deprenyl not only inhibits monoamine oxidase B, an enzyme which is found in glial cells and produces ROS, but also increases longevity in rats[98] and has shown some promise in the treatment of Parkinson's disease.[99] Deprenyl treatment of young rats increases SOD and CAT activities in the brain,[100] whereas deprenyl treatment of Parkinson's patients did not influence free radical status (enzymes, lipid peroxide levels) in RBCs, plasma, or cerebral spinal fluid.[101] PBN is a spin trapping compound which reduces protein oxidation in the brain,[54] and preliminary results suggest that it also increases longevity in mice.[122]

The still rather preliminary results described above implicate oxidative damage as a risk factor for neurodegenerative changes which lead to a variety of neurological diseases, depending on which regions of the brain are most markedly affected. The current need is to develop effective, but selective, antioxidant strategies to prevent or reverse this damage. The data suggest that finding ways to protect the mitochondrial genome from oxidative damage might emerge as a major focus in biomedicine.

4. Osteoporosis

In this important disease, the molecular mechanisms of bone destruction are not well understood. Recent studies have provided evidence for the involvement of ROS. Using rodent *in vivo* and *in vitro* assay systems, Garrett et al.[102] observed that ROS are intermediaries in the formation and activation of osteoclasts. These workers and others[103] provide evidence that free radicals may contribute to bone resorption. A recent study[104] shows that H_2O_2 at 10 nM is a strong stimulator of osteoclastic bone resorption and osteoclastic activity in rats. The authors suggest that H_2O_2 may be generated at the site of osteoclastic bone resorption from the superoxide free radical derived from osteoclasts.

Studies in old animals and persons are now required to determine the extent to which ROS are involved in osteoporosis. Positive results would likely prompt the widespread study of an array of exciting therapeutic approaches, probably involving interactions among the various hormones and cytokines now at the forefront of osteoporosis research and ROS metabolism.

VI. INTERVENTIONS

A popular and sometimes productive approach in gerontology has been the study of interventions aimed at retarding aging processes. Intervention studies are desirable in the context of free radicals in at least two ways. First, a successful intervention should provide a model to study the biology of decelerated aging and the free radical status of such an organism. This results in an experimental situation for testing theories of aging based on free radicals. Second, interventions may prove directly applicable to humans. It may not be all that important if any set of data does or does not support a particular theory, but rather whether or not it identifies critical processes in aging which are amenable to change by diet, chemical or gene therapy.

A. DIETARY RESTRICTION

Based on its capacity to extend a maximum life-span and to keep animals "younger longer" than normally fed controls, most gerontologists share the view that dietary restriction (DR) is the most successful intervention tested to date in mammals.[63,105] As discussed elsewhere in this volume (Chapter 4), several studies describe ROS-related phenomena in rodents subjected to life-span prolonging DR. Because the magnitude of the effect of DR is closely related to the extent of energy intake restriction, explanations of the actions of DR, which are based on energy metabolism, are quite appealing and tie in nicely with current views of significant sources of free radicals. As discussed at length elsewhere,[63] this clearly suggests that major energy-producing and energy-consuming metabolic processes, as well as processes that detoxify noxious by-products of energy metabolism, merit close attention in considering the underlying mechanism of DR.

Robust effects of DR on age-related changes in ROS detoxifying enzyme activities and on "footprints" of oxidative damage have been reported by several laboratories. These include reduced production of ROS,[105] increased activities of radical scavenging enzymes,[106-110] and reductions in age-related increases in oxidative damage.[110-113] It appears that DR results in a situation where detoxification capacities increase, while the generation of ROS does not. This circumstance differs from the more general occurrence of joint increases in production and removal (e.g., in vitamin E deficiency, peroxisomal proliferation, diabetes). These various findings set the stage for future studies on the free radical status of animals and persons on DR and for testing whether these changes are involved in the actions of DR.

The use of DR is advantageous in another critical way. It acts to postpone or prevent the occurrence of the typical diseases of old age in rodent models and allows the opportunity to examine free radicals (or whatever) in life-span-extended, healthier, very old organisms. Thus DR acts to "strip away" the usual pathologies, leaving the investigator an animal offering a clearer view of aging. As studies in gerontology have repeatedly shown over the years, advances in understanding will be strongly linked to the use of appropriate animal models, and it is important to corroborate observations in more than one model.

B. DIETARY ANTIOXIDANTS

A dietary intervention tested with only moderate success in life-span extension has been antioxidant supplementation. Many investigators have hypothesized that if free radical reactions contribute to aging, then treatment with antioxidants should retard aging and increase maximum life-span (i.e., an *in vivo* test of the free radical theory). In general, antioxidants have increased the *average* life-span of mice (particularly in short-lived strains with early incidences of diseases), but not *maximum* species-specific life-span.[114] Logical explanations have been offered to explain these data and still argue for the importance of ROS in aging. For example, Cutler[115] has proposed that dietary antioxidants may disrupt natural antioxidant defenses, with a net zero (or even deleterious) effect on aging. It has also been suggested by several workers that dietary antioxidants fail to increase maximum life-span because they cannot reach needed concentrations at critical sites (e.g., mitochondria). In our view, further aging studies in antioxidant-treated organisms are needed.

C. OTHER POSSIBILITIES

There are several other interventions linked to free radical chemistry and metabolism which require increased investigation. Two such approaches of great potential significance, PBN and deprenyl, were previously discussed herein. Another promising intervention tactic is to inhibit the reactivity of transition metals (especially iron) in an attempt to decrease oxidative stress.[116,117] One agent studied for this purpose is the chelator, desferroxamine. Two other intriguing approaches are treatment with coenzyme Q[118] or acetyl-L-carnitine.[119] Suffice it to say that the possibilities are many, and a clear need exists to test them in appropriate animal models.

VII. CONCLUSIONS

The case for an important role of free radicals in aging and in major geriatric diseases continues to strengthen. Despite these intriguing data, there exists a need to broaden the way we think about free radical reactions to encompass findings in other important areas of gerontology. An example is work from Baynes' laboratory showing an accumulation with age of N^ϵ-(carboxymethyl)lysine and N^ϵ-(carboxymethyl)hydroxyllysine in human skin collagen.[120] This is of interest because these are long-lived molecules which form as a result of both oxidation and glycation reactions. Therefore, the "free radical theory" and the "glycation theory" of aging must be combined in order to understand their presence. Recently, Kristal and Yu[121] have cogently presented a view of aging which does just that, and it is called the "Free Radical-Glycation/Maillard Reaction Theory of Aging". It posits " . . . that age-related deterioration is produced by the sum of the damage induced by free radicals, by glycation, by Maillard reactions, and by their interactions."

An obvious need exists for experiments which either prove or disprove an important role of ROS in aging processes. The challenge is to conduct studies which provide critical insights on the relationships between oxidative stress and aging, rather than projects yielding still more correlative data. Many potentially important research areas were identified in this chapter which concludes with this summary of future directions of free radical research in aging.

- Improved methods for measuring any of the following in biological tissues suitable for aging studies: levels of antioxidants in both the oxidized and reduced state; rate of production of superoxide, H_2O_2, and hydroxyl radical; levels and identification of oxidized products in macromolecules, such as DNA, protein, and lipids; rate of repair of oxidized macromolecules *in vivo*
- The role of heavy metal ions, whether bound or free, in oxidative damage *in vivo*
- Identification of which enzyme activities involved in antioxidant defense are rate-limiting, with an emphasis on age-related changes
- Development of animal models, particularly transgenic ones, to test the effect of altering oxidative damage or antioxidant defense systems on life-span and aging rate
- Determination of how genes involved in antioxidant defense systems are regulated *in vivo;* is this regulation altered during aging?
- The extent to which normal metabolism is responsible for ROS generation, mitochondrial dysfunction, and other expressions of cellular oxidative damage, and how these change with age
- The relationship between oxidative damage and the later development of age-related diseases
- Elucidation of how DR reduces oxidative damage, and whether this is related to life-span extension
- The mechanism of attenuation of oxidative damage by spin trapping compounds and other chemical and dietary interventions
- Development of interventions which reduce oxidative damage through either reduction of the rate of production of ROS, neutralization of ROS, or enhanced repair of oxidative damage

REFERENCES

1. **Sohal, R. S. and Allen, R. G.,** Oxidative stress as a causal factor in differentiation and aging: a unifying hypothesis, *Exp. Gerontol.,* 25, 499, 1990.
2. **Snyder, S. H.,** Nitric oxide: first in a new class of neurotransmitters?, *Science,* 257, 494, 1992.
3. **Stadtman, E. R. and Oliver, C. N.,** Metal-catalyzed oxidation of proteins: physiological consequences, *J. Biol. Chem.,* 266, 2005, 1991.
4. **Chance, B., Sies, H., and Boveris, A.,** Hydrogen peroxide metabolism in mammalian organs, *Physiol. Rev.,* 59, 527, 1979.

5. **Stadtman, E. R.**, Metal ion-catalyzed oxidation of proteins: biochemical mechanism and biological consequences, *Free Radical Biol. Med.*, 9, 315, 1990.

6. **Jesaitis, A. J., Quinn, M. T., Mukhergee, G., Ward, P. A., and Dratz, E. A.**, Death by oxygen: radical views, *N. Biologist*, 3, 651, 1991.

7. **Richter, C., Park, J.-W., and Ames, B. N.**, Normal oxidative damage to mitochondrial and nuclear DNA is extensive, *Proc. Natl. Acad. Sci. U.S.A.*, 85, 6465, 1988.

8. **Wallace, D. C.**, Mitochondrial genetics: a paradigm for aging and degenerative diseases?, *Science*, 256, 628, 1992.

9. **Zhang, Y., Marcillat, O., Giulivi, C., Ernster, L., and Davies, K. J. A.**, The oxidative inactivation of mitochondrial electron transport chain components and ATPase, *J. Biol. Chem.*, 265, 16330, 1990.

10. **Lippe, G., Comelli, M., Mazzilis, D., Sala, F. D., and Mavelli, I.**, The inactivation of mitochondrial F_1 ATPase by H_2O_2 is mediated by iron ions not tightly bound in the protein, *Biochem. Biophys. Res. Commun.*, 181, 764, 1991.

11. **Minotti, G. and Aust, S. D.**, Redox cycling of iron and lipid peroxidation, *Lipids*, 27, 219, 1992.

12. **Hallaway, P. E. and Hedlund, B. E.**, Therapeutic strategies to inhibit iron-catalysed tissue damage, in *Iron and Human Disease*, Lauffer, R. B., Ed., CRC Press, Boca Raton, FL, 477, 1992.

13. **Pryor, W. A. and Godber, S. S.**, Noninvasive measures of oxidative stress in humans, *Free Radical Biol. Med.*, 10, 177, 1991.

14. **Sohal, R. S., Svensson, I., and Brook, U. T.**, Hydrogen peroxide production by liver mitochondria in different species, *Mech. Ageing Dev.*, 53, 209, 1990.

15. **Rikans, L. E. and Moore, D. R.**, Influence of aging on rat liver enzymes involved in glutathione synthesis and degradation, *Arch. Gerontol. Geriatr.*, 13, 263, 1991.

16. **Rikans, L. E., Moore, D. R., and Snowden, C. D.**, Sex-dependent differences in the effects of aging on antioxidant defense mechanisms in the rat liver, *Biochem. Biophys. Acta*, 1074, 195, 1991.

17. **Rikans, L. E., Snowden, C. D., and Moore, D. R.**, Effect of aging on enzymatic antioxidant defenses in rat liver mitochondria, *Gerontology*, 38, 133, 1992.

18. **Ji, L. L., Dillon, D., and Wu, E.**, Alteration of antioxidant enzymes with aging in rat skeletal muscle and liver, *Am. J. Physiol.*, 258, R918, 1990.

19. **Salminen, A., Saari, P., and Kihlström, M.**, Age- and sex-related differences in lipid peroxidation of mouse cardiac and skeletal muscles, *Comp. Biochem. Physiol.*, 89B, 695, 1988.

20. **Vertechy, M., Cooper, M. B., Ghirardi, O., and Ramacci, M. T.**, Antioxidant enzyme activities in heart and skeletal muscle of rats of different ages, *Exp. Gerontol.*, 24, 211, 1989.

21. **Zurlo, F., Larson, K., Bogardus, C., and Ravussin, E.**, Skeletal muscle metabolism is a major determinant of resting energy expenditure, *J. Clin. Invest.*, 86, 1423, 1990.

22. **Ji, L. L., Dillon, D., and Wu, E.**, Myocardial aging: antioxidant enzyme systems and related biochemical properties, *Am. J. Physiol.*, 26, R386, 1991.

23. **Hiramatsu, M., Kohno, M., Edamatsu, R., Mitsuta, K., and Mori, A.**, Increased superoxide dismutase activity in aged human cerebrospinal fluid and rat brain determined by electron spin resonance spectrometry using the spin trap method, *J. Neurochem.*, 58, 1160, 1992.

24. **de Haan, J. B., Newman, J. D., and Kola, I.**, Cu/Zn superoxide dismutase mRNA and enzyme activity, and susceptibility to lipid peroxidation, increases with aging in murine brains, *Mol. Brain Res.*, 13, 179, 1992.

25. **Rao, G., Xia, E., and Richardson, A.**, Effect of age on the expression of antioxidant enzymes in male Fischer F344 rats, *Mech. Ageing Dev.*, 53, 49, 1990.

26. **Nisticó, G., Ciriolo, M. R., Fiskin, K., Iannone, M., De Martin, A., and Rotillo, G.**, NGF restores decrease in catalase activity and increases superoxide dismutase and glutathione peroxidase activity in the brain of aged rats, *Free Radical Biol. Med.*, 12, 177, 1992.

27. **del Rio, L. A., Sandalio, L. M., and Palma, J. M.,** A new cellular function for peroxisomes related to oxygen free radicals?, *Experientia,* 46, 989, 1990.

28. **Radi, R., Turrens, J. F., Chang, L. Y., Bush, K. M., Crapo, J. D., and Freeman, B. A.,** Detection of catalase in rat heart mitochondria, *J. Biol. Chem.,* 266, 22028, 1991.

29. **Simmons, T. W. and Jamall, I. S.,** Significance of alterations in hepatic antioxidant enzymes: primacy of glutathione peroxidase, *Biochem. J.,* 251, 913, 1988.

30. **Huang, T.-T., Carlson, E. J., Leadon, S. A., and Epstein, C. J.,** Relationship of resistance to oxygen free radicals to CuZn-superoxide dismutase activity in transgenic, transfected, and trisomic cells, *FASEB J.,* 6, 903, 1992.

31. **Kinouchi, H., Epstein, C. J., Mizui, T., Carlson, E., Chen, S. F., and Chan, P. H.,** Attenuation of focal cerebral ischemic injury in transgenic mice overexpressing CuZn superoxide dismutase, *Proc. Natl. Acad. Sci. U.S.A.,* 88, 11158, 1991.

32. **Przedborski, S., Jackson-Lewis, V., Kostic, V., Carlson, E., Epstein, C. J., and Cadet, J. L.,** Superoxide dismutase, catalase, and glutathione peroxidase activities in copper/zinc-superoxide dismutase transgenic mice, *J. Neurochem.,* 58, 1760, 1992.

33. **Scott, M. D., Eaton, J. W., Kupyers, F. A., Chiu, D. T.-Y., and Lubin, B. H.,** Enhancement of erythrocyte superoxide dismutase activity: effects on cellular oxidant defense, *Blood,* 74, 2542, 1989.

34. **Góth, L.,** A simple method for determination of serum catalase activity and revision of reference range, *Clin. Chim. Acta.,* 196, 143, 1991.

35. **Jozwiak, Z. and Jasnowska, B.,** Changes in oxygen-metabolizing enzymes and lipid peroxidation in human erthrocytes as a function of age of donor, *Mech. Ageing Dev.,* 32, 77, 1985.

36. **Guemouri, L., Artur, Y., Herbeth, B., Jeandel, C., Cuny, G., and Siest, G.,** Biological variability of superoxide dismutase, glutathione peroxidase, and catalase in blood, *Clin. Chem.,* 37, 1932, 1991.

37. **Perrin, R., Briançon, S., Jeandel, C., Artur, Y., Minn, A., Penin, F., and Siest, G.,** Blood activity of Cu/Zn superoxide dismutase, glutathione peroxidase and catalase in Alzheimer's disease: a case-control study, *Gerontology,* 36, 306, 1990.

38. **Fraga, D. G., Shigenaga, M. K., Park, J. W., Degan, P., and Ames, B. N.,** Oxidative damage to DNA during aging: 8-hydroxy-2'-deoxyguanosine in rat organ DNA and urine, *Proc. Natl. Acad. Sci. U.S.A.,* 87, 4533, 1990.

39. **Stadtman, E. R.,** Protein modification in aging, *J. Gerontol.,* 43, B112, 1988.

40. **Starke-Reed, P. E. and Oliver, C. N.,** Protein oxidation and proteolysis during aging and oxidative stress, *Arch. Biochem. Biophys.,* 275, 559, 1989.

41. **Pacifici, R. E. and Davies, K. J. A.,** Protein, lipid, and DNA repair systems in oxidative stress: the free-radical theory of aging revisited, *Gerontology,* 37, 166, 1991.

42. **Breitmar, L. H. and Lindahl, T.,** DNA glycosylase activities for thymine residues damaged by ring saturation, fragmentation, or ring contractions are functions of endonuclease III in *Escherichia coli, J. Biol. Chem.,* 259, 5543, 1984.

43. **Kasai, H., Crain, P. F., Kuchino, Y., Nishimura, S., Ootsuyama, A., and Tanooka, H.,** Formation of 8-hydroxyguamine moiety in cellular DNA by agents producing oxygen radicals and evidence for its repair, *Carcinogenesis,* 7, 1849, 1986.

44. **Warner, H. R.,** Prokaryotic DNA repair enzymes, in *Enzymes of Nucleic Acid Synthesis and Function,* Vol. 1, Jacob, S. T., Ed., CRC Press, Boca Raton, FL, 1983, 145.

45. **Pegg, A. E. and Bennett, R. A.,** Mammalian DNA repair enzymes, in *Enzymes of Nucleic Acid Synthesis and Function,* Vol. 1, Jacob, S. T., Ed., CRC Press, Boca Raton, FL, 1983, 179.

46. **Hart, R. W. and Setlow, R. D.,** Correlation between deoxyribonucleic acid excision-repair and life-span in a number of mammalian species, *Proc. Natl. Acad. Sci. U.S.A.,* 71, 2169, 1974.

47. **Warner, H. R. and Price, A. R.,** Involvement of DNA repair in cancer and aging, *J. Gerontol.,* 44, 45, 1989.

48. **Cutler, R. G.,** Antioxidants and aging, *Am. J. Clin. Nutr.,* 53, 373S, 1991.

49. **Rothstein, M.**, The alteration of enzymes in aging animals, in *Molecular Biology of Aging*, Woodhead, A. D., Blackett, A. D., and Hollaender, A., Eds., Plenum Press, New York, 1985, 193.

50. **Stadtman, E. R.**, Protein oxidation and aging, *Science*, 257, 1220, 1992.

51. **Oliver, C. N., Ahn, B., Wittenberger, M. E., and Stadtman, E. R.**, Oxidative inactivation of enzymes. Implication in protein turnover and aging, in *Cellular Regulation and Malignant Growth*, Edashi, S., Ed., Springer-Verlag, Berlin, 1985, 320.

52. **Farber, J. M. and Levine, R. L.**, Sequence of a peptide susceptible mixed-function oxidation. Probable cation binding site in glutamine synthetase, *J. Biol. Chem.*, 261, 4574, 1986.

53. **Climent, I., Tsai, L., and Levine, R. L.**, Derivatization of γ-glutamyl semialdehyde residues in oxidized proteins by fluoresceinamine, *Anal. Biochem.*, 182, 226, 1989.

54. **Carney, J. M., Starke-Reed, P. E., Oliver, C. N., Landum, R. W., Cheng, M. S., Wu, J. F., and Floyd, R. A.**, Reversal of age-related increase in brain protein oxidation, decrease in enzyme activity, and loss in temporal and spatial memory by chronic administration of the spin trapping compound N-tert-butyl-alpha-phenylnitrone (PBN), *Proc. Natl. Acad. Soc. U.S.A.*, 88, 3633, 1991.

55. **Dice, J. F.**, Altered intracellular protein degradation in aging: a possible cause of proliferative arrest, *Exp. Gerontol.*, 24, 45, 1989.

56. **Oliver, C. N., Starke-Reed, P. E., Stadtman, E. R., Carney, J. M., Liu, G., and Floyd, R. A.**, Oxidative damage to brain proteins, loss of glutamine synthetase activity, and production of free radicals during ischemia/reperfusion-induced injury to gerbil brain, *Proc. Natl. Acad. Sci. U.S.A.*, 87, 5144, 1990.

57. **Sevanian, A. and Hochstein, P.**, Mechanisms and consequences of lipid peroxidation in biological system, *Ann. Rev. Nutr.*, 5, 365, 1985.

58. **van Kuijk, P. J. G. M., Sevanian, A., Handelman, G. J., and Dratz, E. A.**, A new role for phospholipase A_2: protection of membranes from lipid peroxidation damage, *Trends Biochem. Sci.*, 12, 31, 1987.

59. **Thomas, J. P., Maiorino, M., Ursini, F., and Girotti, A. W.**, Protective action of phospholipid hydroperoxide glutathione peroxidase against membrane damaging lipid peroxidation, *J. Biol. Chem.*, 265, 454, 1990.

60. **Lands, W. E. M. and Merkl, I.**, Metabolism of glycerolipids. III. Reactivity of various acyl esters of coenzyme A with a-acyl glycerol phospherylcholine and positional specificities in lecithin synthesis, *J. Biol. Chem.*, 238, 898, 1963.

61. **Lubin, B. H., Shohet, S. B., and Nathans, D. G.**, Changes in fatty acid metabolism after erythrocyte peroxidation. Stimulation of a membrane repair process, *J. Clin. Invest.*, 51, 338, 1972.

62. **Hansford, R. G.**, Bioenergetics in aging, *Biochim. Biophys. Acta*, 726, 41, 1983.

63. **Weindruch, R. and Walford, R. L.**, *The Retardation of Aging and Disease by Dietary Restriction*, Charles C. Thomas, Springfield, IL, 1988.

64. **Miquel, J.**, An integrated theory of aging as the result of mitochondrial-DNA mutation in differentiated cells, *Arch. Gerontol. Geriatr.*, 12, 99, 1991.

65. **Asano, K., Amagase, S., Matsuura, E. T., and Yamagishi, H.**, Changes in the rat liver mitochondrial DNA upon aging, *Mech. Ageing Dev.*, 60, 275, 1991.

66. **Asano, K., Nakamura, M., Asano, A., Sato, T., and Tauchi, H.**, Quantitation of changes in mitochondrial DNA during aging and regeneration of rat liver using nonradioactive DNA probes, *Mech. Ageing Dev.*, 62, 85, 1992.

67. **Fernandez-Silva, P., Petruzzella, V., Fracasso, F., Gadaleta, M. N., and Cantatore, P.**, Reduced synthesis of mtRNA in isolated mitochondria of senescent rat brain, *Biochem. Biophys. Res. Commun.*, 176, 645, 1991.

68. **Richter, C.**, Do mitochondrial DNA fragments promote cancer and aging?, *FEBS Lett.*, 241, 1, 1988.

69. **Linnane, A. W., Marzuki, S., Ozawa, T., and Tanaka, M.**, Mitochondrial DNA mutations as an important contributor to ageing and degenerative diseases, *Lancet*, i, 642, 1989.
70. **Bandy, B. and Davison, A. J.**, Mitochondrial mutations may increase oxidative stress: implications for carcinogenesis and aging?, *Free Radical Biol. Med.*, 8, 523, 1990.
71. **Demple, B. and Amabile-Cuevas, C. F.**, Redox redux: the control of oxidative stress responses, *Cell*, 67, 837, 1991.
72. **Storz, G., Tartaglia, L. A., and Ames, B. N.**, Transcriptional regulator of oxidative stress-inducible genes: direct activation by oxidation, *Science*, 248, 189, 1990.
73. **Schrech, R., Rieber, P., and Baeuerle, P. A.**, Reactive oxygen intermediates as apparently widely used messengers in the activation of the NF-κB transcription factor and HN-1, *EMBO J.*, 10, 2247, 1991.
74. **Shull, S., Heintz, N. H., Periasamy, M., Monohar, M., Janssen, Y. M. W., Marsh, J. P., and Mossman, B. T.**, Differential regulation of antioxidant enzymes in response to oxidants, *J. Biol. Chem.*, 266, 24398, 1991.
75. **Crawford, D., Zbinden, I., Amstad, P., and Cerutti, P.**, Oxidant stress induces the proto-oncogenes *c-fos* and *c-myc* in mouse epidermal cells, *Oncogene*, 3, 27, 1988.
76. **Fraga, C. G., Motchnik, P. A., Shigenaga, M. K., Helbock, H. J., Jacob, R. A., and Ames, B. N.**, Ascorbic acid protects against endogenous oxidative DNA damage in human sperm, *Proc. Natl. Acad. Sci. U.S.A.*, 88, 11003, 1991.
77. **John, E. M., Savitz, D. A., and Sandler, D. P.**, Prenatal exposure to parents' smoking and childhood cancer, *Am. J. Epidemiol.*, 133, 123, 1991.
78. **Gey, K. F., Puska, P., Jordan, P., and Moser, U. K.**, Inverse correlation between plasma vitamin E and mortality from ischemic heart disease in cross-cultural epidemiology, *Am. J. Clin. Nutr.*, 53, 326S, 1991.
79. **Jeandel, C., Nicholas, M. B., Dubois, F., Nabet-Belleville, F., Penin, F., and Cuny, G.**, Lipid peroxidation and free radical scavengers in Alzheimer's disease, *Gerontology*, 35, 275, 1989.
80. **Diplock, A. T.**, Antioxidant nutrients and disease prevention: an overview, *Am. J. Clin. Nutr.*, 53, 189S, 1991.
81. **Pryor, W. A.**, Cancer and free radicals, in *Antimutagenesis and Anticarcinogenesis*, Shankel, D. M., Hartman, P., Kada, T., and Hollander, A., Eds., Plenum Press, New York, 1986, 45.
82. **Cerutti, P. A.**, Prooxidant states and tumor promotion, *Science*, 227, 375, 1985.
83. **Pitot, H. C.**, Endogenous carcinogenesis: the role of tumor promotion, *Proc. Soc. Exp. Biol. Med.*, 198, 661, 1991.
84. **Trounce, I., Byrne, E., and Marzuki, S.**, Decline in skeletal muscle mitochondrial respiratory chain function: possible factor in ageing, *Lancet*, i, 637, 1989.
85. **Linnane, A. W., Baumer, A., Maxwell, R. J., Preston, H., Zhang, C., and Marzuki, S.**, Mitochondrial gene mutation: the ageing process and degenerative diseases, *Biochem. Int.*, 22, 1067, 1990.
86. **Cortopassi, G. A. and Arnheim, N.**, Detection of a specific mitochondrial DNA deletion in tissues of older humans, *Nucl. Acids Res.*, 18, 6927, 1990.
87. **Cortopassi, G. A., Shibata, D., Soong, N.-W., and Arnheim, N.**, A pattern of accumulation of a somatic deletion of mitochondrial DNA in aging human tissues, *Proc. Natl. Acad. Sci. U.S.A.*, 89, 7370, 1992.
88. **Corral-Debrinski, M., Stepian, G., Shoffner, J. M., Lott, M. T., Kanter, K., and Wallace, D. C.**, Hypoxemia is associated with mitochondrial DNA damage and gene induction, *JAMA*, 266, 1812, 1991.
89. **Hattori, K., Tanaka, M., Sugiyama, S., Obayashi, T., Ito, T., Satake, T., Hanaki, Y., Asai, J., Nagano, M., and Ozawa, T.**, Age dependent increase in deleted mitochondrial DNA in the human heart: possible contributory factor to presbycardia, *Am. Heart J.*, 121, 1735, 1991.

90. **Sugiyama, S., Hattori, K., Hayakawa, M., and Ozawa, T.**, Quantitative analysis of age-associated accumulation of mitochondrial DNA with deletion in human hearts, *Biochem. Biophys. Res. Commun.*, 180, 894, 1991.

91. **Torii, K., Sugiyama, S., Tanaka, M., Takagi, K., Hanaki, Y., Iida, K., Matsuyama, M., Hirabayashi, N., Uno, Y., and Ozawa, T.**, Aging-associated deletions of human diaphragmatic mitochondrial DNA, *Am. J. Respir. Cell. Mol. Biol.*, 6, 543, 1992.

92. **Hayakawa, M., Torii, K., Sugiyama, S., Tanaka, M., and Ozawa, T.**, Age-associated accumulation of 8-hydroxydeoxyguanosine in mitochondrial DNA of human diaphragm, *Biochem. Biophys. Res. Commun.*, 179, 1023, 1992.

93. **Yen, T.-C., Su, J.-H., King, K.-L., and Wei, Y.-H.**, Ageing-associated 5 kb deletion in human liver mitochondrial DNA, *Biochem. Biophys. Res. Commun.*, 178, 124, 1991.

94. **Volicer, L. and Crino, P. B.**, Involvement of free radicals in dementia of the Alzheimer's type: a hypothesis, *Neurobiol. Aging*, 11, 567, 1990.

95. **Taylor, R.**, A lot of "excitement" about neurodegeneration, *Science*, 252, 1380, 1991.

96. **Ozawa, T., Tanaka, M., Ikebe, S., Ohno, K., Kondo, T., and Mizuno, Y.**, Quantitative determination of deleted mitochondrial DNA relative to normal DNA in parkinsonian striatum by a kinetic PCR analysis, *Biochem. Biophys. Res. Commun.*, 172, 483, 1990.

97. **Mortimer, J. A., French, L. R., Hutton, J. T., and Schuman, L. M.**, Head injury as a risk factor for Alzheimer's disease, *Neurology*, 35, 264, 1985.

98. **Knoll, J.**, The striatal dopamine dependency of life-span in male rats. Longevity study with (−) deprenyl, *Mech. Ageing Dev.*, 46, 237, 1988.

99. **The Parkinson Study Group**, Effect of deprenyl on the progression of disability in early Parkinson's disease, *N. Engl. J. Med.*, 321, 1364, 1989.

100. **Carrillo, M.-C., Kanai, S., Nokubo, M., and Kitani, K.**, (−) Deprenyl induces activities of both superoxide dismutase and catalase but not of glutathione peroxidase in the striatum of young male rats, *Life Sci.*, 48, 517, 1991.

101. **Baronti, F., Davis, T. L., Boldry, R. C., Mouradian, M. M., and Chase, T. N.**, Deprenyl effects on levodopa pharmacodynamics, mood, and free radical scavenging, *Neurology*, 42, 541, 1992.

102. **Garrett, I. R., Boyce, B. F., Oreffo, R. O. C., Bonewald, L., Poser, J., and Mundy, G. R.**, Oxygen derived free radicals stimulate osteoclastic bone resorption in rodent bone *in vitro* and *in vivo*, *J. Clin. Invest.*, 85, 632, 1990.

103. **Key, L. L., Jr., Ries, W. L., Taylor, R. G., Hays, B. D., and Pitzer, B. L.**, Oxygen derived free radicals in osteoclasts: the specificity and location of the nitroblue tetrazolium reaction, *Bone*, 11, 115, 1990.

104. **Bax, B. E., Alam, A. S. M., Banjeri, B., Bax, C. M. R., Bevis, P. J. R., Stevens, C. R., Moonga, B. S., Blake, D. R., and Zaidi, M.**, Stimulation of osteoclastic bone resorption by hydrogen peroxide, *Biochem. Biophys. Res. Commun.*, 183, 1153, 1992.

105. **Masoro, E. J.**, Food restriction in rodents: an evaluation of its role in the study of aging, *J. Gerontol.*, 43, B59, 1988.

106. **Lee, D. W. and Yu, B. P.**, Modulation of free radicals and superoxide dismutases by age and dietary restriction, *Aging*, 2, 357, 1990.

107. **Koizumi, A., Weindruch, R., and Walford, R. L.**, Influences of dietary restriction and age on liver enzyme activities and lipid peroxidation in mice, *J. Nutr.*, 117, 361, 987.

108. **Semsei, I., Rao, G., and Richardson, A.**, Changes in the expression of superoxide dismutase and catalase as a function of age and dietary restriction, *Biochem. Biophys. Res. Commun.*, 164, 620, 1989.

109. **Yu, B. P., Laganiere, S., and Kim, J.-W.**, Influence of life-prolonging food restriction on membrane lipoperoxidation and antioxidant states, in *Oxygen Radicals in Biology and Medicine*, Simic, M. G., Taylor, K. A., et al., Eds., Plenum Press, New York, 1989, 1067.

110. **Pieri, C., Falasca, M., Marcheselli, F., Moroni, F., Recchioni, R., Marmocchi, F., and Lupidi, G.,** Food restriction in female Wistar rats. V. Lipid peroxidation and antioxidant enzymes in the liver, *Arch. Geronol. Geriatr.,* 14, 93, 1992.

111. **Laganiere, S. and Yu, B. P.,** Anti-lipoperoxidation action of food restriction, *Biochem. Biophys. Res. Commun.,* 145, 1185, 1987.

112. **Yu, B. P., Lee, D. W., Marler, C. G., and Choi, J.-H.,** Mechanism of food restriction: protection of cellular homeostasis, *Proc. Soc. Exp. Biol. Med.,* 193, 13, 1990.

113. **Youngman, L. D., Park, J.-Y. K., and Ames, B. N.,** Protein oxidation associated with aging is reduced by dietary restriction of protein or calories, *Proc. Natl. Acad. Sci. U.S.A.,* 89, 9112, 1992.

114. **Balin, A. K.,** Testing the free radical theory of aging, in *Testing the Theories of Aging,* Adelman, R. C. and Roth, G. S., Eds., CRC Press, Boca Raton, FL, 1982, 137.

115. **Cutler, R. G.,** Antioxidants, aging and longevity, in *Free Radicals in Biology,* Vol. 6, Pryor, W. A., Ed., Academic Press, New York, 1984, 371.

116. **Chevion, M.,** A site-specific mechanism for free radical induced biological damage: the essential role of redox-active transition metals, *Free Radical Biol. Med.,* 5, 27, 1988.

117. **van Asbeck, B. S.,** Oxygen toxicity: Role of hydrogen peroxide and iron, in *Antioxidants in Therapy and Preventive Medicine,* Emerit, I. et al., Eds., Plenum Press, New York, 1990, 235.

118. **Bliznakov, E.,** Immunological senescence in mice and its reversal by coenzyme Q_{10}, *Mech. Ageing Dev.,* 7, 189, 1978.

119. **Sershen, H., Harsing, L. G., Jr., Banay-Schwartz, M., Hashim, A., Ramacci, M. T., and Lajtha, A.,** Effect of acetyl-L-carnitine on the dopaminergic system in aging brain, *J. Neurosci. Res.,* 30, 555, 1991.

120. **Dunn, J. A., McCance, D. R., Thorpe, S. R., Lyons, T. J., and Baynes, J. W.,** Age-dependent accumulation of N^{ϵ}-(Carboxymethyl)lysine and N^{κ}(Carboxymethyl)hydroxylysine in human skin collagen, *Biochemistry,* 30, 1205, 1991.

121. **Kristal, B. S. and Yu, B. P.,** An emerging hypothesis: synergistic induction of aging by free radicals and Maillard reactions, *J. Gerontol.,* 47, B107, 1992.

122. **Cutler, R.,** personal communication.

INDEX

A